EDIBLEstructures

THE BASIC SCIENCE OF WHAT WE EAT

EDIBLEstructures

THE BASIC SCIENCE OF WHAT WE EAT

JOSÉ MIGUEL AGUILERA

TRANSLATED BY MARIAN BLAZES

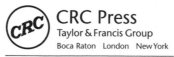

CRC Press
Taylor & Francis Group
Boca Raton   London   New York

CRC Press is an imprint of the
Taylor & Francis Group, an **informa** business

This book is an authorized translation of a book published in Spanish by Ediciones Universidad Católica de Chile, Santiago, Chile, under the title *Ingeniería Gastronómica*, 2011 (http://www.edicionesuc.cl).

CRC Press
Taylor & Francis Group
6000 Broken Sound Parkway NW, Suite 300
Boca Raton, FL 33487-2742

© 2013 by Taylor & Francis Group, LLC
CRC Press is an imprint of Taylor & Francis Group, an Informa business

No claim to original U.S. Government works

Printed in the United States of America on acid-free paper
Version Date: 2012912

International Standard Book Number: 978-1-4398-9890-1 (Paperback)

Visit the Taylor & Francis Web site at
http://www.taylorandfrancis.com

and the CRC Press Web site at
http://www.crcpress.com

CONTENTS

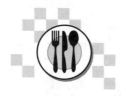

INTRODUCTION

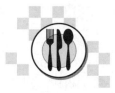

Take a moment to imagine this scenario: you are at home relaxing after a memorable meal in an excellent restaurant. You fall sound asleep and begin to dream, and in your dream you experience everything that had to happen in order for you to achieve this blissful state of satisfaction and well-being.

Molecules, the basic elements of life, first had to organize in such a way so as to give plants, animals, and fish their basic structures (just like those in our own bodies). These structures became the building blocks of foods. Harmful molecules also had to be removed from your food, as well as any microorganisms that might cause illness (though some might have slid through imperceptibly and you may yet discover their detrimental effects in the next few hours or later in life). The vast majority of the molecules entering our mouths are safe and nutritious (some more than others), thanks to trial and error during evolution and the dedicated scientists who work hard to detect unsafe foods and alert the public to any problems in our food supply.

The food industry (which barely existed 100 years ago) played its part by developing technologies like refrigeration that allow us to enjoy perishable fruits and vegetables year round, and by discovering ways to alter natural ingredients to make them more convenient and adequate to our needs, such as the low-calorie sweeteners in soda. Perhaps a small entrepreneur contributed to your meal by ingeniously developing a new seasoning mix. Exotic ingredients from around the world brought interesting flavors to the meal as well, and getting them to the table required the processing and packaging that protect perishable goods during long-term transport.

The restaurant chef combined familiar and new flavors in creative ways. In the kitchen, molecules and structures underwent spectacular changes, each in their own rhythm, regulated by well-known chemical and physical principles. These cooked "structures" were broken down in your mouth to release delicious aromas and flavors that you enjoyed (and may have even caused you to recall past experiences), and the brain played its role.

You discussed all of this with your dinner companions, because this meal was a social occasion. You and your friends are health conscious, and though you recognized that the meal may not have been nutritionally perfect, you enjoyed it immensely anyway, which is also important. You discussed how you still take pleasure in preparing traditional meals at home with your families, even though the busy rhythms of modern-day life are intruding upon this ritual.

At a certain point during the meal, your body signaled that you were full and you stopped eating. And although you could have polished off your dessert, you left half on the plate with some difficulty, proud of your willpower. The bill for the meal was steep, but you understand that, like it or not, in order to have access to food in this world we must pay for it. Meanwhile, hundreds of millions of people on this planet, especially children, suffer from hunger and the illnesses associated with living on less than a dollar a day. Many others overeat almost unconsciously and suffer from obesity and its associated complications, a paradox of the twenty-first century that must be addressed.

But now, as you sleep, your body is busily breaking down flavorful food structures and sending molecules to your cells, where genes create the machinery that repairs your tissues and brings just the right amount of energy to them (or maybe too much, which would cause you to gain weight). At this point there's not much for you to do. And tomorrow? Tomorrow you will have to burn those excess calories and eat less than usual to make up the difference. Some fortunate people have occupations requiring physical activity, but those of us with sedentary jobs must opt to walk to work, climb the stairs, or go for a jog. The rules of thermodynamics imply we must also cut back on sedentary activities like watching television, surfing the Internet, and playing video games, because any calories we don't burn as fuel will accumulate as fat. Before you wake from your dream, you remember that each day brings new and better information on what we eat and how food affects our health and well-being. You promise yourself that you will pay more attention.

Certainly the world of food and eating food is fascinating. Humanity now has access to the best variety, quality, and quantity of food per person than ever before in history, though this food is very poorly distributed throughout the world. Some eat too much while many are at the brink of starvation. For the first time, basic scientific relationships are being established between what we eat and how we feel (and between nutrition and the risk of certain diseases). Today there are hundreds of research labs where scientists generate better understanding of raw materials and food products. Bookstores have many books on cooking and nutrition, while newspapers and TV offer articles and programs dedicated to nutrition, health, and gastronomy. Despite all of this information, we still don't know how to feed ourselves. Obesity has become the most prevalent disease in the world, so much so that the problem has been coined *globesity*, and has surpassed tobacco use for its negative effects on public health. Unfortunately this phenomenon typically affects the poorest and least educated people in society. Food should be our friend, but because we don't know our friend well enough, we have transformed it into an enemy. We need a much better understanding of what we eat, including the important role food has played in the development of humanity, the science behind nutrition, and the ways food can be manipulated to bring us better nutrition, health, well-being, and pleasure. This knowledge is essential if we are to guide our eating habits in an informed way.

The central objectives of this book are to address the pressing food trends of this century, among them: (a) the growing evidence that flavorful food structures are as important as the nutritious and healthful food molecules of which they are made; (b) a need to understand and control how these food structures are created and presented as products that respond to nutritional requirements; (c) the empowerment of consumers and the appearance of the axis that connects the brain, digestive system, and the cells in our body after foods enter our mouth; (d) the separation between a knowledgeable gourmet "elite" and the rest of the population who simply want to eat quick meals as cheaply as possible; and (e) a reasonable and widespread concern with health and well-being, and in advanced societies, with the environment as well. For this reason I have made an effort to contextualize much of the information on the subject into one single book, drawing from diverse disciplines such as physical and engineering sciences, food technology, nutrition, and gastronomy. This book is far from a specialized reference for any of these subjects. Instead, it attempts to explain certain concepts of physics, chemistry, engineering, and the science of food in an entertaining but sufficiently rigorous way. I have chosen to use certain scientific terms in order to facilitate the communication between those who create the knowledge in these fields and the educated public, especially those who are curious, love to cook, and want to enjoy good food. The language and concepts presented in this book should give the reader some access to specialized texts and scientific journals, and above all, to the best and most current information available on the Internet and other media.

This book is formatted into short sections on specific themes (thematic "appetizers"), some of which can be read as opinion columns. Some sections can be read independently from the rest, and there are many cross-references within the book to facilitate comprehension. You will be surprised at how much knowledge already exists about the foods we eat each day and yet how much there is left to discover and understand. What makes this book novel is that it examines the importance of food structures—the supramolecular assemblies and matrices that are created by nature and when we cook—rather than the basic chemical compounds that are the more traditional focus of study. After all, we buy, cook, eat, and digest food structures, and we use spoons, tongs, pots, and pans to explore and develop these food structures, not pipettes and test tubes.

In recent decades the idea has emerged that the structures or matrices that contain food molecules are what is most responsible for the acceptability (taste and texture) of our food, as well as for a large part of its nutritional and healthful benefits. The ability of certain molecules to protect us from certain illnesses depends on how the molecules are structured in the food, for example. These helpful molecules must be successfully liberated, absorbed, digested, and sent to the cells. Food technology must expand to include other scientific disciplines, and as it does, certain myths will begin to fall by the wayside.

The cooks in cafeterias and casinos as well as chefs in restaurants together with food scientists and technologists in industry are responsible for most of what that we eat today. In order to continue to develop palatable foods in the future, their kitchens and laboratories must become places for experimentation, where they can create food structures that, above all, taste good. This is a main characteristic, *sine qua non*, of food that nourishes the soul. But the molecules we eat should also be safe, they must help protect us against preventable chronic diseases, help us to maintain a stable weight, and contribute to our vitality and well-being. And all of this must be accomplished on a finite planet with scarce resources, so the creation and consumption of these food structures must be sustainable for future generations.

The schematic in Figure I.1 illustrates the scope of this book. Nature converts molecules into edible food structures, most of which are then transformed into products in factories and the kitchens. Tasty food structures enter our mouths and different sensations invade our body. When these structures finally reach our cells, they have been broken back down into molecules helping our body to function. All of this is happening on our limited and fragile planet Earth.

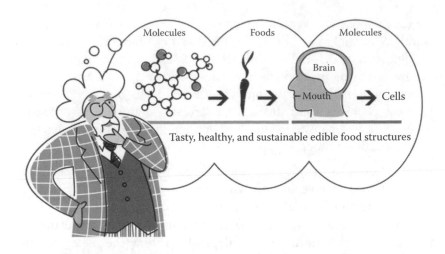

FIGURE I.1   THE ORGANIZATION AND CONTENTS OF THE BOOK.

I teach food engineering and have researched the processes and micro-structures of raw materials and food products for nearly 35 years. Over my years as a professor I have explained the basic principles of science and engineering by often using cooking processes as examples, as they are such familiar subjects to the students. In the last five years I have also invited young chefs into my laboratory, to the surprise of my engineering colleagues, and have enjoyed the joint culinary experimentation that results.

Everyone has to develop a certain individual relationship with food and how to eat properly, so there are no universally applicable guidelines about how to think about food, regardless of what some diet gurus tell. Today it is not easy to establish a healthy relationship with food, especially for the millions of people who live in urban settings, and who must balance the time spent in preparing and consuming their meals with the demands of transportation, work, and multiple distractions. The 1967 Nobel laureate in Literature, Miguel Ángel Asturias (1899–1974), summed it up very well:[1]

> From the kitchens fled the loving hours of preparation that went into meals and pastries, and the sadness disguised as concern for weight, figure, sin, cost, and

timeliness ended what had once been pleasant and enjoyable: eating food. (*Comiendo en Hungría* [*Eating in Hungary*], Ediciones Universidad Católica, Chile, 2009)

I am grateful to have witnessed the "other side" of food engineering—what happens on the "micro" level—and to be able to propose some interpretations that may be controversial, but are at least original and provocative.[2] Why else dedicate oneself to academia? My gratitude goes to my students who have accepted my challenges and responded with elegant, rigorous, and intelligent propositions, many of which are in this book. I am also grateful to various people who have contributed their suggestions to different parts of the text and to Marian Blazes who has done a superb translation of the revised Spanish text (*Ingeniería Gastronómica*, Ediciones UC, Santiago, Chile). Finally I thank my wife Astrid, and my children Carolina, Sebastián, and Magdalena, who endured a few long explanations at lunch and dinner on the foods we were eating, without ever requiring empirical proof for my arguments.

NOTES

1. The ceremonies honoring the recipients of the Nobel Prize include a grand banquet whose history and menus are described in the book Soderlind, U. 2005. *The Nobel Banquets*. World Scientific, New Jersey.
2. See also Aguilera, J.M. 2012. The engineering inside our dishes. *International Journal of Gastronomy and Food Science* 1, 31–36.

ABOUT THE AUTHOR

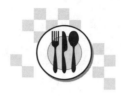

José Miguel Aguilera is a professor in the College of Engineering at the Pontificia Universidad Católica de Chile (PUC). A chemical engineer (PUC, 1971), he earned a master of science degree from MIT (1973), a doctorate from Cornell University (1976), both with specialization in food technology, and an MBA from Texas A&M University (1983). He has been the head of the Department of Chemical and Bioprocess Engineering at PUC, Associate Dean for Development and Director of Research and Postgraduate Studies in the School of Engineering. He is the author or editor of 13 books, 25 book chapters, and more than 170 articles on food technology and food engineering in international journals. He has been or is on the editorial committee of six international science journals, including *Journal of Food Science*, *Food Engineering*, and *Trends in Food Science and Technology*. He has been a visiting professor at the University of California at Davis, Cornell University, and Technical University Munich, a technical consultant for the Food and Agriculture Organization of the United Nations (FAO), and a scientific advisor for the Nestlé Research Center in Switzerland for more than 12 years. Among his most significant awards are fellowships from the Fullbright Commission (1989) and the Guggenheim Foundation (1991), and the Alexander von Humboldt Prize for Research (Berlin, 2002). In the United States he has received the International Award (1993), Research and Development Award (2005), and the Marcel Loncin Research Prize (2006), all from the Institute of Food Technologists (IFT). He was appointed a commander in the Order of Orange-Nassau by the Dutch government, and is a Fellow of the IFT and the International Association of Food Science and Technology. In 2008 he was awarded the National Prize for Applied Science and Technology, the highest scientific honor in Chile, and in 2010 was the first Chilean to become a foreign associate member of the U.S. National Academy of Engineering, for his contributions to the understanding of the role of food structures and their properties.

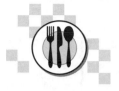

CHAPTER 1

Nutritious and Delicious Molecules

Just like our bodies, all of our food is made up of molecules, and it's important to know what to call them. Chemical nomenclature can be cumbersome, but nowadays there's no way around it: words like "trans" fatty acids, dioxins, and antioxidants are part of our vocabulary. We are going to learn about the molecules that form the building blocks of food structures (good and bad), including their origins and how they function in our lives. But this molecular tour is full of revelations including the risks involved when we eat and the fact that although there are enough food molecules in this world, many do not get a fair share of them.

1.1 WE EAT MOLECULES AND WE ARE MOLECULES

It is often said that you are what you eat, and from a chemical point of view this is quite true—our bodies are formed of molecules that

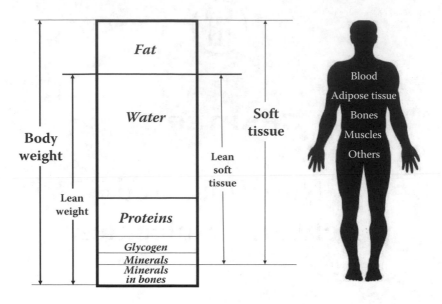

FIGURE 1.1   THE MAIN TYPES OF MOLECULES (AND MINERALS) AND THEIR RELATIVE DISTRIBU-
TION IN THE HUMAN BODY. THE HUMAN BODY IS MADE UP OF AN ARRAY OF MOLECULES THAT
COME FROM THE MOLECULES IN OUR FOOD. BOTH THE FLUIDS AND TISSUE STRUCTURES IN OUR
BODY ARE MADE UP OF MOLECULES.

primarily come from the food that we eat (Figure 1.1). After we enjoy
the sensory experience of eating a food, our body digests it into simple
molecules, which are absorbed and transported to different tissues.
Our body is like a giant LEGO® creation made of many cells assembled
together, and each cell contains tiny specialized chemical "factories"
called *organelles* that power the cells, and together power our body. But
just like a car, we need a fuel source to function, and our fuel (energy)
comes from the oxidation of food molecules. In addition to fuel, our
diet must provide certain molecules that our bodies cannot synthesize,
such as minerals, some vitamins, and particular amino acids and fatty
acids. People sometimes need to take nutritional supplements when
they are not getting enough of these essential molecules from their diet.
Finally, not all the molecules in our food are equally beneficial.

It all starts when solar energy flowing from the sun to the Earth is
captured by plants (as well as some algae and bacteria) and converted
to molecules. Less than 3% of the solar energy that hits the Earth is

captured by chlorophyll in plants through a process called *photosynthesis*. This energy is stored in the molecules that make up all the Earth's biomass. During photosynthesis, solar energy is used to convert carbon dioxide and water into sugars and oxygen:

$$nCO_2 + nH_2O + energy \rightarrow (CH_2O)_n + nO_2$$

This process begins the food chain that allows for life on our planet. Most food molecules were once part of another organism. Humans are heterotrophic—we depend on these foreign food molecules because we cannot perform photosynthesis and convert solar energy directly into energy for our cells. Once food reaches our cells, our mitochondria (one of the tiny organelle "factories" in the cell) reverse the work of photosynthesis and convert sugar and oxygen back into the energy we need to build and break down tissues and make our bodies function. These chemical reactions that occur in our cells are together called *metabolism*.

From all of this information we can extract three important facts. First, our survival depends on other organisms with which we share this planet. Second, the molecules that our body consumes as food come in the form of organized structures derived from photosynthesis. And third, we must understand the natural chemical origin of our food, because our body is also a chemical array of molecules. And so we arrive at our first dilemma. If our body is just a collection of molecules, does it make any difference whether we ingest a molecule of ascorbic acid (vitamin C) from a pill made by a pharmaceutical company or from a glass of orange juice? This is not an insignificant question, but rather the fundamental point of difference between advocates for natural foods versus "artificial" or "synthetic" foods. I will address this topic further later in the book, after a few "warm up" discussions.

1.2 THE BUILDING BLOCKS

The molecular makeup of our food and the role of these molecules in human physiology and nutrition require us to consider chemistry, although very superficially. The following section is a very general introduction to the vocabulary associated with the molecular principles that will appear late in the book, and is a tribute to the nineteenth century chemists who developed the field of *bromatology* (from the Greek *broma* = food) or the study of the chemistry of food. As it turns out, the first groups of molecules studied were ultimately the most important—proteins, fats, and carbohydrates—which today appear (or should appear) on the nutritional information of all packaged foods.

Proteins are macromolecules or polymers (large and long molecules) constructed by the bonding together of many small units (monomers) called *amino acids*.[1] Twenty-two amino acids are important in human nutrition, all of which have an amino group ($-NH_2$) and an acid group ($-COOH$).[2] Nine of these amino acids (histidine, lysine, methionine, tryptophan, threonine, phenylalanine, isoleucine, leucine, and valine) are known as the essential amino acids, because the human body cannot synthesize them so they must come from the diet. The number of amino acids that make up a protein chain can vary from just a few (as in peptides of soy sauce), to hundreds (as in the whey proteins of milk), to thousands (as in the milk protein casein). The sequence of the different amino acids determines the folding of the protein chain in space and its interaction with more complex structures, and therefore establishes much of the physiological and biological properties of the protein. In their natural state, proteins adopt a special conformation called the *native structure*. Some proteins appear rolled up like a ball of yarn and are called *globular proteins*, while others are elongated in shape and are called *fibrous proteins*. Often when proteins undergo a change in their environment, such as an increase in temperature, or an exposure to acidity (change in pH), they lose their original or native structure and take on other characteristics and properties. *Enzymes* are proteins that accelerate certain specific chemical reactions (a role of chemical entities called *catalysts*), like the enzyme papain, which is used to tenderize meat by cutting down proteins. The molecules that we call vitamins are not all "vital amines," as erroneously suggested by the name Casimir Funk assigned to them in 1812. He was the Polish biochemist who is credited with recognizing the importance of these essential nutrients.

Lipids are a varied group of molecules that store energy and have the unusual characteristic of being insoluble in water. Fats and oils are the most abundant lipids in food, and they contain molecules called *fatty acids* (FA), which are made up of chains starting with a $-CH_3$ group and ending in an acid group (-COOH).[3] If in between both ends are only $-CH_2$- monomers linked together, the FA is said to be *saturated*; however, if there are some double bonds (i.e., -CH = CH- groups) in the chain, then the FA is unsaturated (see below). Most fats and oils are actually *triglycerides* (also called triacylglycerides) or molecules where three fatty acids are combined with a glycerol molecule (a 3-carbon alcohol). In turn, triglyceride molecules can be displayed as "fork" (trident) or "chair" (one back and two legs) structures which play an important role in how fats solidify into semi-crystalline structures (Section 3.9). There are also monoglycerides and diglycerides that contain one or two fatty acids, respectively, attached to glycerol. Saturated fats are generally more solid at a given temperature than unsaturated ones. The double bonds found in unsaturated fats can be broken by adding hydrogen atoms (in a process called *hydrogenation*), which results in a fat that melts at a higher temperature. Margarine is an example of a hydrogenated fat. As mentioned, one of the most remarkable properties of fats and oils is their hydrophobicity—they dislike mixing with water. They can also maintain their molecular integrity up to temperatures of 190°C, which makes them ideal for frying foods. Another relevant class of lipids with technological applications is the *phospholipids* like lecithin (which are similar to fatty acids but have a phosphate group attached) that exhibit polarity, with a polar (electrically charged) head and a long apolar (no electrical charge) tail. These molecules like to position themselves at the junction between water and oil or water and air (as emulsions and foams, respectively), with their polar heads immersed in water and their apolar tails extended into oil or air. Phospholipids are essential components of the biological membranes that surround cells and organelles. These membranes have two layers (bilayer structure), with the polar ends of the molecules facing outwards toward the aqueous phase and the apolar tails hidden in the middle.

Unsaturated fats (although it's the fatty acids that are unsaturated) deserve further comment regarding their nomenclature because some of them are important in nutrition. Unsaturated fatty acids receive a chemical name based on the total number of carbon atoms and number and position of double bonds in the chain. For example, C20:5 ω3 is called eicosapentaenoic acid (EPA)—it has 20 carbon atoms, five double bonds, and the first double bond is in the third carbon counting from the -CH$_3$ end. Thus, it is an omega-3 fatty acid (ω represents the Greek letter omega). The presence of a double bond (-CH = CH-) imposes an extra alternative to the FA chain; in *cis* unsaturated fatty acids, the two hydrogen atoms adjacent to a double bond are on the same side, while in *trans* unsaturated fatty acids, they are on opposite sides. In general, *trans* FA are considered by doctors as bad for your health. Box 1.1 shows the terminology used to refer to some famous unsaturated fatty acids, and in the Appendix some chemical formulas of lipids are explained.

Carbohydrates are cheap and abundant molecules, and as their name suggests they have a composition of $C_x(H_2O)_y$ but they don't actually contain water. In biochemistry, the molecules for which x and y equal 6 or 12 are called sugars (from the Greek *sákkharon* = sugar). Carbohydrates can be small monosaccharides (such as glucose, abundantly present in plants, and fructose, the main sugar in honey) or disaccharides (like sucrose or table sugar, formed from the union of glucose and fructose, and lactose, the sugar in milk, made of galactose and glucose). Carbohydrate polymers or *polysaccharides* are important larger molecules, composed of the same or different types of sugars joined together in a long and linear chain, sometimes with branching chains. One interesting chemical feature of these polymers is that the same sugars can be attached in different ways to form polysaccharides with very distinct properties. For example, the linear chains of glucose in amylose, one of the polymers present in starch, are easily broken down during digestion, while the glucose chains in cellulose are insoluble and indigestible. In both cases, the chemical formula is the same. *Starch* is one of the most important polysaccharides in food and will be discussed in Section 2.1. Glycogen, the branched polysaccharide produced in the body and stored in the liver and muscles, will be addressed in Section 6.4. Gums (or hydrocolloids) such as pectins, which come from the cell walls of fruits (Figure 1.2), or alginates, agar, and carrageenan from algae are also polysaccharides. Other edible gums can be extracted from legumes (guar gum) or are secreted by trees (gum arabic and tragacanth) and microorganisms (xanthan gum). Because these molecules are very large, they produce very viscous solutions at low concentrations and can thicken enough to form gels in some cases (see Box 11.1). There are some plant polysaccharides that our bodies

**BOX 1.1   SHORT GLOSSARY OF
THE TERMINOLOGY FOR CERTAIN
UNSATURATED FATTY ACIDS AND OTHER
LIPID MOLECULES (SEE APPENDIX)**

Polyunsaturated fatty acids (PUFAs). This is the generic name for fatty acids that have more than one double bond in the FA chain. In general, they are known to provide certain health benefits, including protection against heart disease and hypertension, and contribute to good brain development and cerebral growth.

Long-chain PUFAs. Omega-6 LC-PUFAs (linoleic acid, C18:2 ω6) and omega-3 LC-PUFAs (alpha linolenic acid, C18:3 ω3) are considered essential fatty acids and must be obtained from our diet, as the human body cannot synthesize them. Diets high in omega-6 LC-PUFAs are not recommended, while omega-3 fatty acids exhibit anti-inflammatory effects (so they're good).

Very long-chain PUFAs. Eicosapentaenoic acid (EPA) (C20:5 ω3) and docosahexanoic acid (DHA) (C22:6 ω3) are important fatty acids both nutritionally and physiologically (see Appendix for formula). Fish and microalgae are good sources. A consumption of 250 to 500 mg of EPA and DHA per day is recommended (i.e., two servings of fish per week). We can convert alpha linolenic acid into EPA and DHA.

Conjugated linoleic acid (CLA). These are variations of linoleic acid (C18:2) that are present in nature having the two double bonds in *cis*-9, *trans*-11 and *trans*-10, *cis*-12 positions (the name conjugated comes from the double bonds being separated by one single bond). CLA appears to be involved with reducing body fat, increasing muscle mass, and reducing levels of cholesterol and triglycerides in the blood. Found in milk, butter, cheeses, and meats from ruminant animals.

Tocopherols. Also known as vitamin E, tocopherols (and tocotrienols) are antioxidants in cell membranes and plasma lipoproteins (see below). They are found in vegetable oils, leafy vegetables, and carrots.

Cholesterol. This is a molecule structurally different from tri-glycerides that is needed for membrane formation and synthesized in the body or provided by the diet. An elevated concentration of cholesterol in the blood plasma (the aqueous fraction devoid of blood cells) is a risk factor for atherosclerosis and heart disease.

Sterols and stanols. Also known as *phytosterols* and phytostanols when derived from plants, these molecules are similar to cholesterol. They are thought to have beneficial antioxidant and hypolipidemic effects (reducing the level of cholesterol in the blood).

Plasma lipoproteins. These are complex protein and lipid macro-molecules that allow water-insoluble lipids to be transported in the blood plasma. In this group are high-density lipoproteins (HDLs), which remove cholesterol (and are good), and low-density lipoproteins (LDLs), which can contribute to plaque formation in the arteries or atherosclerosis (bad). *Trans* fats raise your LDL cholesterol and lower your HDL cholesterol.

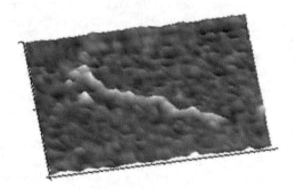

FIGURE 1.2   NOWADAYS MOLECULES CAN BE "SEEN" WITH POWERFUL MICROSCOPES: THREE-DIMENSIONAL (3-D) IMAGE OBTAINED BY ATOMIC FORCE MICROSCOPY OF A PECTIN MOLECULE SITTING ON MICA (DARK BACKGROUND). THE SCALE IS 109 × 160 NANOMETERS (NM). THE LENGTH OF THE MOLECULE IS ~70 NM AND THICKNESS ~0.6 NM. (COURTESY OF DR. VIC MORRIS, INSTITUTE OF FOOD RESEARCH, NORWICH, UK. WITH PERMISSION.)

cannot digest—they are what nutritionists call *dietary fiber.* Insoluble fiber (cellulose, hemicellulose, and lignin) promotes intestinal mobility, while soluble fiber (gums, mucilages, pectins) is supposed to reduce cholesterol and glucose levels. Starch that is not digested by intestinal enzymes is also considered a form of dietary fiber (Section 7.7).

In addition to the molecules we eat for energy and protein, we need minerals and vitamins from our food, as our bodies cannot synthesize them. Minerals perform structural functions (like calcium and phosphorous in bones and teeth) as well as participate in metabolic regulation. Vitamins are organic nutrients that also contribute to various metabolic functions.

We have left water for last, though going by number of molecules it is the main component of our food, even in dehydrated foods like raisins or noodles. Water is a key reactant in many chemical reactions and functions as a solvent that allows other molecules to move and disperse among the food matrices. Water is also essential for the growth of microorganisms and is responsible for the texture of food (e.g., whether it is soft or hard). Interestingly, water is the only component in nature and in food that exists in three states: as a solid (ice), a liquid, and a vapor. But be aware that "tap water" is not pure H_2O but varies from place to place, and even minimal amounts of chemicals dissolved in tap water can affect its culinary properties (more on water in Section 2.2).

1.3 MOLECULES THAT CHANGE

Although the emphasis of this book is more on food structures than on molecules, it's important to discuss some of the main molecular reactions that occur in our foods and during food preparation which can affect their quality as well as our health (listed in Box 1.2). If some food molecules were not constantly changing and others were not reacting during cooking or processing, we would not be able to enjoy the aroma of fruits, wine, or roasted coffee, or the texture of a Camembert cheese or a ripe avocado. But we must also be aware that some molecules produced by these reactions can cause health risks (Section 1.11).

BOX 1.2 SOME OF THE IMPORTANT CHEMICAL REACTIONS THAT AFFECT THE COLOR AND TASTE OF FOODS

Lipid oxidation. Produced by the interaction of unsaturated fatty acids with oxygen, generating highly reactive intermediates called free radicals that trigger a chain reaction. An example of oxidation is the formation of unpleasant odors in fatty fish.

Nonenzymatic browning. A collection of reactions between reducing sugars (mainly glucose) and the free amino groups in proteins, resulting in the development of caramel colors and aromas. This reaction is responsible for the dark beer and the flavor of roasted coffee, among many other things.

Enzymatic reactions. Mediated by the enzymes intrinsic to foods (e.g., the oxidation of legumes by lipoxygenase) or by enzymes added to foods (the coagulation of milk by rennin). They can result in changes to the physical properties or organoleptic properties (perceived by the senses) of the food.

Enzymatic browning. A browning reaction in vegetables produced by enzymes called polyphenoloxidases or peroxidases, like when raw sliced potatoes turn brown.

Maillard reaction. See nonenzymatic browning.

Some foods suffer undesirable changes when exposed to oxygen because of a chemical reaction generally termed *oxidation*. Unsaturated fats are very susceptible to oxidation and produce unpleasant odors and flavors, which is the reason why oxygen is often removed from the packages or antioxidants are added. Oxidation of fat in foods occurs very quickly once the very reactive intermediate compounds called *free radicals* form (Section 7.9). There are other kinds of oxidations, like those that affect the color of meat by involving the muscle pigment myoglobin. Fresh cuts of meat have an attractive red color, but given time the iron atom in myoglobin will oxidize and the meat will turn brown (but nothing is wrong, so far).

Many food molecules are either purposely modified or naturally transformed to produce desirable changes in food texture and taste. Enzymatic reactions are mediated by *enzymes* that break specific chemical bonds and release smaller molecules. Enzymes that break down proteins, starches, and fats are called proteases, amylases, and lipases, respectively. Hydrolysis or hydrolytic reactions are very important in the food industry. Hydrolyzed proteins are used for flavor, and the products of starch hydrolysis are prized for their solubility and sweetness (Section 1.2). As cheese ripens, molds and bacteria produce lipases that cleave fatty acids from the triglycerides in the milk fat, producing powerful aromatic molecules. Enzymes normally cleave large molecules into smaller ones, but they can also catalyze the opposite reaction, and under special conditions (outside of normal food preparation) add small molecules onto larger ones. Enzymes are normally inactivated by heat treatments such as blanching or cooking. There is more about this in Sections 1.13 and 2.2.

The speed with which these reactions occur is as important as the changes they produce. In general, chemical reactions occur more slowly at lower temperatures (the reason why we store some foods in the refrigerator), when enough water is removed from a food (which is why dried products do not spoil), if one reactant is in short supply (like when oxygen concentration is reduced by dipping cut potatoes in water), or when specific inhibitors are added (e.g., adding sulfur dioxide to prevent cut apples from turning brown. Chemists tend to study chemical reactions in their labs using test tubes and pure reactants in dilute solutions (a technique also known as wet chemistry), but it can be frustrating to extrapolate those results in order to see what happens with real foods. To start, there are various other food components in real food that may interfere with the reaction. But a major effect is that the reacting species are inserted in a matrix that precludes their free movement, unlike when they are dissolved in pure water (Section 7.2). Some reactants may be in cellular compartments or linked to other components, or the food structure may restrict the movement of molecules, all of which can affect reaction rates. Note that foods are multicomponent, structured materials. See Section 5.4 for more discussion about the chemical reaction rates in foods.

1.4 THERE IS AN ADDITIVE IN MY SOUP!

You need only glance at a label to appreciate the large number of molecules added in tiny proportions to the formulations of processed foods, for many different purposes. In technical jargon, the term *food additive* includes all the natural or artificial substances intentionally added to food in small quantities in order to preserve or intensify its qualities, protect it from microorganisms, enhance the taste or color, or improve its texture.[4] Even a food as basic as commercial salt contains an anti-caking additive (usually magnesium carbonate or silicon dioxide) that prevents moisture from causing clumps that could clog the holes in a salt shaker. Most food additives are natural or synthetic colorants and flavorings (see Section 1.6 on food color). There are many textbooks that cover the chemical traits of food additives, including the classic *Food Chemistry* by H.-D. Belitz and collaborators.[5] The subject is so extensive and specialized that extremely interested readers should consult original sources.[6]

Certain natural additives like smoke and salt have been used since ancient times. Some additives are derived from the spices that Marco Polo brought back from the Orient in the fourteenth century, or from the spices that the Arabs introduced to the West, like saffron, as well as from ingredients discovered in the Americas, like vanilla. Some spices, such as thyme and rosemary, are used to season traditional dishes but also have antioxidant properties that prevent the formation of undesirable flavors. Moreover, some spices are commonly used as natural antimicrobial agents in foods. The next step was to extract from these natural ingredients the most important molecules, refine them, and concentrate them for use as potent extracts.

Natural additives are used in many different ways, and their classification is similarly diverse (some examples are in parentheses): preservatives to prolong shelf life ("weak" acids such as lactic, acetic, tartaric, and citric acids), colorants (turmeric, saffron, etc.), flavors (various types of essential oils, vanilla, etc.), antioxidants (ascorbic acid, alpha tocopherol), texturizing thickeners (starches, hydrocolloids), emulsifiers or emulsifiers that help to make mixtures more homogeneous (lecithin), humectants to retard moisture loss (sorbitol, glycerol), and flavor enhancers (monosodium glutamate, disodium inosinate, etc.), among others.

Scientists discovered over time that certain molecules were the active agents in natural food additives, and that some of these molecules could be produced in a laboratory, and thus artificial colorings and flavors were born. Some industrially produced molecules worked better or were less expensive than natural ones, like the antioxidants butylated hydroxyanisole (BHA), butylated hydroxytoluene (BHT), and the propyl gallate that we see on some labels.[7] In the twentieth century the food industry developed rapidly, resulting in massive increases in the use of food additives for preservation of quality, safety, and attractive presentation of processed foods. Today the long list of additives on the packages of some foods can cause anxiety, because it is difficult to understand why so many are there and what they actually do. To give an idea of how many chemicals can be legally added to foods, the Food Code in Spain contains over 400 permitted additives, many of which are synthetic. The food industry is under pressure to eliminate some of them, reduce their use, or replace them with additives of "natural" origin. A variety of natural preservatives called *bacteriocins*, which kill or inhibit the growth of undesirable bacteria, are naturally produced by microorganisms present in food. One of them, nisin, has been an approved food preservative in more than 50 countries for 30 years.

Food additives are obviously strictly regulated by food safety agencies, which set the uses and doses for each application. In the United States, one very important category of additives are the GRAS (Generally Recognized As Safe) additives, which have proven their safety over a long period of use (from before 1958 at least) or have been proven harmless from the scientific viewpoint. European food additives are identified by the letter "E" followed by a number (e.g., citric acid, used to preserve the color of fresh fruits and vegetables, is E330).[8] The manufacturer of a new food additive must test it extensively in animals, using large doses. From these experiments scientists can "infer" that the additive will not cause harmful effects in humans when used in reasonable doses. As might be expected, the results of these kinds of studies and the extrapolation of the results from animals to humans are unconvincing to some (as well as unethical to others).[9]

If the reader is feeling a little uncomfortable at this point with so much molecular nomenclature (and there is a little bit more to come in the following sections), Box 1.3 provides a list of some of the common ingredients on a variety of grocery store food labels and their uses. Requiring companies to fully list all food additives on product labels, which provides buyers relevant information about their food at the time of purchase, has been a great victory of consumer advocacy organizations.

Obviously, the use of these additives is permitted only within certain limits, though the label "natural and artificial flavorings" doesn't give us much information and can be misleading. If we care so much about what we eat, are we capable of knowing what every food additive does?

BOX 1.3   SOME OF THE UNUSUALLY NAMED INGREDIENTS FOUND ON A VARIETY OF FOOD LABELS

Dehydrated soups. Maltodextrin, monosodium glutamate, disodium inosinate and guanylate, nature-identical flavoring, whey

Salad dressing. Whey, glucose-fructose syrup, modified starch, guar gum, xanthan gum

Flavored cookies. Antioxidant BHT, whey, fructose, ammonium bicarbonate, sodium stearoyl lactylate, nature-identical flavoring, lecithin, sodium, sodium metabisulfite

Orange drink. Citric acid, guar gum, ascorbic acid, gum arabic, nature-identical flavoring substances, beta-carotene

Frozen breaded shrimp. Bleached wheat flour, modified corn starch, sodium acid pyrophosphate, whey, partially hydrogenated soybean oil, sodium tripolyphosphate

Strawberry low-fat milk. Nature-identical flavoring (strawberry), disodium phosphate, carrageenan, food dye Ponceau 4R

Dessert-style yogurt. Stabilized corn starch, gelatin, whey, nature-identical flavoring, potassium sorbate, carmine

Table salt. Sodium silicoaluminate and silicon dioxide, potassium iodate

There are about 25 additives listed in Box 1.3, so we can test ourselves on how many we know.

Recognize 20 to 25 of them?: excellent, you should be a Director of Food Safety (or perhaps sell food additives); 15 to 19: very good, feel proud that you know what you are eating at least 70% of the time; 10 to 14: good, but keep reading this book to learn about the other half; 5 to 9: you have cooked a few meals and passed a basic chemistry course; 0 to 4: careful about drinking sulfuric acid, it makes you sick!

1.5 SWEET MOLECULES

Sweetness is greatly valued in food. Candy, jams, desserts, cake, and ice cream owe their great popularity to the sweetness of sugar or sucrose (Section 1.2). Sugarcane has been commercially used since the eighteenth century, and the first European factories built to process sugar from beets appeared around 1813. Before the eighteenth century, honey was a primary sweetener in foods. Some of the problems associated with the abundance of sugar in our diets, such as its high caloric content, its association with the increased incidence of diabetes, and its cariogenic (cavity-causing) effects, have inspired the search for substances that can provide the sweetness of sugar without the negative effects. It is difficult to completely replace the sugar in desserts and ice cream because it makes up such a large proportion of the ingredients and it plays an important physicochemical role by binding water. In many products sugar contributes to caramelization reactions that give them flavor and color (Section 2.4). Sugar refined from both sugarcane and sugar beets is 99.95% sucrose, so both provide the same amount of sweetness, but to connoisseurs they do not taste exactly the same. The tiny remaining 0.05%, a mixture of minerals and proteins that survive the refining process, can make a difference in *crème brûlées*, cookies, and cakes.[10]

Not all sugars are equally sweet. The sweetness of a 5% sucrose solution is equivalent to that of solutions containing 8.3%, 4.2%, and 15.7% glucose, fructose, and lactose, respectively. For the past half century, corn syrups have been widely used in commercial foods, especially in soft drinks. As stated, cornstarch is formed of chains of many glucose molecules, which if broken with enzymes change to a glucose syrup (regular corn syrup) that is almost half as sweet as a sucrose syrup of similar concentration. Another enzyme can convert some of the glucose to fructose, resulting in a high-fructose corn syrup (HFCS, as known in the trade) containing 24% water and either 55% fructose and 42% glucose (HFCS 55, mostly used in soft drinks) or 42% fructose and 53% glucose (HFCS 42 used in beverages, processed foods, cereals, and baked goods). HFCS 42 is approximately 80% as sweet as sucrose. Because table sugar (sucrose) is 50% glucose and 50% fructose, consumption of these products does not significantly increase the intake of fructose (review Section 1.2).

A sweetener is a natural or artificial substance other than sugar that gives a sweet flavor to foods. Sweeteners are measured by comparing their sweetening power to sugar. Among the most well-known natural sweeteners are sorbitol, mannitol, isomalt, and xylitol. Xylitol, an ingredient in certain chewing gums, is particularly interesting because it is said to prevent tooth decay while tasting similar to sugar, but it has also been known to cause a laxative effect in some cases.

Some zero calorie artificial sweeteners are saccharin, cyclamate, aspartame, sucralose, acesulfame potassium, and neotame. Three of these sweeteners were discovered by accident.[11] In 1879 a chemist at Johns Hopkins University accidentally spilled the substance he was preparing onto his hand, and so he tasted it and noted that it was quite sweet (apparently chemists at that time were much more inclined to smell and taste the materials they worked with). Realizing its potential usefulness, he patented the substance and named it *saccharin* (from the Latin *saccharum* = sugar). Saccharin is the most potent approved artificial sweetener: 300 times sweeter than an equal weight of sugar. In 1937 a graduate student in chemistry at the University of Illinois noticed a sweet taste in the cigarette he was smoking (a forbidden practice in modern laboratories) which he attributed to the drug he was trying to synthesize. These compounds are now known by the generic name *cyclamate*. In 1956 *aspartame* was discovered in the laboratories of the pharmaceutical company G.D. Searle & Co., the by-product of a search for ulcer remedies. Aspartame is a dipeptide composed of the amino acids phenylalanine and aspartic acid, and it is 200 times sweeter than sugar.

What is remarkable about these three sweeteners is that their chemical formulas are totally different from natural sugars (chemically, they are not actually sugars), but they have similar physiological effects (a sensation of sweetness). While saccharin and the cyclamates contain nitrogen or sulfur, aspartame and neotame are peptides, and both are metabolized like any other protein. (See Section 1.11 for a discussion of the risks associated with these sweeteners and Section 6.4 for their effect on caloric intake). Aspartame is not recommended for people with the genetic disease phenylketonuria, as they are unable to metabolize phenylalanine.

If *Stevia rebaudania* had been discovered before sugarcane and beets, it is likely that many of the nutritional problems associated with the overconsumption of calories from sugar would not exist today. This plant grows in the tropical regions of South America and produces a noncaloric natural sweetener called *stevial glycoside*. Its leaves have been consumed by the natives of Paraguay since time immemorial. The commercial extract of stevia is 200 times sweeter than sugar and is currently used in many countries, including Japan and the United States (since late 2008).

Most of these nonsugars can have bitter or metallic aftertastes when ingested at high concentrations, but their lack of calories is well worth the small unpleasantness to many people.

1.6 THE COLOR OF FOOD

It has been said that we eat with our eyes, and that's true to a certain extent. The perception of the color of a food is sometimes crucial for its initial acceptance and later it may influence the perceived flavor and palatability. In addition, color helps us to ascertain the quality of food. For example, bananas are judged for their ripeness according to the color of the skin: green for unripe, yellow for ripe, and the emergence of small dark dots signals the initiation of over-ripening. The presence of a large dark blemish on the skin indicates a damaged fruit.

Color is the result of the interaction between electromagnetic radiation and specific molecules which upon excitation emit waves. The reflected waves (those that are not absorbed), having the wavelengths of 400 to 700 nanometers, are perceived by the eye as colors resulting in a progressive color range from violet to blue to green to yellow to orange and to red. *Chlorophyll*, located mainly in cell chloroplasts (which also contain carotenoids), is the pigment responsible for the characteristic green color of many fruits and vegetables. When degraded by enzymes or heated in a weakly acidic media, chlorophylls (in fact, there are two types) change into another molecule, resulting in unappealing olive-brown pigments. *Carotenoids* (so named because they were isolated from carrots) are responsible for the red, yellow, and predominantly orange color of fruits and vegetables. Interestingly, some carotenoids can be converted into vitamin A in our intestinal wall. *Anthocyanins* are pigments that vary in color from red to purple and blue. Anthocyanins belong to the group of phenolic compounds (which include the tannins) and are found in many berries, red grapes, and eggplant. Anthocyanins are also water soluble, unlike chlorophyll and carotenoids, which are fat soluble. Related compounds called *antoxanthines* give foods a creamy white color.

Many natural colors derived from plants were used as dyes for textiles in ancient times, so it is not surprising that some of the natural food colorants also come from plants. Examples include annatto, a yellow oil extracted from the plant *Bixa orellana*; saffron, the aqueous extract from the pistils of the flower *Crocus sativus*; turmeric, a deep orange-yellow pigment obtained from the plant *Curcuma longa*; and betalains extracted from red beets. There are also nine synthetic colors used in foods in the United States, which have all been subjected to rigorous safety certification processes prior to their approval. Most of these colors are easily recognized on labels by the code "FD&C," followed by the color number (e.g., FD&C Red No. 40).[12] If you want to avoid them, just read the labels.

Natural colors are relatively stable as long as the structure of the food remains intact. Fruits and vegetables suffer discoloration when cut or bruised due to the release and subsequent action of the enzyme polyphenol oxidase (a reaction called enzymatic browning). As we learned in Section 1.2, the activity of this enzyme decreases at higher temperatures (but heat also changes texture and flavor), with changes in pH (which may affect taste), at lower temperatures (an easy one),

with limited exposure to oxygen (e.g., by putting peeled or cut potatoes under water or vacuum packing them), and by the addition of
preservatives (like sulfur dioxide). Freshly butchered meat gets its
purple-red color from the presence of myoglobin, and with a short
exposure to oxygen it develops an attractive bright red color. The
brown pigment metmyoglobin forms during cooking. Cured meats
owe their pink coloration to the addition of nitrites or nitrates. They
release nitric oxide that combines with myoglobin to produce a stable
pigment, which also prevents the growth of *Clostridium botulinum*,
a highly pathogenic microorganism. Mention should also be made
of the addition of a type of carotenoid called *asthaxantin* to the feed
of reared salmon, which enhances the bright orange-pink color of
salmon fillets.

A colored surface can be dull or shiny, and a food's "glossiness"
depends on how much light is reflected from its surface.[13] Those who
swear they would never eat an insect or any part of one should prepare
for a big surprise. Shellac is a resin secreted by the lac beetle (*Coccus
lacca*), which feeds on certain trees in India and southern Asia. Shellac
is approved for use in food applications by the U.S. Food and Drug
Administration (FDA), and many confections are coated with shellac
in order to make them glossy and eye-catching. If you are concerned
about this, beware: the use of shellac may appear on the label as "res-
inous glaze" or "confectioner's glaze."

1.7 SALT FOR ALL TASTES

Ordinary table salt or *sodium chloride* (NaCl) is the most widely used
additive in the world. "Can that which is tasteless be eaten without
salt?" asks Job in the Bible (Job 6:6), and Plutarch concedes that "salt
is the most noble of foods, the best seasoning." In ancient times salt
was scarce—in fact the word *salary* comes from the Roman practice
of paying its militia with salt. Saltshakers were status symbols in the
Middle Ages. A large, richly ornamented saltshaker indicated great
wealth. More recently low cost iodized salt has been an important
treatment for iodine deficiency, which is still a problem in many parts
of the world.

When salt makes contact with water, two chemical species are formed: the chloride ion with a negative charge (Cl^-) and the sodium ion with a positive charge (Na^+). This molecular disassociation that occurs in a liquid is called a *solution*. A solution is different from a dispersion, which is when small particles rather than molecules scatter in a liquid medium. A sodium chloride molecule weighs very little, so a small quantity of salt produces lots of ions. Chemically, a salt solution behaves very different from pure water. The ions migrate rapidly to opposite charges on other molecules, "shielding" their electric effect. This comes in handy when hard boiling eggs—if you add a pinch of salt to the cooking water, any egg white protein that escapes through cracks in the shell is quickly coagulated by the salt ions and any further leaks are blocked.

Throughout history salt has been used to preserve food in two ways: the salt curing of meat and fish (by covering them with granulated salt), and the brining of macerated fruits and vegetables. The salt extracts water from the tissues of the food through osmosis (the passage of water across cell membranes), and any salt that enters the cells reduces the multiplication of microorganisms. The use of salt to preserve foods like anchovies and cod has had an important economic and culinary role in many civilizations, from the Iberian Peninsula throughout Europe and the Americas. Table salt is not only of great interest to cooks, but also to food technologists, chemists, doctors, and nutritionists. Salt affects the flavor and texture of foods (e.g., salt gives bread a finer texture and milder taste). But salt also helps to protect food from microorganisms, and it affects the chemical "environment" in foods, in which other molecules are dispersed.

The sodium content in salt (40% of its weight) is essential for maintaining the equilibrium of the fluids in our bodies. Adults need only 2.3 grams of sodium per day (the equivalent of 5.8 grams of salt); in fact, some experts recommend a daily sodium intake as low as 1.5 grams. However, U.S. adults consume on average around 3.5 grams (or 3,500 mg) of sodium per day, an estimated 77% of which is "hidden" in processed and restaurant foods, and only about 10% comes from table salt and cooking. There is ample evidence that excess sodium leads to elevated blood pressure (hypertension), which increases the risk for stroke, coronary heart disease, and renal disease. One bouillon cube may contain over 660 milligrams of sodium, 10 potato chips have around 150 milligrams, one slice of processed cheese or a frankfurter around 500 milligrams, and a French bread roll may have as much as 1 gram. Fresh chicken sold in supermarkets is often "pumped" with a saline solution, increasing its natural salt content several times over.

Thus, at present the challenge in the processing of these types of foods is to figure out how to reduce the salt content without losing flavor, texture, and shelf life (if possible, without decreasing sales!). In order to perceive the taste of sodium chloride, it must be ionized (i.e., dissolved into solution by saliva). Normally only 20% of the salt in a potato chip dissolves on the tongue before swallowing, so the remaining 80% does not contribute to flavor and only causes problems later on. There are already companies developing microscopic salt crystals that can be more effectively dissolved in the mouth, which could help decrease the amount of undissolved salt that is absorbed into the digestive system without ever being tasted. This replacement may reduce the sodium levels in snack foods by as much as 25%.[14] There are also versions of table salt made of "spongy" crystals containing air, which simply deliver less actual salt per unit of volume.

The most common salt substitute is potassium chloride (also a salt), which has potassium in place of sodium and can maintain the salty flavor when used to replace up to 25% of sodium chloride. But potassium chloride often leaves a bitter aftertaste. Potassium chloride is commercially available as a salt substitute or mixed with sodium chloride as a low sodium choice. Another salt alternative is the partial substitution of salt with savory flavor enhancers like yeast extracts, hydrolyzed vegetable protein, or specific compounds like monosodium glutamate, disodium guanylate, and disodium inosinate.

The food industry must play a very important role in reducing the added salt in foods, which has become a significant public health problem. The consumers who brandish saltshakers at will must be aware of the health risks associated with the overconsumption of salt. And part of the solution must come from science, by developing our understanding of taste and by discovering ways to "trick" the palate in a healthy way with lower doses.

1.8 MOLECULES FOR GOOD HEALTH

In addition to the molecules that form food structures (Chapter 2) or are sources of energy, the body also needs to obtain small quantities of a variety of nutrients from food, the micronutrients. Some of the devastating diseases of the past century were due to dietary deficiencies in these micronutrients, and are completely preventable by adding them to the diet. *Vitamins* are a heterogeneous group of molecules that perform various functions. We must obtain them from our diet, as our bodies cannot synthesize them from other nutrients. Some vitamins are soluble in oil or fat (like vitamins A, D, E, and K) and are better absorbed in the intestine in the presence of lipids. Others are water soluble and can be partially lost when food is cooked in water. There are some vitamins that are thermolabile, which are destroyed at higher temperatures, like vitamin C (ascorbic acid) and vitamin B_1 (thiamine). *Minerals* are the other group of micronutrients, of which 16 are "essential" in that they perform vital bodily functions and must be obtained from the diet. Some important minerals include calcium and phosphorous (for bones and teeth), iron (a component of hemoglobin in red blood cells), sodium and potassium (participate in transmission of nerve impulses and muscle contraction), iodine, magnesium, and zinc. Many of the minerals that we need are in the plants that we eat because plants get minerals from the soil. A varied diet from diverse sources should prevent any micronutrient deficiencies though iron is a special case because it must be supplied in an absorbable form.

Functional foods provide beneficial physiological effects beyond the intrinsic nutritional value of the food.[15] This additional effect can contribute to maintaining health and well-being, or disease prevention. *Nutraceuticals* are substances found in food that have demonstrated health benefits. Functional foods and nutraceuticals can be consumed as food, or taken separately as tablets or capsules.

It is likely that the concept of functional foods came from the work of Ukrainian scientist Elie Metchnikoff (1845–1916), who received the Nobel Prize for Medicine in 1908 for his research in the field of immunology. Metchnikoff was curious about the longevity of Bulgarians, who

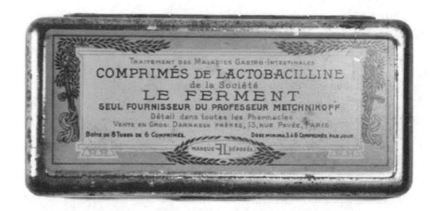

FIGURE 1.3   SMALL METAL BOX FROM THE EARLY TWENTIETH CENTURY CONTAIN-
ING "ACIDOPHILUS" TABLETS PREPARED UNDER THE DIRECTION OF ELIE METCHNIKOFF.
(PHOTOGRAPH BY A. BARRIGA A.)

consumed great quantities of foods that were fermented with *lactobacillus* bacteria, such as yogurt. He suggested that these beneficial microorganisms were replacing harmful microbes in the intestine. He even developed tablets containing these microorganisms, though it is unclear if they were living microbes, which would have been necessary to provide the beneficial effect (Figure 1.3). Today these and other microorganisms that benefit the intestinal flora are known as *probiotics*, and are even present in breast milk (having come from the mother's intestine).

There is growing scientific evidence that certain compounds found in small quantities in plants, generically called *phytochemicals*, have positive health benefits. This is not so surprising as Chinese medicine has a long history of using food as therapy, and Hippocrates considered food the same as drugs. In fact, in many languages the word *recipe* is used interchangeably to mean the prescription for a pharmacist and the directions for the preparation of a dish, which indicates a possible common origin. Popular medicine also attributes preventive and curative properties to certain foods.

The modern history of functional foods began in Japan around 1950, and today this country regulates those products known to provide health benefits, identifying them by the acronym FOSHU (Foods of Specified Health Use). The regulatory aspects of functional foods are becoming more important, because if the claim is that a certain product can treat a disease, it then falls into the category of medications, the sale and use of which are strictly regulated. If a product is said to promote health, then it is considered a food and is subject to different regulations. It is difficult to estimate the global market for functional foods as there is still so much uncertainty about the wide range of products that could be included in this category, but it is clear that sales of these types of products are growing by about 10% every year.[16]

Table 1.1 shows the diversity of raw materials, bioactive compounds, and health benefits attributed to certain functional foods. Raw ingredients include fruits, vegetables, leaves, seeds, algae, and microorganisms. Bioactive molecules range from those that give color to fruits and vegetables (carotene, for example) to a heterogeneous group of macromolecules called *fiber*. The benefits attributed to these products vary widely, but the most common is an antioxidant effect.

Except for the probiotics, which are living bacteria, the bioactive compounds listed in Table 1.1 perform their beneficial effects on a molecular level, so not only must they be present in our food, but they must be available as molecules for our bodies to assimilate them. These molecules must be liberated and recovered from the extracellular matrices of plant and animal tissues where they are naturally located, and the efficiency of this process can influence their bioactivity, or condition for their absorption by our body (see Section 7.8).

Lycopene is one of the antioxidants that has been extensively studied. It is a carotenoid that is partly responsible for the intense red color of tomatoes and that appears to protect against a series of cancers, including prostate cancer. Several events that happen during the industrial processing of tomatoes are relevant to the beneficial action of lycopene. First, when tomatoes are pureed to make juice and sauce, the walls of the tomato cells are broken, freeing lycopene from the tissue matrix, making it more bio-accessible in the gut (see Section 7.8). Second, the heating that occurs when making tomato sauce and tomato concentrates transforms the natural *trans* configuration of the lycopene molecule to a *cis* configuration, which is more rapidly absorbed by our cells.[17] Although some might find it hard to accept, taking these facts

TABLE 1.1
Some Components of Functional Foods and Their Potential Benefits

Class/Component	Origin	Claimed Benefit
Beta-carotene	Carrots	Neutralizes free radicals that can harm cells
Lutein	Green vegetables	Contributes to healthy vision
Lycopene	Tomatoes	Reduces the risk of prostate cancer
Insoluble fiber	Wheat bran	Prebiotic and reduces risk of colon cancer
Beta-glucan	Oatmeal	Reduces risk of cardiovascular diseases (CVDs)
Omega-3 fatty acids	Fish oils	Reduce risk of CVDs and improves other functions
Catechins	Tea	Neutralize free radicals, can reduce cancer risk
Plant sterols	Corn, soy, wheat	Reduce blood cholesterol levels
Isoflavones	Soy	Can reduce menopause symptoms

Continued

TABLE 1.1 (*Continued*)
Some Components of Functional Foods and Their Potential Benefits

Class/Component	Origin	Claimed Benefit
Polyphenols	Wine, apples	Neutralize free radicals, can reduce cancer risk
Lactobacilli and Bifidobacteria	Yogurt	Probiotics, improve gastrointestinal health

into consideration means that cooked pasta sauce can be better for you than eating fresh tomatoes.

The beneficial action of probiotics, such as inhibiting certain pathogens, stimulating the immune system, assisting in vitamin syntheses (like vitamin K), happen while these organisms are living in our intestine, which means they must survive their journey through the upper digestive system and colonize the intestine. For this to happen efficiently, it is sometimes necessary to protect them with artificial capsules before they are added to foods, in a process called *microencapsulation*. Probiotics should not be confused with prebiotics, which are indigestible ingredients added to foods (like fructo-oligosaccharides and inulin) which stimulate the proliferation and activity of probiotic bacteria in the colon.

There are still those who dismiss the many health benefits attributed to functional foods as panacea, and maintain that these foods cannot substitute for a balanced diet, which is and will remain the cornerstone of good nutrition. The case of functional foods differs from that of vitamins and minerals that alleviate specific nutritional deficiencies. For example, the ability of vitamin C to cure scurvy or iodine to cure goiter can be easily demonstrated. Although some functional foods and nutraceuticals can exhibit positive effects for some people, they are certainly not equally beneficial for all (see Section 5.3). Before venturing into the world of functional foods, consumers should research any clinical trials of their claimed beneficial effects, become well informed of any risks associated with the consumption of these foods, and take into consideration their own personal health situation.

1.9 GENES A LA CARTE

Naturally occurring genetic changes in plants and animals have been occurring since there has been life on this planet, either as spontaneous mutations (errors in copying of genetic material during cell division) or by crosses between individuals of the same species. In food production, genetic selection has occurred for millennia in the form of plant and animal breeding by selecting the plant or animal varieties that are more productive, give the best quality products, are most resistant to pests and abiotic factors (water, temperature, etc.) or diseases in the case of fauna. Since 1960, various improved species of wheat and rice that produced yields three times higher than traditional crops have been introduced to the Third World. Plant geneticist Norman E. Borlaug (1914–2009) won the Nobel Peace Prize in 1970 for his Green Revolution, temporarily silencing any Malthusian prophecies (Section 4.2).[18] But it was not all good news, especially for the developing world. The new seeds needed better soil to germinate, with plenty of irrigation and stronger fertilizers, factors often out of reach for small, poor farmers. Another criticism of modified seeds is that they are engineered to provide higher yields and better disease resistance at the expense of the excellent flavors and textures found in traditional seed varieties.

In fact, 99% of agricultural production is concentrated in 24 plant species. Of these, rice, wheat, and corn make up the majority of the calories that we consume. Conventional genetic modification of these and other plants is slow and cannot always keep up with new developments in agriculture and nutrition. In the early 1970s, scientists discovered how to cut pieces of deoxyribonucleic acid (DNA) that contained specific genetic information and insert them into other organisms. By the end of the decade, this recombinant DNA technique was being used to produce insulin and interferon in bacteria (DNA and genes are discussed in Section 12.2). *Genetic engineering* is a technology that manipulates and transfers DNA from one organism to another for commercial purposes. The term *genetically modified organisms* (GMOs), or more specifically, genetically modified food (GM foods), refers to microorganisms, plants, and animals (or products derived from them) that we eat as food that have been altered by genetic engineering. These alterations are called *transgenic* when the new genes come from a different organism or species than the host DNA. The new genes give the plant information on how to make proteins that provide tolerance for pests or diseases, improve its amino acid balance, change its fatty acid profile, and so forth. In practice, however, transgenic soybean, cotton, and corn crops have so far only demonstrated improved agricultural traits. Approximately 80% of the harvested soybeans worldwide are genetically modified, while this figure drops to about 26% for corn. Table 1.2 shows some of the possible benefits and risks associated with transgenic crops.

Although North American consumers appear mostly unconcerned about the use of GMOs in food (the United States does not require special labeling on the products that contain them), Europeans and New Zealanders are very skeptical. New Zealand does not allow any genetically modified crops in the food supply, and their experimental use is tightly regulated. Paradoxically, many justify the genetically modified foods not because they can increase the world's food supply and fight hunger, but because they could help to significantly reduce the use of pesticides and insecticides, which is also the reason for much of the strongest opposition to GMOs. With regard to biodiversity, cisgenic plants are an interesting alternative to GMOs, as the genes introduced are from wild varieties of the same species and are not found in domesticated plants.

There are other nuances involved with GM foods. The genetic alterations cause the plants to make new proteins, which may intervene directly or indirectly with the synthesis of basic components of the food. Vegetable oil from a transgenic plant that has been genetically modified for better resistance to herbicides will be the same as vegetable oil from an unmodified plant, because the proteins that are directly involved with oil synthesis don't change. Obviously the residue left behind after the oil is extracted (which normally becomes animal feed and is consumed by humans in only a few cases) will contain proteins synthesized by the introduced genes.

TABLE 1.2

Some Benefits and Risks Associated with Transgenic Crops

Benefits	Risks
Higher yields; transgenic crops can help feed the developing world	Spread of altered genes to wild relatives and other species, and alteration of biodiversity
Significant decrease in spraying of chemicals to kill insects and weeds; resistance to herbicides	Greater resistance to pesticides and herbicides on the part of insects and weeds
Improved resistance to abiotic stress (such as dry soils, high temperatures, etc.) that will result from climate change	Some of the possible principal beneficiaries (e.g., inhabitants of sub-Saharan Africa) may not be favored
Higher content and better quality of protein and incorporation of micronutrients and bioactive compounds into widely consumed crops[a]	Allergenic potential of new proteins expressed by altered genes

Source: Ackerman, J. 2002. Food: How safe? How altered? *National Geographic* 201, 2–51.

[a] Rice with higher levels of beta-carotene is the best known example of a transgenic crop with improved nutrition. Two genes were introduced to cause beta-carotene accumulation in the grain rather than in the leaves. To date there has not yet been any commercial production of this "golden rice."

It is a different case when the foreign protein becomes an integral component of the food and therefore is likely to be ingested. One recent study from Argentina found trace quantities of the protein CryIA(b) (from genetically modified Bt corn to protect it from pests) in certain commercial products, including raw and precooked polenta, corn snacks, and breakfast cereals (corn flakes).[19] Since consumers cannot detect these foreign proteins when they eat something, foods that contain them should be labeled. One major criticism of GM foods is that those who want to avoid them have no idea whether they are eating them or not.[20] But the presence of both foreign DNA and expressed proteins in grain or food can be detected and quantified in any molecular biology lab, using techniques like polymerase chain reaction (PCR) analysis, DNA chip technology, and mass spectrometry analysis.[21]

As we enter the twenty-first century, it is impossible to ignore the enormous potential of food biotechnology in the areas of agriculture production, vaccine development, diagnostic tests, and so forth. It is hopeful to think that this technology will enable agriculture to confront the challenges of climate change such as drought and increased ambient temperatures, and help feed the ever-growing world population. But consumers also need assurance that scientists, producers, and regulatory agencies are working together to establish the necessary controls for safe and appropriate use of these technologies in our food production.

1.10 UNWANTED GUESTS

Microorganisms or microbes are very small (microscopic) unicellular organisms (bacteria, yeasts, and some algae), viruses, fungi, and other types of living entities, found everywhere in the world. They are often the unwanted guests in our food and for sure in this chapter, as they are certainly not molecules. We admitted them into this section under the subterfuge that they produce both toxic molecules (the *Clostridium botulinum* toxin, for example) as well as beneficial molecules (like acetic acid in vinegar, and ethanol in beer). Microbes are like living factories and participate in important chemical reactions during the *fermentation* of foods (transformations produced by microorganisms like bacteria, yeasts, and molds). They also entered by force, because the number of microbes in our large intestine is 10 times larger than the number of cells in our body, weighing about 1 kg in an adult, and they play an important role in nutrition and health. Finally, they do not fit anywhere else in the book.

The air that we breathe contains thousands of microorganisms per cubic meter and thousands more cover the surfaces with which our food comes in contact (as well as our hands). So it's not so strange that microorganisms (colloquially known as germs) are ubiquitous in food, though they are only welcome in fermented foods. The vast majority of the food we eat contains microorganisms that are harmless to our health or at most cause some decomposition of the food. *Pathogenic* microorganisms are the dangerous ones—they can cause infections (when the microorganism is the pathogenic agent) or can poison us by producing toxins (intoxications). Some bacteria form *spores* (a latent state of encapsulation, desiccation, and dormancy of the microorganisms) that are very resistant to heat and chemical agents, and from which they can return to an active metabolic state and reproduce.

In 1810, when Napoleon needed nonperishable food for his troops, the French chef Nicolas-François Appert (1752–1841) developed a method for preserving food in closed containers by heating them in a water bath. But it was the chemist Louis Pasteur (1822–1895), who made numerous other contributions to science, who proposed that certain diseases were caused by pathogens entering the body. Since that time, methods of canning food (though sometimes in containers other than cans) and other thermal processes have been developed to keep harmful pathogens and spoilage microorganisms out of our food. The most common method of ridding food of harmful microorganisms is to use heat (and high pressure will also be used in the future), but restricting the amount of water can also inhibit their growth (except for spores), as can the presence of certain molecules (Section 5.5). *Pasteurization* is a process that eliminates pathogenic microorganisms by heating food to a certain high temperature for a very short period of time. However, some microorganisms that cause decomposition of the food survive pasteurization. A drop of pasteurized milk (treated at 70 to 75°C for 15 seconds) does not contain a single pathogen but can harbor some 500 living microorganisms per cubic centimeter and must be refrigerated to prevent decomposition. This method preserves most of the organoleptic characteristics, such as color and taste, and nutritional quality of the food (some vitamins are also destroyed by high temperatures), while still killing the harmful bacteria.

Commercially sterilized foods (e.g., canned foods) are heated in auto-claves to temperatures of 121°C for several minutes and become essentially microorganism-free, so they can be stored at room temperature. Under these process conditions there is often a negative effect on vitamins such as vitamin B_1 and vitamin C. Modern processes tend toward higher temperatures and shorter times as is the case of shelf-stable UHT milk (heated for 2 to 3 seconds at 135 to 145°C). The ultra high temperature (UHT)–short time combination reduces the extent of chemical reactions that affect color, taste, and nutrient losses while accomplishing the same killing effect on bacterial spores. Once a commercially sterilized product is opened, it must be refrigerated because it is exposed to new organisms from the air that can cause decomposition.

There are several ongoing challenges to keeping foods safe from harmful pathogens. One problem is the infinite capacity of microorganisms to mutate and adapt to unfavorable environments. A problem is that heat and antibiotics can eliminate the weakest genotypes and select for the most resistant microorganisms. In addition, new microorganisms find "ecological advantages" (niches where they can compete favorably with other microorganisms) and can develop into emerging pathogens. Such is the case of *Listeria monocytogenes*, a pathogen that is widely distributed in the environment but that only recently colonized our refrigerators as demand grew for convenience foods that require little or no cooking. Nowadays food processing plants are likely sources of *Listeria* contamination, where the bacteria can hide even in odd places like drains. Our increasing appetite for fresh-appearing convenience foods is steering the food industry toward more minimal processing with milder preservation treatments, which come with a greater risk for contamination.

As noted above, microorganisms are the guests of honor in the production of fermented foods like yogurt, cheese, sauerkraut, *tempeh*, salami, wine and beer, among others. Korean meals would not be the same without their 300 types of *kimchi*, a mix of fermented cabbages and radishes, combined with herbs, spices, and other seasonings. Bacteria (sauerkraut), yeast (wine, bread), and molds (some ripened cheeses and *tempeh*) have "contaminated" our foods for many centuries, and the results have proven to be both healthy and delicious. This is the case of microbial enzymatic activity that occurs during cheese fermentation, breaking down molecules, generating flavors and aromas, as well as modifying the molecular structures and altering texture.[22] There are also various microorganisms used as "mini factories" for the industrial production of metabolites such as chemicals, pharmaceuticals, biofuels (bioethanol and biodiesel), plastics, and fragrances.

1.11 THERE IS ALWAYS RISK

We understand *risk* to mean the possibility that a chosen action may cause an undesirable (and possibly harmful) result. In this sense we take a risk each time we put a bite of food in our mouth. The British (who are good at keeping statistics) have calculated that approximately 80 people, mostly children, die each year in the United Kingdom from choking on otherwise perfectly healthy food. Besides, there are more than 160 foods that, though harmless to most people, can produce allergic reactions in others, some severe enough to cause death.[23]

An individual consumes around 30 to 40 tons of food during his or her lifetime, yet only rarely does this food cause real harm. According to a U.S. study from 20 years ago, eating was not considered a risky act among those surveyed, unlike driving a car or motorcycle, smoking, drinking alcohol, and using firearms, to name a few. Nuclear energy was perceived as more dangerous than ingesting artificial food coloring.[24] The fact that a danger is documented and even avoidable does not necessarily mean that people will pay attention. That is what the 1.3 billion remaining smokers in the world, according to the World Health Association (WHO), are doing—ignoring the risk—as are the millions of sunbathers who lie out in the sun without a sunblock, despite knowing that sun exposure increases their chance of skin cancer.

Keep in mind that the presence of hazardous substances in food is almost inevitable. To start, there are thousands of chemical substances in food, even in those considered perfectly "natural" and "healthy" (see Table 1.3). Spinach contains oxalic acid that can cause kidney stones, cassava root (also known as yuca or manioc) has cyanogenic compounds that attack the nervous system, many beans have enzyme inhibitors that act as antinutritional factors, potatoes can contain toxic

TABLE 1.3
Some Hazardous Agents and Food Contaminants

Possible Agents	Example	Some Common Carriers
Bacteria	*Campylobacter jejuni*	Poultry
	Echerichia coli	Ground beef, fresh produce
	Salmonella enteritidis	Chickens and eggs
	Listeria monocytogenes	Soft cheeses and processed meats
	Vibrio parahaemolyticus	Raw seafood
Algae	Algal bloom (red tide)	Raw seafood
Contaminants	Pesticides	Fruits, vegetables, juices
	Aflatoxins	Peanut butter, milk, animal feed
	Various chemicals	Migration from plastic packages
	Polychlorinated biphenyls (PCBs)	Animal fats and fish
	Lead	Contamination from cans and from the environment
	Cadmium	Fish, shellfish, and seaweed
	Dioxins	Chicken and other meat, milk

TABLE 1.3 (*Continued*)
Some Hazardous Agents and Food Contaminants

Possible Agents	Example	Some Common Carriers
Formed during processing/ cooking	Nitrosamines Polycyclic aromatic hydrocarbons Heterocyclic amines Acrylamide	Some cured meats Smoked fish, grilled meats Grilled meats Some fried and baked products
Natural substance	Allergens Hemagglutinins Alkaloids	Milk, eggs, fish, shellfish, peanuts, wheat, soybeans, etc. Beans, soy Some lupins, immature potatoes

alkaloids, and so forth. Fortunately some of these compounds are deactivated or eliminated during processing and cooking and are drastically reduced by selective breeding.

A few of the food processing procedures that have been in use for centuries produce harmful chemical precursors or generate substances that have been proven toxic under laboratory conditions and in high doses. A case in point is heterocyclic amines, molecules that can increase the risk of cancer, which are found in meats that have been smoked or cooked at high temperatures. Nitrosamines, which are produced in the stomach from the nitrates used to cure meat, are another example. Lately the news is about acrylamide, which has also been linked to cancer, and which forms when a food containing the amino acid asparagine is heated in the presence of sugars, like in certain baked and fried products.[25] But there are also potential risks associated with mostly beneficial molecules, such as the artificial sweetener cyclamate

(Section 1.5), which has been shown to produce bladder cancer in rats, or aspartame, which when given in large doses can cause brain damage in people with phenylketonuria.[26] Other harmful molecules can be ingested unconsciously, like those that migrate into food from some plastic containers. Persistent organic pollutants like dioxins and polychlorinated biphenyls (PCBs), among others, are found in the environment and accumulate in meat and milk (Table 1.3). New threats come to light as research progresses, more sensitive and specific detection methods are found, and new evidence accumulates. Certain pathogenic microorganisms that are currently problematic and hit the press from time to time, like *Campylobacter jejuni, Escherichia coli O157:H7*, and *Listeria monocytogenes,* were not even on our radar a few decades back.

In the sixteenth century, the Swiss physician Paracelsus stated: "all substances are toxic, only the dose differentiates between a remedy and a poison."[27] This is an important idea to keep in mind when assessing the risk of harmful substances in food. For example, the recommended daily dose of iron for children is about 10 to 15 mg, but an intake of 600 mg of iron could be lethal, as could an overdose of vitamin A.[28]

It's important to distinguish between the hazardous effects of a harmful substance and the actual risk of exposure. For example, the damage from a meteorite hitting the Earth could be immense, but the risk of that happening is very low. For this reason it is necessary to set limits to the levels of toxicity that protect health and provide a baseline for evaluating risk. The basic criterion for tolerable exposure limits in foods is the *acceptable daily intake* (ADI), which represents the quantity of a compound (expressed in mg/kg of weight) that can enter the human body daily without harmful effect. Unfortunately, the ADI is difficult to calculate and must be determined based on animal studies. Another important parameter used by toxicologists is the *median lethal dose* (LD_{50}) of a substance, or the quantity necessary to kill half the members of a tested population, which depends on genetic characteristics as well as environmental factors.

As mentioned above, there is always the possibility that food is contaminated with unsafe or toxic molecules that were not introduced intentionally. There are many potential sources: the environment, waste from agriculture and animal husbandry, packaging materials, and so forth. Normally the quantities are very small and are measured in ppb (parts per billion), or the equivalent of one divided by one billion. To give an idea of this magnitude, think of a drop of ink dispersing in the water of an Olympic pool. With constant improvements in the sensitivity of analytical techniques for detecting chemical compounds, our ability to find traces of toxic ingredients in food improves each day.

A recent outbreak of E. *coli* infection in Germany killed at least 16 people and sickened hundreds more. The contamination was traced to otherwise harmless raw lettuce, cucumbers, and tomatoes. Statistics show that in developed countries, one out of every four to five people are hospitalized each year for illnesses related to microbiological contamination of food. It is estimated that around 5,000 people die each year in the United States from food poisoning (Table 1.3). Most of these infections are caused by *Salmonella* or *Campylobacter* bacteria. Many times the contamination occurs because of poor food handling practices at home, and only 1 in 10 incidents are associated with chain restaurants.[29] The actual risk of acquiring food poisoning at a franchise of a global food chain or a fast food restaurant is much lower than what most people consider it to be. Why? The answer may have to do with the fact that people associate risk with the memory of a bad experience. Each time someone falls ill after eating at a fast food restaurant, a lot of people hear about it in the news, comment on it, and remember it. Returning to the example of sun exposure, we only hear about skin cancer–related deaths when they happen to someone we know or to someone famous, even though skin cancer kills around 12,000 people annually in the United States. Though some of the symptoms of food poisoning can begin almost immediately, in other cases the consequences manifest over time and the evidence is less obvious (e.g., the consumption of heavy metals or carcinogenic agents).

The best way to protect ourselves against these risks is to follow the basic rules of food sanitation, to eat food from a variety of sources, and to stay well informed. Research performed by industry, academia, and government about potential risks should be disseminated quickly to the public (constituency or stakeholders) in a way that is easily understood and internalized. But it is also very important for people to be able to understand the information correctly. Risk analysis is the responsibility of national authorities charged with food safety. The three-part process includes estimating any health risks (evaluation), applying appropriate measures to control them (management), and communicating the risks and measures implemented to all those who are affected (communication).[30] One final word: In general, we tend to ignore the fact that being overly risk-averse has a cost and many possible consequences. Those who are afraid to try new things and who lack confidence never get their "square meal."

1.12 WHO CAN PROTECT US?

How can we be sure that most food molecules we consume each day are healthy and safe? This is a very pertinent question as food-borne illnesses can be severe, even life threatening in some cases. There are five vectors of disease that have the greatest impact on food safety: pathogenic microorganisms (which are not molecules, of course), chemical contaminants, certain natural components that are toxic or allergenic, chemicals produced during processing and cooking (see Table 1.3), and to a much lesser extent, some of the approved synthetic food additives (Section 1.11). Unfortunately, we are typically unable to detect any of these vectors by sight, smell, or taste, because they occur in such small amounts (unless you eat spoiled food). In the past it was only after people suffered traumatic outcomes from contaminated food that doctors could prevent further illness, but today modern science enables us to detect most cases in a timely fashion as well as warn consumers of possible problems (like allergens).[31]

It is important to understand the difference between food safety and food security, as the two terms are not interchangeable. *Food safety* ensures that the food supply (consumed by both people and animals) is safe and not harmful to our health.[32] Food safety is essential for a healthy society. When there is *food security*, individuals have continuous access to sufficient food to meet their nutritional needs in order to maintain a healthy and active lifestyle.

The complexity of modern life is such that certain large tasks, like ensuring food safety, are best left in the hands of government and industry, rather than individuals. The mission of governmental food safety agencies (or Ministries of Health) is to establish regulations that protect consumers, ensure that the food supply meets the established standards, and to carry out the assessment, management, and communication of any threats to food safety (as seen in Section 1.11). In the United States, the FDA (www.fda.gov) is responsible for regulating foods and beverages for humans and animals, as well as nutritional supplements.[33] Since 2002, the European Union has relied on the European Food Safety Authority (EFSA) (www.efsa.europa.eu) for risk assessment in relation to food safety and the security of the European food supply. According to their Web site, "(the EFSA acts) in close collaboration with national authorities and in open consultation with interested parties (stakeholders) to provide independent scientific advice and clear communication on existing and emerging food safety risks."[34] It would take many pages to describe the procedures that these and other agencies use to evaluate and re-evaluate (when necessary) food safety and to approve new food additives, but they are well described in publicly available documents.[35] EFSA recently announced that it is willing to reassess the safety of all previously authorized food additives by 2020, taking into consideration the latest available scientific evidence.

Exposure to pathogenic microorganisms, environment contaminants, and natural allergens is inevitable with the consumption of food. But there are also synthetic molecules designed for a particular purpose, such as improved appearance and flavor (colorants and flavorings) or to reduce the calorie content of widely consumed foods (sweeteners, fat substitutes). One emblematic example in recent years has been the introduction of *Olestra®* (see Section 1.13), a synthetic, no caloric fat substitute that is a polyester of sucrose (a sugar molecule attached to various fatty acids) that does not exist naturally in food. The synthetic molecule is not reactive and is passed through the digestive system without being absorbed, so no calories are ingested. Olestra can cause diarrhea in some cases and may affect absorption of fat-soluble vitamins. It took Procter and Gamble 30 years and $200 million of research and development to convince the FDA that Olestra was safe and could reduce fat consumption, particularly in snack foods. If you want to keep away from these molecules, read the labels.

Another notable example of extreme action on the part of the food regulatory agencies involves the case of food irradiation, a technology that has been studied since the early twentieth century, designed to destroy pathogenic bacteria and parasites in food. Foods are treated with ionizing radiation (a form of energy having short waves that can penetrate a food) in the form of x-rays, electron beams, and gamma rays, which is powerful enough to break molecules and produce ions.[36] This causes irreversible damage to the DNA of microorganisms, insects, and plants, but does not affect other molecules or raise the temperature of the food. Irradiation has been extensively studied and evaluated for safety, with results demonstrating that in appropriate doses irradiation is as safe as alternative methods of food preservation. Since the mid-1980s food irradiation has been more widely used, replacing less effective measures, and is currently approved in authorized doses in more than 50 countries for specific products (including ground beef, spices, chicken, fish, and seafood). An important application is as replacement of certain harmful chemicals used as fumigants in fresh fruits and vegetables. For consumer awareness foods that have been irradiated are required to be labeled with an internationally recognized symbol as well as with the phrase "treated by irradiation."

Industry and the academic sector also participate in the safety of our food. The food industry as well as fast food chains implement preventive protocols to detect microbiological contamination and monitor food hygiene, which are collectively known as Hazard Analysis and Critical Control Points (HACCP). Big multinational companies have their own research laboratories dedicated to food safety, where chemists, toxicologists, and microbiologists work together. In universities, food microbiologists are very active in the food science departments and perform research in the areas of emerging infections, techniques for rapid microbiological analysis, and applications of molecular genetics for pathogen identification. There are toxicologists in academia as well, who study the properties and detection of toxic substances in food and their harmful effects on the body. The Academies of Science in various countries and the FAO (UN Food and Agriculture Organization) convene from time to time so that experts can discuss various issues and produce public reports.37 But it is today's informed consumers who increasingly demand safer and healthier food. There are many organized consumer groups as well as NGOs concerned with food safety in the developed world, and these groups have easily accessible Web sites.[38]

1.13 DESIGNER MOLECULES

It is quite logical to wonder how there could be molecules that are nutritionally healthier than those available from natural food. The actual fact is that our planet is somewhat imperfect. The Periodic Table shows us that certain chemical elements exist and can be part of molecules but they cannot be found anywhere in this world. According to some scientists, these missing elements could have surprising applications.[39] You might think that through the slow but effective process of evolution, nature has rarely failed to provide solutions to real-world problems. But with everything changing now so rapidly in relation to the times of biology, isn't nature's stride a bit slow? As we've seen, some of the molecules naturally present in food are not that good, and we have learned to transform or eliminate them over time. We don't hesitate to introduce pharmaceutically produced molecules into our bodies (sometimes so many that we need special pillboxes to carry them) when they have been proven to be much more effective than the "natural" alternatives. But we have not progressed as far with food, and molecules that are designed (using chemical, physical, or enzymatic methods) to overcome the functional limitations or nutritional properties of natural food molecules are still regarded with suspicion. Biotechnology allows us to make very controlled changes to the molecules directly in the plant or organism that synthesizes them, but some people are not willing to eat GM foods because they do not trust the technology or regard them as "non-natural." As expected, in all cases the production and use of some beneficial designer molecules will be extensively investigated and regulated by food safety agencies.

To the list of synthetic molecules that already includes artificial sweeteners and other synthetic additives like colorants and flavors, you can add molecules with important benefits like lower caloric content and improved culinary properties. All of these molecules are part of our processed food, but they tend to be displaced by natural ingredients. The following paragraphs deal with the chemical nature of these transformations and the resulting products, which we already consume in a variety of foods.

Modified starches are designed to overcome some of the limitations found with natural starches, such as excessive physical degradation during cooking, instability with exposure to heat or acid pH, retrogradation (recrystallization) upon storage, and syneresis (exudation of water) after thawing from the frozen state. Chemically modified starch molecules are quite common in the processed food industry, and some of the most frequently performed modifications are the creation of derivatives in the form of ethers, esters, and oxidized compounds (i.e., natural molecules with modified segments), and the cross-linking or hydrolysis (breakdown) of amylose and amylopectin chains (Section 2.1). For example, oxidized starches (starches that have been treated with sodium hypochlorite, the same chemical used to bleach clothes) allow mayonnaise and salad dressings to have low viscosities, while preventing retrogradation (the formation of hard crystals) and the formation of opaque gels.[40] Starch ethers, often found in the fruit fillings of frozen desserts and pastries, provide greater stability to frozen products, making them more resistant to freeze-thaw cycles. Some modified starches are not digested as well as natural starches, so they produce less glucose and are effectively lower in calories, which is good for dieters and the diabetic (Section 7.7). The hydrolysis (breakdown) of starches by acid under conditions of low humidity (<15%) and high temperatures (150 to 200°C) produces a yellowish powder made of short glucose polymers called *dextrins*. Because of their solubility and viscosity, dextrins are used in instant foods and baby foods that don't need to be cooked. By adjusting the size of the resulting polymers, hydrolysis allows the food industry to obtain attractive combinations of viscosity and solubility.

Structured lipids are lipid molecules that have been "tailored" for a specific nutritional or technological function, by selecting the fatty acids that make up the triglycerides and placing them in the exact position within the glycerol molecule. Many of these structured lipids are uncommon or do not exist in nature. Enzymes can both cleave apart and attach molecules together, and under particular conditions a lipase enzyme can add a fatty acid to a glycerol molecule in a particular place to form a new triglyceride (Section 1.2). Structured lipids are used as cocoa butter substitutes, low calorie fats, in infant formulas, and in enteral and parenteral nutrition products. One of the most interesting commercial applications for structured lipids is a triglyceride called *Betapol®* that has the same structure as the main triglyceride in human milk. Betapol is used in infant formula and adds superior nutritional benefits compared to any other known fat. Noncaloric fat substitutes are produced by reaction of several of the -OH groups in sucrose with medium-chain fatty acids (C8:0 to C12:0), forming a new molecule called an ester, which results in a product that has no flavor and is heat stable. *Olestra®* is the most famous of these noncaloric sucrose esters and can be used for frying and in baked products.

Acids and enzymes can also cleave proteins, producing peptides and amino acids with savory meat flavor which are used in soup bouillons and meat sauces. These molecules are labeled on packaging as "hydrolyzed soy protein" or "hydrolyzed corn." As mentioned previously, it's possible also to enzymatically join peptides and amino acids (in a chemical reaction called plastein) to create new proteins with a higher nutritional value. Proteins can also be used to mimic the mouthfeel of fats, but with fewer calories. These wet microparticles of protein between 100 nm and 3 microns in size, seem to "melt" in the mouth and provide a sensation of creaminess. Microparticulated whey protein (e.g., *Simplesse®*) is used in ice creams and other desserts, where they can replace enough of the fat to lower the caloric content by up to 85%.

Development of these engineered "designer" food molecules can be thought of as a form of food pharmacology (pharmafoods), because these molecules can play an important role in public health by reducing the caloric content of foods without greatly impairing their taste. The future use of designer molecules depends on many things: specific health needs, quality and effectiveness, and the ability of chemists, biochemists, and biotechnologists to design molecules that perform as close to natural ones as possible in products. Evidently, the potential risk of designer molecules must be evaluated and regulatory approval will be mandatory. Moreover, unlike pharmaceuticals, which cost hundreds of millions of dollars to develop but are profitable when very effective, designer food molecules need to be inexpensive and produced in large quantities. Besides having to overcome many safety concerns and suspicions from some users, foods containing these molecules will face highly competitive markets.

1.14 BITTERSWEET

Verjuice is the sour juice obtained from unripe grapes that was commonly used in the Middle Ages to flavor dishes. It leaves a slightly bitter taste in the mouth before swallowing. The Spanish word for verjuice, "agraz," is used colloquially to denote something that leaves a feeling of bitterness and sorrow. One might feel sad and bitter when contemplating certain recent traumatic experiences with dangerous food products that entered the market and caused great harm. One of the more serious cases occurred in 1981 in Spain, where some canola (rapeseed) oil that had been denatured with aniline and was intended for industrial use, was released into the food market. The resulting "toxic oil" syndrome resulted in over 24,000 poisonings and 580 deaths.

The first cases of "mad cow disease," or bovine spongiform encephalopathy (BSE) were detected in the United Kingdom in 1986. BSE is caused by *prions*, which are transmitted to humans through infected animal parts, especially nervous system tissue. Prions are aggregates of certain proteins that are normally harmless cell components, but which have the capacity to become stable particles that cause various brain diseases in humans and animals. Symptoms can include loss of muscle control and memory loss. The English scientist Stanley B. Prusiner (1942–), a professor at the University of California, San Francisco, received the 1997 Nobel Prize in Physiology or Medicine for his discovery of this new class of infectious agents, adding to the long list of bacteria and viruses.[41]

Dioxins are highly toxic substances that are formed during thermal processes at very high temperatures (200 to 600°C) in the presence of chlorine. Dioxins are widely distributed in the environment and can be found concentrated in the fat of animals that have been exposed to them. The first documented case of dioxins entering the food supply occurred in Belgium in 1999, when stock animals were fed feed that was contaminated with dioxins and other chlorine compounds, which then passed into the human food chain. A few months later, health problems began to appear which were linked to contaminated chicken, and eventually dioxins were determined to be the cause, a reflection of the progress science has made in detecting the precise source of these types of episodes. This embarrassing and unfortunate incident, in which many people were affected, eventually led to the fall of the Belgian government administration at that time.

Milk contaminated with melamine in China has been another unfortunate recent event that resulted in the death of at least six babies and sickened more than 30,000 with still unknown long-term effects. Melamine is used in the production of plastics, fertilizers, and cleaning products. Because of its high nitrogen content, melamine can be used to adulterate milk, making it appear to have more protein.[42] This incident had large commercial repercussions as well, causing the New Zealand company Fonterra, which owned 43% of the Chinese company involved, to lose more than $150 million.

Bird and swine flu are indirectly related to the food supply. The most recent swine flu pandemic caused around 12,000 deaths and the culprit was a virus, a piece of RNA or DNA surrounded by a protein coat that is unable to replicate without a host cell. The flu virus has existed in wild bird populations for thousands of years and usually did not cause harm. But if it passes to humans it can cause pandemics like the "Spanish flu" epidemic of 1918 that killed more than 50 million people worldwide. To date, there is no scientific data to suggest that viral diseases can be transmitted to humans through food when it is cooked properly. But intensive farming of poultry and pigs in overcrowded conditions can be a breeding ground for the selection and replication of a highly virulent virus.[43] The European Union has launched a series of initiatives to improve the conditions in the housing and transportation of animals for food production. In another case, the infectious salmon anemia (ISA) virus, which is not contagious to people, is believed to have spread in Chile (the world's second largest producer of salmon after Norway) due to the overcrowded conditions of farmed salmon there.

At least three causes or conclusions can be drawn from these tragic episodes related to food consumption. First is the problem of greed and unscrupulous individuals eager for profit at any cost. Second, the amount of contaminants recirculating through the food supply chain is increasing. Finally, part of our food industry lacks the scientific knowledge and respect necessary to maintain the stability of the very fragile biological systems on which it is dependent.

1.15 MISALLOCATED MOLECULES

This chapter would not be complete without a discussion about the fact that there are still many people who are undernourished in the world, despite all of the technological advances that allow for more and better food production. It is a paradox that we can produce enough food to feed the 7 billion people in the world, yet there are 1,200 million people who are overfed, 850 million who do not have an adequate diet, and 250 million who are starving. As this book is written, there are famines affecting as many as 12 million people across the horn of Africa. In southern Somalia nearly 3 million people are facing starvation, and childhood malnutrition in Somalia has escalated to 55%, while infant mortality is up to six deaths per day.[44]

The world produces enough food to feed every human being on this planet. According to FAO, by 2002 the agricultural output was enough to provide the entire world population with at least 2,720 kilocalories per person per day, which is 17% more calories per person than 30 years before, despite a 70% population increase across the same period.[45] Back in 1994, U.S. farmers produced enough food to meet almost one and a half times the nutritional requirements of the entire U.S. population, even with subsidies that discouraged farmers from growing certain crops.[46] The amount of grains fed to livestock in the United States is enough to feed about 840 million people who follow a plant-based diet.[47] In Europe, almost one third of food available at supermarkets cooked at home goes to the trash container.

Article 25 of the Universal Declaration of Human Rights states that "everyone has the right to a standard of living adequate for the health and well-being of himself and his family, including food." An estimated 6 million children in the world die each year as the direct or indirect result of hunger or malnutrition. This is often a difficult problem of economics, as most of these people are living on less than a dollar a day and are too poor to buy food. This flagrant violation of human rights is occurring around the world. Unfortunately no one is charged with finding those responsible and bringing them to trial in international courts.

There is a more subtle deprivation buried within the issue of food scarcity—that of micronutrient deficiencies. Although they may not cause death, these deficiencies can greatly reduce quality of life and limit human potential. Enzymes, hormones, and other compounds essential for growth and development of our bodies need micronutrients to function properly. In poorer countries, vitamin A deficiency is the primary cause of preventable blindness in children and pregnant women, and also increases the risk of complications and death from infections. This is a problem in more than half the countries around the world, especially in Africa and southwest Asia, where an estimated 250,000 to 500,000 people go blind due to vitamin A deficiency each year. Iodine insufficiency is the most common cause of brain damage and mental retardation worldwide. The solution, iodized salt, costs less than 5 cents per person per year. Despite the affordable solution, iodine deficiency is still prevalent in more than 50 countries. Iron deficiency is the most widespread deficiency of all. It is estimated that some 2 billion people, or 30% of the world population, suffer from some degree of anemia. The solution, iron-fortified foods, is not as simple as adding iodine to salt, because the iron must be in a form that the body can absorb.[48] Cultural factors are another limitation to combat deficiencies, as pills and tablets are still not well accepted in some parts of the world.

NOTES

1. The size of the molecules is not expressed by their length or volume, but by their molecular weight (MW), and in the case of polymers, by the number of monomers (basic units) in their structure. For example, the beta-lactoglobulin in whey (from cow's milk) is a small protein (measuring a few nanometers), consisting of 162 monomers (amino acids) with a MW of 18.4 kDa (kiloDaltons).
2. The hyphen (-) next to the NH_2 symbol represents a possibility that this group (or any other group) bonds or links to another atom or molecule.
3. Fats are solid and oils are liquid at room temperature, but both are lipids and have the same type of triglyceride molecules.
4. A good definition of *additive* is that of the European Union: "a food additive is any substance that is not itself normally consumed as food nor used as a characteristic ingredient, whether or not it has nutritional value. They are added to perform a technological purpose during the manufacture, processing, preparing, treating, packaging, transport or storage of a food, and the additive or its products become a component of the food,

directly or indirectly." (For a full definition see Article 1(2) of Directive 89/107/EEC.)

5. Belitz, H.-D., Grosch, W., and Schieberle, P. 2004. *Food Chemistry*, 3rd revised ed. Springer, New York, pp. 434–472.

6. There are many sources on food additives, but keep in mind that the regulation changes periodically and is different in different countries. A good encyclopedia is accessible on the Internet: FoodinCanada.com. 2006. Encyclopedia of Food Additives. www.bizlink.com/foodfiles/PDFs/apr2006/food_encyclopedia_food_additives_apr06.pdf. You can also consult Burdock, G.A. 1996. *Encyclopedia of Food & Color Additives*. CRC Press, Boca Raton, FL.

7. Butylated hydroxyanisole (BHA), butylated hydroxytoluene (BHT), the tertiary butyl hydroquinone (TBHQ), and propyl gallate (PG) are synthetic antioxidants authorized for food use.

8. You can access a list of the food additives that are permitted in the European Union here: European Food Safety Authority (EFSA). Food additives. www.efsa.europa.eu/en/topics/topic/additives.htm (accessed February 14, 2012). Information for the United States is available at U.S. Food and Drug Administration (FDA). Food ingredients and colors. 2010 (revised). www.fda.gov/food/foodingredientspackaging/ucm094211.htm#types (accessed February 14, 2012).

9. There are several books discussing potential risks associated with the consumption of additives, such as Simontacchi, C.N. 2000. *The Crazy Makers: How the Food Industry Is Destroying Our Brains and Harming Our Children*. Tarcher/Putnam, New York.

10. According to a March 31, 1999, article in *The San Francisco Chronicle*, sugar processed from sugarcane and sugar processed from beets act differently in the kitchen, even though they share the same chemistry.

11. Roberts, R.M. 1989. *Serendipity: Accidental Discoveries in Science*. Wiley Science Editors, New York, pp. 150–154.

12. The nine synthetic colors approved by the U.S. Food and Drug Administration (FDA) are FD&C Blue Nos. 1 and 2, FD&C Green No. 3, FD&C Red Nos. 3 and 40, FD&C Yellow Nos. 5 and 6, Orange B, and Citrus Red No. 2.

13. More about shiny foods and how to measure gloss can be found in Mendoza, F., Dejmek, P., and Aguilera, J.M. 2010. Gloss measurements of raw agricultural products using image analysis. *Food Research International* 43, 18–25.

14. Complete information in: PepsiCo develops designer salt to chip away at sodium intake. *The Wall Street Journal*, March 22, 2010.

15. The subject of functional foods has been extensively covered in recent years in books and scientific papers. A good overall reference to the subject of this section is Webb, G.P. 2006. *Dietary Supplements and Functional Foods*. Blackwell, Oxford.

16. Information and market projections are available for a variety of functional foods. Jeya Henry, Director of the Functional Food Centre in Oxford, United Kingdom, estimates that the market for functional foods will be around 500 billion dollars per year in 2010 (personal communication). Menrad, K. 2003. Market and marketing of functional food in Europe. *Journal of Food Engineering* 53, 181–188, suggests a figure closer to 30 billion dollars annually. Part of the problem is what is considered a functional food.

17. When there is a double bond joining two carbon atoms in a long molecule, it restricts the rotation of the ends of the molecule. The hydrogen atoms can then either end up on the same side (*cis*) or on opposite sides (*trans*). This also applies to fatty acids (Section 1.2). The molecules in *cis* and *trans* configurations have the same chemical formula (and therefore the same name), but they have different properties.

18. It is interesting to note that this is the only Nobel Prize ever awarded for food-related research. See www.nobelprize.org.

19. Margarit, E., Reggiardo, M.I., Vallejos, R.H., and Permingeat, H.R. 2006. Detection of BT transgenic maize in foodstuffs. *Food Research International* 39, 250–255.

20. Read more on the views of those opposed to GM foods in Teitel, M., and Wilson, K.A. 2001. *Genetically Engineered Food: Changing the Nature of Nature*, Park Street Press, Vermont, which has a foreword by Ralph Nader.

21. Polymerase chain reaction (PCR) analysis is a technique that allows millions of precise DNA replications to be created from a single sample of DNA. The enzyme DNA polymerase builds a new strand of DNA that is a template of the original DNA, and a chain reaction occurs whereby this template is amplified many times.

22. It is estimated that there are more than 500 varieties of cheese in France and about 2,000 in the world. Former President Charles de Gaulle complained about how difficult it was to lead the French, who could not even agree on a cheese.

23. Reactions to the consumption of certain foods that do not involve an immune response are called *intolerances*, such as lactose intolerance. An immune system reaction that occurs soon after eating certain foods is called allergy.

24. Slovic, P. 1987. Perception of risk. *Science* 236, 280–285.
25. For example, see Stadler, R.H., Blank I., Varga, N., Robert, F., Hau, J., Guy, P.A., Robert, M.C., and Riediker, S. 2002. Acrylamide from Maillard reaction products. *Nature* 419, 449. All these researchers worked at the time of publication at the Nestlé Research Center in Switzerland.
26. Mead, P.S., Slutsker, L., Dietz, V., McCaig, L.F., Bresee, J.S., Shapiro, C., Griffin, P.M., and Tauxe, R.V. 2000. Food-related illness and death in the United States. *Journal of Environmental Health* 62, 9–18, is a widely cited article on food-borne diseases (3,581 citations on January 30, 2010). This article argues that more than 200 known diseases are transmitted by food (at the time of publication of the article) including diseases caused by viruses, bacteria, parasites, toxins, metals, and prions. Symptoms of food-borne illness range from mild gastroenteritis to potentially life-threatening illnesses involving neurological, liver, and kidney damage. According to the article, food-borne diseases affect between 6 million and 81 million people in the United States, and cause up to 9,000 deaths each year.
27. It is interesting that poison is technically a toxic substance that is used intentionally.
28. Data obtained from Ribas, B. 2000. The importance of iron in food. In *Food and Health* (B. Sanz Pérez, ed.), Real Academia de Farmacia, Madrid, pp. 237–264. The toxic overdose of vitamin A for children is 1,500 IU/kilo of body weight per day.
29. See Spain, W. 2007. MarketWatch. Less danger in dining out? www.marketwatch.com/story/it-may-be-statistically-safer-to-eat-at-chain-fast-food-joints (accessed March 14, 2011).
30. Two of many documents on food-related risks: FAO. 2007. Food Safety Risk Analysis: A guide for national food safety authorities. FAO Food and Nutrition paper 87, Rome, and Winter, C.K., and Francis, F.J. 1997. Assessing, managing and communicating chemical food risks. *Food Technology* 51(5), 85–92.
31. The warning "made in a facility that processes peanuts, almonds, other grains, wheat protein, milk and egg protein" can be found on the packaging of many products, especially candy and snacks. This warning is necessary because the presence of only tiny amounts of these ingredients (which may have been inadvertently introduced by not properly cleaning the equipment, for example) can cause allergy symptoms in susceptible individuals.
32. Part of a statement by President Barack Obama on March 14, 2009: "We are a nation built on the strength of individual initiative. But there are certain things that we can't do on our own. There are certain things only a government can do. And one of those things is ensuring that the foods we

eat, and the medicines we take, are safe and don't cause us harm" www. whitehouse.gov/blog/09/03/14/Food-Safety (accessed June 19, 2012).

33. It is not so simple. The U.S. Department of Agriculture (USDA) is also involved in controlling food safety through the Food Safety and Inspection Service (FSIS) (www.fsis.usda.gov), a public health agency responsible for overseeing the commercial supply of meat, poultry, eggs, and products derived from these, and the Animal and Plant Health Inspection Service (APHIS) (www.aphis.usda.gov), which is the agency charged with protecting agriculture, which therefore monitors agricultural imports (e.g., fresh fruit) to the United States.

34. The European Union countries each maintain their own agencies responsible for food safety and regulations.

35. This article reviews in detail the approval process for food additives by the FDA, and discusses some specific cases: Rulis, A.M., and Levitt, J.A. 2009. FDA'S food ingredient approval process: Safety assurance based on scientific assessment. *Regulatory Toxicology & Pharmacology* 53, 20–31.

36. For more information about food irradiation visit U.S. EPA. Food irradiation. www.epa.gov/radiation/sources/food_irrad.html.

37. In December 2008, the Institute of Medicine (one of the U.S. National Academies of Science) hosted a discussion panel on the role of nanotechnology in food. The results are published in the book *Nanotechnology in Food Products*. The National Academies Press, Washington, DC (2009). There you will find my chapter entitled "Where is the nano in foods?"

38. *Consumer Reports* provides consumer alerts on its Web site concerning reported cases involving food safety (http://blogs.consumerreports.org/safety/food/). *Greenpeace* has an active Web site as well, mostly dedicated to its opposition to genetically modified foods.

39. Since 1981 six chemical elements have been discovered with atomic numbers from 107 to 112. The latter has been named *Copernicium* (Cp) In early April 2010 a team of Russian and American scientists reported discovery of an element with atomic number 117, which had an average life span of 78 milliseconds.

40. At this point it might be worth a trip to the refrigerator to check the list of ingredients in *light* mayonnaise. Obviously, no label will say carboxymethyl starch or hydroxypropyl starch, which is what some of these compounds really are. On ingredient labels they are more elegantly described as "modified starches."

41. Nobelprize.org.   http://nobelprize.org/nobel_prizes/medicine/laureates/1997/press.html (accessed August 20, 2009).

42. The routine analysis of protein content in food is based on determining the nitrogen, then multiplying the percentage of nitrogen by a factor of

6.25 (or other similar factor, depending on the type of protein) to calculate the percentage of protein. This value is called the *crude protein value*, as not all of the nitrogen in food is in protein molecules.

43. Wuethrich, B. 2003. Chasing the fickle swine flu. *Science* 299, 1504–1505. This article states that a virus will have more opportunities to replicate and spread on a large farm with 5,000 animals than in a smaller group of 100 pigs raised on a small farm.
44. Editorial published in *The Washington Post* on August 2, 2011. See entire article here: WP Opinions. Somalia's hunger: A man-made crisis requires action. www.washingtonpost.com/opinions/somalias-hunger-a-man-made-crisis-requires-action/2011/08/02/gIQA3sCTqI_story.html (accessed August 18, 2011).
45. Data from the paper FAO. Reducing poverty and hunger: The critical role of financing for food, agriculture and rural development, www.fao.org/docrep/003/Y6265e/y6265e00.htm (accessed January 12, 2012).
46. Kantor, L.S., Lipton, K., Manchester, A., and Oliveira, V. 1997. Estimating and addressing America's food losses. *Food Review* 20(1), 2–12.
47. Pimentel, D., and Pimentel, M. 2003. Sustainability of meat-based and plant-based diets and the environment. *American Journal of Clinical Nutrition* 78, 660S–663S.
48. The problem of vitamin A deficiency and its global impact is described on the World Health Organization Web site (World Health Organization. Nutrition health topics. www.who.int/nutrition/topics/en/).

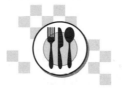

CHAPTER 2

Food Materials
and Structures

Nature is in charge of transforming molecules into edible structures, and the kitchen turns them into delicious meals. In this sense, ingredients are building materials and we can describe them as such: hard or soft, smooth or fibrous, crisp, and so forth. The science of food materials provides a framework for the conversion of these raw materials into structures that we can appreciate with our palate, as well as the development of potentially amazing new structures yet to come.

2.1 NATURAL STRUCTURES

Foods come from tissues that serve certain purposes in nature. Over time humans have chosen to domesticate certain edible plants, selecting those that are easiest to cultivate, with the best flavors and textures. Thus, we eat flowers (cauliflower, broccoli, and artichokes) or their parts (stigmas like saffron), leaves (lettuce, endive, and spinach), and even stems (palms and asparagus). There are also the sweet fruits that we all love in our desserts and juices, and those we consider vegetables like cucumbers, tomatoes, and avocados, and olives from which we also harvest oil. The dried fruits called cereals or grains, such as wheat, corn, and rice, have an important culinary and nutritional role. Our menus are enriched with seeds such as legumes and pseudo-roots like carrots, beets, and radishes, as well as thickened stems that grow underground like potatoes.[1]

To simplify, the "natural structures" that make up the raw materials of our food can be classified into four major groups: (a) tissue structures that are assembled from smaller molecules (glucose, amino acids) or macromolecules (starch, proteins) which have a specific function, like the bundles of cellulose present in vegetable cell walls or the muscle fibers in meat; (b) the fleshy parts of plants that are made of groups of cells which retain water and have cell walls that allow turgidity, such as tubers, fruits, and vegetables; (c) encapsulated embryos that contain discrete packages of starch, proteins, and fat, like grains, legumes, and eggs as well; and (d) a complex and specific liquid called milk, the nutrition for infant mammals, which has basic nutrients in a state of colloidal dispersion or in aqueous solution.

Nature creates functional structures from a limited number of small molecules by associating them into macromolecules or polymers, which in turn are assembled into increasingly complex hierarchical structures like organelles, cells, tissues, organs, and ultimately organisms (Figure 2.1). For example, the elasticity of tendons comes from a chain of structures ranging from collagen molecules to the fiber bundles that make up the tendon. Those molecules that don't have a functional purpose in cereals, legumes, and oil seeds accumulate as reserves in small structures such as starch granules, protein bodies (small sacks of proteins), and oil globules. Starch and the proteins in wheat (called gluten), which are so important to our food supply, play a different role in food than in plants—as a thickener and an elastic matrix, respectively. Clearly, nature did not design plant tissues and organs with our culinary delight and nutrition in mind, but humans discovered these side benefits in a slow process of trial (literally) and error.

Nature often keeps groups of molecules separated from other groups as a control mechanism—otherwise these molecules might react with one another out of turn. Some reactive molecules are kept in a nonreactive

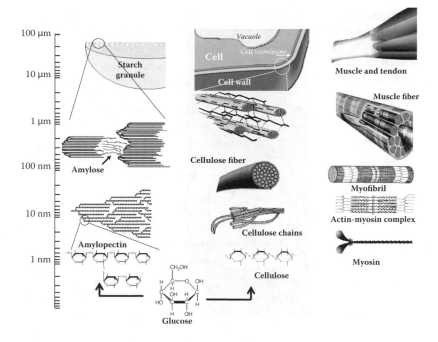

FIGURE 2.1   HIERARCHICAL STRUCTURES IN STARCH GRANULES, PLANT TISSUES, AND MUSCLE TISSUE. NATURE FABRICATES INCREASINGLY COMPLEX STRUCTURES FROM RELATIVELY SMALL MOLECULES, AND THESE STRUCTURES PLAY A FUNDAMENTAL ROLE IN WHAT HAPPENS DURING FOOD PROCESSING AND COOKING. THE DIMENSIONS ON THE VERTICAL AXIS ARE APPROXIMATE.

form but can be activated when needed, such as enzymes as well as their substrates (the molecules on which they act). For example, garlic cells have microcompartments inside of them, separated by thin biological membranes. Some compartments contain the enzyme alliinase, while others hold the chemical alliin, an inoffensive amino acid compound. Breaking open a garlic clove destroys the compartmentalization and the enzyme alliinase comes into contact with the alliin and produces another compound called *allicin*, which gives garlic its familiar pungent smell.

Although we eat the molecules in our food, we don't actually chew them. The molecules in our food are part of the natural plant and animal tissue structures, and by processing or cooking our food we form other structures from them. Food structures will be further addressed in later sections of this chapter, but it's important to realize how nature organizes molecules into complex hierarchical structures to fulfill various functions, and how in turn, these structures give rise to the unique culinary characteristics of different foods. We will consider three examples: starch, the cell walls of plants, and muscle tissues (Figure 2.1).

Starch is not a molecule but rather a tiny granule assembled from two types of polymers, both made of glucose monomers: *amylose*, which is composed of a few thousand glucose units in the form of a helical strand, and *amylopectin*, which is a large branched macromolecule made of several thousand glucose monomers. Because the main function of starch is to store energy, nature designed these polymers so that lots of them can be stored compactly inside the starch granule, forming ordered crystalline layers that alternate with less-organized amorphous layers (Figure 2.1, left). This is why native starch is often referred to as a semi-crystalline material. Under the microscope, starch granules look like small pieces of solid granite, the largest of which are smaller than the thickness of a single hair (Figure 3.3). All natural starch is in the form of these dense granules that are between 5 and 50 microns in size and round to ellipsoidal in shape. Commercial potato starch and corn starch are produced by grinding potatoes or corn and then dispersing the mash in water. Centrifugation or filtration of the aqueous dispersion can separate out the dense and small granules (respectively) from the rest of the tissue debris, which are then dried to a powder and used for many purposes, from making sweeteners to preparing biofuels.

When nature cannot obtain the desired properties from one single material, it combines the material with others so that the resulting structure has superior qualities. In the field of engineering, a *composite* structure is one that consists of a continuous matrix containing diverse elements embedded within it that together provide superior properties. Corrugated plastic roofing sheets that are reinforced with fiberglass for added strength are an example of a composite structure. *Cell walls* are the analogous structures in plants. The "bricks" of the plant are cells, about 100 microns in size that have semi-rigid walls that surround the *cytoplasm* or the entire contents of the cell. Inside the cytoplasm there is a vacuole (or balloon) confined by a cell membrane, containing a water solution. The cell wall is a composite structure composed of an amorphous matrix reinforced by pectin molecules (35%), cellulose (30%), hemicellulose (20%), and some proteins (Figure 2.1, middle). On the outside of the cell wall is the middle lamella, a kind of cement that holds adjacent cells together and plays a role in the softening of plant tissue that occurs during ripening and cooking.

Cellulose is made of a linear chain of glucose units just like amylose in starch. Unlike starch, however, the glucose molecules attach with a different bond that favors a lateral association between chains, causing them to form into long and resistant strands or fibers about 3.5 nm in diameter (Figure 2.1, middle). These cellulose fibers are difficult to break with heat or by enzyme action. This property allows nature to build large and flexible structures that defy gravity like the stems of plants and the hard, tough shells of nuts. The cell walls of plants accumulate lignin over time, which is a three-dimensional polymer mesh that does not dissolve or break easily, and is associated with the stiffness of tissues. You can easily appreciate lignification in asparagus, which becomes tougher and more fibrous over time. Lignification is also involved when older vegetables won't soften with cooking (see Section 3.8). The cell walls of wood contain cellulose and lignin, both hard and indigestible, which allow trees to live many years and withstand the various onslaughts of weather and nature. The cells of fresh vegetables are young cells with soft, hydrated cell walls (which later function as dietary fiber in our bodies). The water contained in the membrane-enclosed sacs or vacuoles of these young cells has many solutes that collide with the surrounding membrane exerting an outward pressure. This *osmotic pressure* is responsible for the cell turgor resulting in the firmness characteristic of fresh fruits and vegetables. We already discussed the cell membrane that surrounds the cytoplasm. Biological membranes are complex structures that self-assemble into thin lipid bilayers with inserted proteins here and there. Cells have different separate organelles surrounded by these membranes, which are used to control the transport of molecules in and out of the compartments. Maintaining functional cell membranes, which are easily destroyed by heat, is important in order to preserve the metabolism of fruits and vegetables after harvest. There is also a technological advantage to keeping cell walls and membranes intact, as this preserves their ability to filter out large molecules while allowing liquids to pass through. This is the case with the extraction of sugar from beets. The tubers are cut into long ribbons containing many intact cells in their interior. These cells release the sugar when immersed in water while retaining undesirable material in their interior. After the sugar is extracted, these beet "noodles" called *cossettes* are dried to become excellent animal feed.

Skeletal *muscle tissue* of animals is formed of elongated thin cells arranged into fiber bundles. Each of these fibers is surrounded by connective tissue (mostly collagen) that holds the bundle together. These cells, unlike those of plants, do not have cell walls. The ability of muscle to contract and relax is based on the assembly of two protein molecules belonging to the group of myofibrillar proteins, *actin* and *myosin*, which make up more than 20% of the weight of muscle cells and around 60% of the total protein. Both proteins are contained in myofibrils (around 1 micron in diameter) where they overlap and slide past each other in a parallel formation that allows the muscle to stretch and contract. In turn, myofibrils in muscle fibers are immersed in a fluid called *sarcoplasm*, which contains another portion of the proteins (20% to 30% of the total), the sarcoplasmic proteins, including the red pigment myoglobin. Figure 2.1 (right) illustrates the hierarchical structure of muscle tissue.

Fiber bundles can be separated easily with a fork in well-cooked poultry and fish. These fibrous structures are held together by connective tissue, composed mainly of the protein collagen. The connective tissue converges into tendons that attach the muscle tissue to bone (Figure 2.1, top right). Collagen consists of three protein chains that are wound into the shape of a helix that is stabilized by intermolecular bonds. The collagen of older animals has more of these cross-linking bonds, making the connective tissue more resistant to cooking, and the meat is consequently tougher. When collagen is heated (e.g., above 60 to 65°C in meat), parts of the helix are destroyed and the disrupted fractions are soluble in water. Upon cooling they become reordered, forming gelatin gels. Gelatin is also extracted from the hydrolysis of the collagen in hides and bones, dried and sold commercially.

From all of this we can conclude that the known nutritional components of our food are not distributed evenly but are part of complex structures within plants and animals, and these structures give them properties that we can remember and recognize with our senses. The dedicated work that food biochemists and food microscopists have done to provide a more accurate understanding of these arrangements has allowed the development of better technologies for food processing. We also know that our digestive system must be able to somehow release the nutrients from these structures if we are to be able to absorb them. This process is discussed in Section 7.6.

2.2 MOLECULAR SOCIOLOGY

We have discussed molecules and structures, but not how the first transforms into the latter. The interactions between neighboring molecules, which can be attractive or repulsive, can be compared to the interactions between people, which is how the term *molecular sociology* came about. We often talk about the "chemistry" between people, and the sociological concept of "human chemistry" analyzes the "reactions" that form and break the bonds between people and the social structures that derive from those relationships.[2] It may seem strange to make these analogies between human and molecular interactions, but it works well here as a way of using daily experience to explain a complex concept.

Some people come together and never separate, like a marriage. In chemistry, neighboring molecules can be attracted to one another, with a range of attraction from strong to weak. The closest and most permanent bond between molecules is the covalent bond, in which the outer electrons are shared by two or more atoms. Covalent bonds join the monomers together that form polymers like proteins and polysaccharides. Enzymes are used to break these bonds in our food, like the amylase that breaks down starch molecules into simple sugars (Section 7.7), and rennin (or rennet) that cleaves part of the milk protein casein which results in the formation of cheese curds (Section 2.12).

But in the higher levels of biological structures, the interactions between molecules are less specific than covalent bonds. Weak interactions, based on specific properties of the molecules, become more important. Jean-Marie Lehn (1939–), Nobel Laureate in Chemistry 1987 (see Section 10.6) proposed the name *supramolecular chemistry* for the study of the noncovalent interactions between molecules.[3] These interactions are crucial in the formation of food structures. Electrostatic interactions occur between molecules that carry an electric charge. They can be attractive (between oppositely charged molecules) or repulsive (between molecules with the same charge). Hydrogen bonds occur between a positively charged atom (H^+) and negatively charged molecules, have only 1% of the intensity of a covalent bond. The hydrogen bonds that occur between water molecules (H^+-$O^-$$H^+$) give this molecule many of its properties, including its interaction with charged groups of other molecules, such as in the hydration (water binding) of proteins and polysaccharides. Van der Waals interactions are the attractive and repulsive forces between molecules due to permanent or temporary weak electrical charges. There is much more to know about molecular interactions, but this should be enough information to proceed for now.

Polymer chains with localized electrical charges, like some polysaccharides, can join with an oppositely charged ion to form stable macromolecules such as carrageenan or alginate gels (Section 2.8). But lack of electrical charge can also cause molecules to associate with one another, especially if they are in a highly "charged" environment like an aqueous medium. Groups of uncharged molecules cluster together and hide from the charged environment, forming hydrophobic attractions (disliking contact with water), just as people who experience discrimination join together to form separate and close-knit groups. Some protein gels are stabilized largely through this mechanism. As already mentioned, it would not be an exaggeration to say that these and other kinds of weak interactions are fundamental to the formation of the food structures obtained in the kitchen and to the development of new food structures in the future.

The breakup of a relationship is a painful event. Hydrolytic enzymes are the divisive elements that break big molecules like proteins, carbohydrates, and fats into smaller molecules. But under certain conditions these enzymes can also act as matchmakers and create new bonds between molecules. Many chemical reactions are reversible, and some enzymes can form polymers from monomers (synthesizing proteins from a soup of amino acids, for example). Certain lipases link specific fatty acids to form triglycerides that are called *structured lipids* and have unique properties (Section 1.13). Enzymes can be used to build rings of six or nine glucose units called *cyclodextrins* which have a hydrophobic interior and a hydrophilic core. These rings can harbor water-insoluble compounds like aromatic molecules, pigments, or vitamins, allowing these compounds to be dispersed into an aqueous medium.

The concept of molecular self-assembly refers to a spontaneous and reversible association of molecules to form a structure determined by certain "chemical information" contained within the molecules. This association results in a jump from the molecular scale to larger structures that can be tens or hundreds of nanometers in size. There are examples of these self-assembled associations in food, such as the milk protein casein that measures 200 to 400 nm (Section 2.1) and is formed by hundreds of smaller subunits, and the biological membranes in plant and animal cells where lipids align to form layers. It is fascinating that depending on the conditions of the medium in which they are dispersed, monoglycerides and phospholipids (lipid molecules with a polar head and apolar tail) can self-assemble spontaneously into a multitude of nanostructures including extended layers called lamellae (like biological membranes), micelles (compact spheres), vesicles (hollow spheres), and even ordered phases that extend in three dimensions.

It has been understood for some time that several protein molecules form various types of semi-spherical aggregates, some of which continue to associate further and form gel networks like tofu or yogurt (Figure 2.5). Other proteins like the beta-lactoglobulin in whey join to form fibrils several nanometers in size, which can be transformed into fibrous structures. In summary, the sugar, lipid, and protein molecules that we consume can all form supramolecular structures under certain conditions by various mechanisms that we are just beginning to understand. There is great interest in the possible technological applications that could develop from this research, such as the ability to build and create food structures starting at the molecular level.

Attractive and repellent forces between macromolecules lead to other associative mechanisms at the supramolecular level, covering an extensive portion of the space called a phase (Section 2.3). The sociological equivalent of a phase might be the giant conglomerates that join to form left and right political parties, or the fans of Real Madrid and Barcelona soccer teams. When molecules of two different types of polymers form a concentrated solution in water, they separate into two immiscible aqueous phases, each enriched with a single type of polymer (much like the fans of Real Madrid and Barcelona who stay at opposite ends in a soccer stadium). This type of phase separation is different from that of oil and water, because water is the common solvent for both polymer phases after separation. In a dilute solution there are relatively few molecules of each polymer and plenty of water to surround them. But when conditions are more crowded (concentrated solution), each polymer chain is more comfortable surrounded by its own class (a common experience among humans as well). For example, a mixture of the polymers casein and alginate in water will separate into two phases when the total concentration of the polymers exceeds approximately 3%. But it takes time for each type of polymer to reach the final separation in the top or bottom phase (i.e., to reach equilibrium). Meanwhile pockets of one phase can form and be dispersed in the other phase, forming microstructures on the scale of microns. It is possible to "freeze" these structures at any stage of separation, for example, making them form gels (a process that will be discussed later on). These heterogeneous mixed gels have unusual textures, but so far they are only a food lab curiosity. Another form of separation occurs when polymer molecules carry an opposite charge that allows them to group and form complex polymers that separate from the solvent (water), like when gum arabic is mixed with whey proteins. These two phenomena (phase separation and complex formation) are hidden mechanisms behind many of the structures in processed foods.[4,5] The formation of polymer networks that lead to macroscopic structures like gels will be addressed in Section 2.8.

The reason why polymers have different properties than smaller molecules when they are in solution can be explained by an analogy to human behavior. Polymers have very long chains (think of a piece of spaghetti several meters long) and when they are submerged in a solvent, they turn quickly in all directions, occupying a lot of space. Other polymer chains (which are doing the same thing) then "see" less available space in the solvent because they cannot interfere with the crazy movement of other chains. This phenomenon does not occur with small molecules that are the size of solvent molecules. These long-chain polymers are similar to a skier who walks around erratically with the skis on his shoulders and poles sticking out in all directions. The skier wrongfully occupies a much larger volume than someone without skis, and everyone else must keep their distance as any sudden turn may be dangerous.

The molecules in a gas phase are special. They are very distant from each other and more independent, interested only in arranging themselves uniformly in space. If too many of them are placed in one zone they quickly and spontaneously spread throughout the available volume. Well, unless they are attracted to a high energy surface. People are also attracted to enticing surfaces, like when they surround the buffet table loaded with fancy sandwiches and delicious pastries and refuse to leave. In chemical terms, we would say that the tables become "saturated" with the fastest and most greedy people. A second layer of people might get some food by reaching in with their arms, but not as much, and finally there is a large erratic mass of people circulating around the tables as if they were simply taking a walk and not realizing that the food was there.

Water molecules in the air behave the same way as they approach the surface of dry food. A first layer or monolayer of molecules adheres firmly to the surface and is very difficult to remove. Additional molecules form multilayers with decreasing levels of adhesion energy, but they still do not behave as molecules in liquid water. This type of interaction occurs when a dry cracker is exposed to humid air and becomes soft yet no water can be expelled from the piece. In the case of fresh fruits, vegetables, and meats there is so much water (on the order of 3 grams of water for each gram of solid) that the amount bound to surfaces becomes a minute fraction of the total water. We can even expel the free water from them in the form of abundant juice.

This spectrum of hydration, from dry to wet, is defined by a parameter known as *water activity* or a_w, and describes how water interacts with food. The a_w varies between 0 for a dry material and 1 for pure water. Low a_w values mean less water available for the growth of microorganisms and for the diffusion of molecules that could participate in chemical reactions. Foods with low a_w values are therefore generally safer and more chemically and structurally stable. Foods with high a_w values (foods that contain lots of water) require heat treatments, pH adjustments, the use of preservatives, and refrigeration to remain in a stable form. Honey and dry pasta have a_w values of 0.75 and 0.3, respectively, representing the range of a_w values in foods that have been stabilized by keeping humidity at intermediate or low levels, removing some or most of the water, and adding small solutes like sugar or salt (to control microorganism growth). Jams are a typical example of a food that is stabilized at intermediate water activity (around 0.80) by the addition of sucrose. There is more on water in foods and their stability in Section 8.1.

2.3 THE SCIENCE OF CHEWABLE STRUCTURES

So far we have seen how nature provides food structures in the form of fruits, vegetables, meat, and so forth, which are the basis of our diet. Over time these structures have been transformed through processes like drying (beef jerky and raisins, for example), fermentation (in the case of cheese and yogurts), and heat (a cooked potato). All of these structures are still considered to be natural foods, despite the physical and chemical changes that accompany the processes above. Processed foods have became more elaborate and complex due to the addition of refined ingredients and food combinations (like ice creams and jam), as well as mass-produced preservation technology and packaging (frozen and canned food). All of this has increased the spectrum of food structures significantly.

Twenty years ago, food scientists realized that the chemical and mechanical behavior of both natural and processed foods was just like other materials found in daily life. In fact, Henry Ford used the same soy proteins that are used to make *tofu* to construct the handlebars of his Model T in the 1930s, and casein from milk was molded and made into buttons and combs for centuries. Recently, food engineers have transformed solutions of starches and other polysaccharides into transparent films similar to polyethylene, cellophane, or PVC (polyvinyl chloride) sheets used as wrappers. Many vehicles are fueled by bioethanol made from sugarcane or cornstarch or by biodiesel made from vegetable oils. There is even talk of biorefineries where plants or plant waste could be processed into products similar to those derived from petroleum and thus create a "greener" economy.

Food structures must be tasty and easily broken down. Our mouths anticipate receiving these structures in a way that produces agreeable sensations. The recognition that food is made up of structures with desirable properties (e.g., taste and nutrition) diverges from the purely chemical approach that was prevalent in the last century, and opens the door to the *Science of Food Materials*. This new approach can irritate those who regard food as more than just a material, and who believe that food is an essential part of human culture and tradition. Their perspectives are valid and are an important part of the discussion.

Food technology has harnessed the abundance of scientific and technologic knowledge available in material science research, diverting food science away from the empiricism that has characterized it in the past. Given the abundance of proteins and polysaccharides in most foods, the science of synthetic polymers is a good place to begin. Unlike synthetic polymers or "plastics" (as they are commonly known), polymers in foods are usually mixed with other components that can affect their behavior, complicating things. But if the presence of multiple components was an excuse to give up, there wouldn't be any basic studies on food. It could be said that study of food materials began in the late 1980s when two scientists, working for Nabisco, presented research applying known concepts about the physics of polymers to certain food products.[6]

Solids present themselves in different states of aggregation called *phases*. Water has a solid phase (ice), a liquid phase (tap water), and a gas phase (water vapor). Although there are two simultaneous phases in a glass of ice water or in a boiling kettle, in equilibrium (which occurs over time) water is in liquid form at room temperature and under atmospheric pressure, as shown in the phase equilibrium diagram in any thermodynamics class. This means that the ice will eventually melt and if you remove the kettle from the fire it will stop making steam and in both cases liquid water will be the only phase present.

In material science there is a form of matter called a *metastable state* that takes place when the molecules of a material are restricted from moving freely and spontaneously, making the material appear momentarily stable though it is not in an equilibrium phase. A parachutist who is caught in a tree during a fall is in a metastable position and will not reach equilibrium until he touches the ground (hopefully without injury). The point is that materials in foods are rarely in equilibrium and most often are found in a metastable state, primarily if dehydrated or frozen (more on this in Section 8.1). Leave the jar of dairy creamer open on a hot and humid day and see how the metastable particles move to equilibrium. The result is a sticky mass.

Many foods leave the liquid state and end up as a solid. Think of molten sugar as it cools to become icing, or molecules dispersed in complex liquids like milk that become powders when the water is removed through dehydration. The change from liquid to solid must be traumatic for molecules because they lose their freedom to move quickly and haphazardly. In the solid state they are trapped and immobile. A key variable in the transition from the liquid to the solid state is how rapidly the cooling of a pure liquid occurs, or how quickly water is removed from a solution containing a solute.

Did you know that the glass windows and glass bottles broken in Hollywood films are often made from sugar? A glass is formed when a pure liquid (e.g., sugar melted over 150°C) cools so rapidly that the molecules cannot organize themselves and are trapped in the solid form almost exactly as they were arranged in liquid form. Some solutes in solution (lactose in liquid milk, for example) also change to a glass-like solid form when water is removed very rapidly by dehydration, as happens when producing milk powder. Sugar molecules in the glassy state (also referred to as amorphous or vitreous state) become trapped in a random fashion and not arranged in a regular lattice as found in a crystal of table sugar. A glass is in a metastable condition, much the same as the parachutist hanging from the tree, and given a chance it will move to equilibrium where molecules adopt an ordered structure. Remember that in high school window glasses were defined as "super-cooled liquids"? Now we know why. The molten mixture of silica and other components of glass is cooled so rapidly that molecules "freeze" as a solid much in the same position as when they were in the hot liquid condition. An interesting conclusion is that since glasses are technically liquids they have viscosity (Section 2.5), but it is so high that they look like solids and their flow would not be visible even if we wait all our life.[7] In a cotton candy machine the hot syrup of molten sugar (a viscous liquid) rapidly becomes fine threads (a glass) as they cool down to ambient temperature after being spun by the rotating disc. The viscosity of the cotton candy threads is millions of times higher than that of the molten sugar inside the machine. Various types of food molecules form glasses, like almost all of the sugars (including sucrose and lactose), some proteins (especially if they have been hydrolyzed) and small starch derivatives like dextrins. Next time you bite into a fresh cracker remember that you are eating a glass.

For a pure liquid such as water to turn into glass, it would have to be cooled extremely rapidly. Not even liquid nitrogen which is at −195°C will do it. Under normal conditions, the water molecules spontaneously and quickly order themselves into regular positions forming a *crystal* called ice, which represents a final state of equilibrium. When a glass forms, this equilibrium state is not reached, which is why the glassy state is called a metastable state (in between liquid and crystal). Eventually, under the right conditions for molecules to move and according to the law of thermodynamics (Section 6.2), the molecules in a glass organize and become crystals, which are the most ordered and least complex structures of all. This produces one of the most incredible paradoxes in the material world. Although under given conditions the crystalline state is the equilibrium state (e.g., 0°C and atmospheric pressure for water) and the molecules should achieve that state spontaneously, the transition from liquid to this condition is not easy. Under controlled conditions in a laboratory, extremely pure water can be kept in a liquid state by *supercooling*, achieving temperatures up to −40°C even though equilibrium says it should form ice below 0°C (like in a home freezer). You can prepare sugar solutions in the kitchen that are more concentrated than normal saturation or equilibrium (67% sucrose at 20°C) without forming crystals, which is called *supersaturation*. For ice or a sugar crystal to form there must first be a nucleus or tiny crystal template onto which the other molecules can quickly and orderly attach. Very seldom a small group of molecules spontaneously get together and become this nucleus, in a process called *homogeneous nucleation*. It is more frequent to find that nuclei form by *heterogenous nucleation* when molecules get ordered around small surface imperfections or contaminating particles. Now we understand that supercooling and supersaturation are possible metastable states of freezing and crystallization, respectively, due to the absence of nuclei onto which the molecules can grow a crystalline structure. There will be more about this and equilibrium in Sections 6.2 and 6.3.

There are many culinary situations in which the cooking process is conducive to the formation of glass and crystalline states. Confectionery is largely based on the fact that sucrose does not crystallize and remains in a glass state, like in hard candy. Conversely, during the production of table sugar, the supersaturated syrup in the sugar factory is "seeded" with small crystals of powdered sugar so that the sucrose will crystallize more rapidly. In the production of powdered milk, lactose finishes in a glassy state due to the rapid removal of water from the drops of milk that are dispersed during the spray-drying process.

But materials science is full of surprises. There is another metastable state called the *rubbery state*. In material science terminology, a rubber is the state in which the molecules (large or small) of a solid can move enough to slide past one another. While a glass is hard and brittle, a material that is in the rubbery state is soft and flexible. A PVC pipe is so rigid because its molecules are prevented from moving (in fact, the pipe is a glass), while a hose made of the same material is flexible because an added plasticizer—a small molecule that occupies positions between polymer chains—works as a lubricant and enables the molecules to move. Therefore, a hose is literally and technically a rubber.

The change from glass to crystalline state is a time-dependent process, and the material must pass through the rubbery state, as the molecules need to be able to move in order to arrange themselves in the ordered manner required to become a crystal (Figure 2.2). In nature, and therefore in food, there is a plasticizer that can transform materials from glass to rubber: water. Dried seaweed is as rigid as a PVC pipe but softens after soaking in water and becomes as flexible as a hose. As a matter of fact, heat can also make glasses turn into rubbers, and this is exactly what the plumber does when he wants to bend a rigid plastic pipe.

The boundary line between the glass and the rubbery states is determined by the *glass transition temperature* or Tg, which is unique to each material (just like its melting and boiling points), but it depends on the moisture content (Section 8.1). As moisture of a glassy material increases, Tg decreases. However, Tg does not signal a phase transition

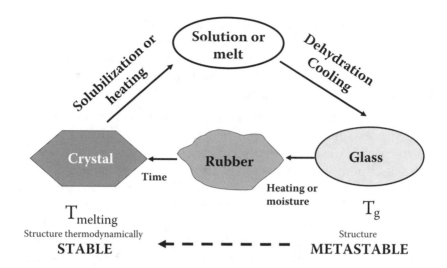

FIGURE 2.2   CHANGES OF A LIQUID TO SOLID STATES IN FOODS. DEPENDING ON THE COOLING RATE, EITHER A METASTABLE AMORPHOUS GLASS OR A STABLE ORDERED CRYSTAL CAN FORM. THE CHANGE FROM GLASS TO CRYSTAL OCCURS SPONTANEOUSLY ONCE THE CONDITIONS ARE REACHED FOR THE MOBILITY AND ORGANIZATION OF THE MOLECULES (RUBBER STATE).

(because it refers to two states and not two phases) and does not require any heat to occur (as the latent heat for a change of phase). Once the temperature of a material that forms crystalline structures exceeds Tg, the transit from glass to a crystal through the rubbery state is just a matter of time (Figure 2.2).

Perhaps an analogy with foods may help. In spaghetti that has just been cooked and is warm (let's say, it's above a fictitious Tg), the long strands can slide over one another and can fit into many shapes, so they are in a "rubbery state." However, when the spaghetti cools down (e.g., it gets below Tg) the strands begin to stick to one another and the spaghetti becomes fixed in the shape of the bowl and it is "glassy" (and less tasty).

Why do food scientists worry so much about Tg? Stability is the answer. A cookie just taken out of its packaging will crunch noisily when you take a bite, typical of its glassy state. But if left sitting out, the cookie will absorb water molecules from the humid air and it will become soft enough to eat silently, as it will have passed into its rubbery state (Figure 2.2). Water has "plasticized" the starch in cookies in the same way that chemical plasticizers converted a rigid PVC pipe into a flexible hose. In summary, Tg is a fundamental parameter for amorphous or glassy foods with low humidity, and is an essential criteria for determining their structure, texture, and chemical reactivity with other molecules in the system. More on Tg and its effect on food stability is discussed in Section 8.1.

The rubbery state should not be confused with rubber elasticity. A gum, like the rubber in car tires, is a randomly cross-linked network of polymers with elastic properties. A rubber band can stretch to several times its length without breaking, and when the stretching force is removed, it returns to its original length. This happens because when long polymer chains are stretched, they momentarily order themselves, but when the stretching force is removed they spontaneously return to a less orderly state or a state of higher entropy (a concept discussed in Section 6.2). Elastin is the principal elastic protein in vertebrates and with collagen it forms part of the ligaments and joints. There are few natural food materials that exhibit the remarkable elasticity of rubber, except for chewing gum of course, wheat gluten,[8] some melted cheeses, and in a limited way, abalone meat.

2.4 TRANSFORMING
STRUCTURES WITH HEAT

The most common way to transform food structures is to heat them. At low temperatures the heat destabilizes the weaker molecular interactions (like hydrophobic interactions), but eventually enough energy accumulates to break covalent bonds and produce various chemical reactions (see Section 2.2). Figure 2.3 shows the changes that occur in different food components when heated.

When proteins are heated they progressively lose their native structure, unfold, and pass to a less orderly state, but the chemical bonds holding amino acids together are not broken. The complete process is called *thermal denaturation*. When they are denatured, protein molecules lose their solubility, retain less water, become more viscous in solution, and so on, which in culinary terms means they coagulate, aggregate, and gel. Normally the denaturation of proteins occurs within a range of

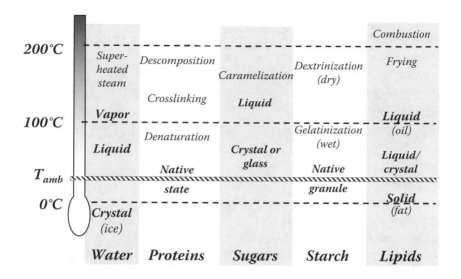

FIGURE 2.3 THE EFFECTS OF HEAT ON PHASE CHANGES, TRANSITIONS BETWEEN
STATES, AND SOME OF THE PRINCIPAL CHEMICAL REACTIONS IN FOOD COMPONENTS
(T_{AMB} = AMBIENT TEMPERATURE).

temperatures and depends on many factors like water content, pH, and the presence of ions, for example. Proteins in living beings can withstand temperatures over 40°C, but denaturalization almost never begins below 60°C. For example, egg whites begin to denature at 63°C, make a smooth gel at 65 to 70°C, and become a firm gel around 77°C. The yolk begins to denature at 65°C, turns into a thick paste around 73 to 75°C, and is completely firm at 80°C. Heating squid to 100°C for 1 minute makes the muscle collagen fibers become soluble and softens the composite structure, providing a chewable texture.

At higher temperatures there is enough energy for new bonds to form between the protein molecules through *cross-linking* reactions. The chemical bonding between the stretched molecules in soy protein, which occurs around 140 to 169°C, allows us to obtain a meat-like texture that retains its fibrous structure when cooked (Sections 4.8 and 8.4). At even higher temperatures, proteins decompose. Proteins can also become denatured by changes in pH (as when adding lemon juice to milk), by being at the interface between two phases (e.g., when forming extended films around gas bubbles in foams), and by the addition of salts (as in the coagulation of egg albumin with NaCl). As long as no permanent bonds are cleaved from between the long unfolded chains of a denatured protein, the process may be reversible—that is, the protein can return to its native state. Irreversible denaturation takes place when interactions between unfolded chains stabilize the molecule (as occurs with egg proteins during boiling).

At room temperature sucrose is in crystalline form (and sometimes in an amorphous state like glass, see Section 2.3). We consume other kinds of sugars, like fructose in honey and fruits, and lactose in milk. Heating sucrose above 160°C melts the crystals and triggers a series of complex reactions known as caramelization that produce the aromatic compounds and brown pigments associated with roasting and caramel candy. Sucrose crystals melt into a colorless liquid at 154°C, which begins to turn amber in color at 168°C, and burns at 190°C, creating bitter flavors and an intense brown color. Liquid sucrose between the temperatures of 155 and 165°C is an excellent heating medium and can be used in a novel way to "fry" foods in sugar. Certain sugars called reducing sugars (glucose, fructose, maltose, and lactose) participate in a reaction known as the *Maillard reaction* when heated in the presence of proteins, peptides, amino acids, or amines. This reaction is named for the French biochemist Louis Camille Maillard (1878–1936). The Maillard reaction produces brown color (typical of the surface of seared meat and the crust of bread) and volatile compounds that are very important in cooking, baking, and frying, as well as bitter flavors. Some of the compounds produced from this reaction have a potential mutagenic activity, though we have eaten them for centuries.

In nature, starch is in the form of granules between 5 and 50 microns in size, which are like tiny grains of sand in the sense that the two polymer components of starch, amylose and amylopectin, are densely packed inside the granule, rendering it insoluble (Section 2.1). If starch is heated in the presence of abundant water, the starch granules begin to hydrate and swell between 55 and 65°C, a phenomenon known as the *gelatinization* of starch. Figure 3.3 in Chapter 3 shows the swelling of a grain of starch under a light microscope. Gelatinization of starch is not to be confused with gelation or gelification, which is the formation of gels by proteins and polysaccharides and will be discussed in Section 2.8. During heating, the suspension becomes more viscous as the swollen granules break and release amylose and amylopectin molecules. You can appreciate this when you add starch or flour to a hot broth to make a thick sauce. Too much agitation during this stage reduces the viscosity, and if this is followed by cooling, a weak gelification occurs, and eventually a partial crystallization of the liberated polymers if left standing for a long period. Gelatinization of starch not only changes its culinary properties but also makes it digestible in the gut (Section 7.7). Starch can also undergo *dextrinization*, in which the amylose and amylopectin molecules are cut by enzymes or by friction and dry heat, like in the case of extruded products (extruded corn snacks have dextrinized starch, for example). Dextrins are short glucose polymers (and therefore relatively soluble) that are used, among other things, to make infant formulas and porridges.

Lipids crystallize and become solid at low temperatures. If oil is stored in the refrigerator, harmless white particles sometimes settle in the bottom—these are triglycerides that have crystallized. In the form of oils or melted fats, lipids are liquids that can be heated to around 190 to 200°C at atmospheric pressure without undergoing major chemical changes. This allows many different foods to be heated in a liquid medium at high temperatures, a process called frying (Section 8.7). At around 200 to 230°C, these lipids begin to decompose, and the temperature at which this happens for a particular fat is called its *smoke point*. At atmospheric pressure there aren't many liquids that can cover the range of temperatures between the 100°C of boiling water and the 180 to 190°C of hot oils. In terms of handling and storage, lipids can be exposed to two deterioration reactions: hydrolytic rancidity and oxidative rancidity (Section 1.3). The first reaction is caused by enzymes found in food that release free fatty acids, which cause unpleasant odors and flavors (like butyric acid in rancid butter). Fat oxidization (oxidative rancidity) is a reaction between oxygen and the unsaturated fatty acids, which can be partially controlled using antioxidants or removing fats from exposure to air.

2.5 STRANGE LIQUIDS AND SOLIDS

From the point of view of a physicist, foods are soft materials, a form of condensed matter, that is, deformable solids or liquids that flow under low force and whose molecules remain very close together by multiple interactions (see Section 2.2). Just open the refrigerator door and you will see the diversity of materials that fulfill this definition: mayonnaise, milk, soft cheese, jelly, egg yolks and whites, and so forth.

Engineers like to make simple references about material behavior which are easy to explain and model, but these may only exist in their imagination. The ideal solid and the ideal liquid (see Section 5.2 for definitions) are at the opposite ends of the spectrum of mechanical behavior of all the real forms of condensed matter that we know (i.e., almost everything except gases). The physical behavior of real materials, like most of the "liquids and solids" making up our foods, is more complicated than these ideal behaviors.

Liquids have no fixed form and adopt the shape of their container. The property called *viscosity*, which is equivalent to consistency or fluidity, describes how liquids spontaneously flow under the application of a force. When a liquid flows, the molecules must slide past one another, so that liquids composed of smaller molecules have a lower viscosity. Liquids that have large molecules (like polymers) that can become entangled with one another or those that contain irregular particles that hinder movement have a higher viscosity. The viscosity of water is 100 and 1,000 times less than the viscosity of oil and syrup, respectively.

Viscosity is not constant for some liquids that contain polymers or fibers (e.g., fruit juices and purees) that when rapidly deformed (like when mixed with a whisk or inside a blender) can appear less thick. These liquids are called *pseudoplastic fluids*. In these cases the structure of the liquid changes and the polymer molecules or fibers align in the direction of the deformation, which decreases the resistance to flow, and makes the liquid less viscous than when it is still. When the agitation stops, the liquid returns to its original higher viscosity. If you mix a solution of 1% carrageen in a blender that turns at 50 revolutions per second, the apparent viscosity is almost a fifth of what it is when the solution flows slowly. This is important in the case of salad dressings that must flow out of the bottle when shaken and poured but also still stick to and cover the salad leaves. The strange behavior of ketchup provides more evidence that complex liquids have structure. To get ketchup out of the bottle, it is necessary to overcome the force that prevents its flow which is produced by cross-linking between the tomato paste molecules. Shaking the bottle generates cutting or shear forces on the material, beginning the flow and continuing until the bottle empties if necessary. Squeezing a plastic bottle also overcomes the action of cross-linking by driving the fluid toward the mouth of the bottle. Some mayonnaises and mustards exhibit this same strange behavior, as does toothpaste.

One intuitive way to describe a solid is that it can withstand the application of force without losing its shape or deforming. This is what is expected of car bumpers and building rafters, but not of a piece of meat, an apple, or jelly. Hard candies and nutshells behave almost like ideal solids in that they can resist large forces and do not deform before suddenly breaking. Other foods that seem solid, like cheeses, show a plastic deformation before breaking apart, or lose their shape appreciably but in a slow manner without flowing. Many foods exhibit behavior that is not quite what is expected of a solid, largely because they contain a lot of water, but they don't flow easily either. These materials are called *viscoelastic*. They show some viscosity and tendency to flow, but at the same time they have some ability to resist a force and recover like an elastic solid (some cheeses, jello, mayonnaise, etc.). Temperature is the main variable that transforms solids into liquids but its effect is only apparent if certain components melt, like the cocoa butter in chocolate or ice in frozen foods. All these subtleties in the behavior of materials are perceived to a greater or lesser degree in the mouth and are part of the sensory properties in food.

2.6 LOVE/HATE RELATIONSHIPS

Water and oil do not mix spontaneously and separate into two phases (Section 2.2). If they are mixed together and agitated, one will disperse itself within the other in the form of droplets, but over time these drops rejoin and the phases separate again. An *emulsion* is the dispersion of two liquids that are immiscible, one of which becomes the dispersed phase (droplets) while the other is the surrounding medium or continuous phase (Figure 2.9D). The most common food emulsions have two components: water (W) and oil (O). Consequently, there are emulsions in which oil droplets are suspended in water (O/W), typically mayonnaises and sauces, and vice versa (W/O) like butter. The droplets in an emulsion generally vary in size from 1 to 50 microns (see Figure 2.9D). Creams and many sauces are emulsions with soft, creamy, palatable consistencies that have the advantage of bringing together colors, flavors, and aromas that are water soluble, oil soluble, or soluble in both phases.

To form an O/W emulsion, energy is needed first to disperse the oil in the form of drops (a blender, for example) and then the droplets need to be stabilized so they don't rejoin together, which is achieved by positioning special molecules at the interface between oil and water. The chemical agents that do this last job are called *emulsifiers* or *surfactants*. They work by reducing the surface tension (or surface energy) that attracts the molecules in the interface to the interior of the droplets. A lower surface energy also decreases the amount of energy needed to form the emulsion. Commercial surfactants are molecules with polar heads (that point toward water) and apolar tails (that are immersed in oil). The relationship between the polar and apolar effects is known in technical jargon as the HLB value (hydrophilic-lipophilic balance). The HLB value ranges between 1 and 20 and is used to select surfactants. The type of emulsion depends greatly on the type of emulsifier and its solubility in the continuous phase. Emulsifiers that are oil soluble have low HLB values (3 to 6), and those soluble in water have high HLB values (10 to 18). These technical criteria can be used to search for food-grade emulsifiers to make a particular emulsion. The other general rule for creating stable emulsions is that the material that makes up the continuous phase should be present in larger proportion to the material that is dispersed within it, but this is not always the case.

Surfactant molecules are not the only stabilizers for emulsions; polymers and fine particles can also do the job. Unfolded (denatured) proteins and some polysaccharides position themselves at the interfaces with their hydrophilic and hydrophobic parts pointing toward the aqueous and oil phases, respectively. Their large size prevents the droplets from touching one another, and the presence of a net electrical charge (positive or negative) causes repulsion. Fine particles that manage to locate themselves in the interface of the droplets help to keep the droplets apart, like when finely ground mustard grains are added to mayonnaise to stabilize the emulsion.

A recent science development that may have unexpected possibilities are double emulsions. A thick mayonnaise is composed of 80% to 90% droplets of pure oil around 20 microns in size, tightly packed into an aqueous phase (Figure 2.9D). What would happen if inside each oil droplet there was an even smaller droplet of water? This would be a double emulsion: the water droplets inside the oil droplets make a water-in-oil (W/O) emulsion, and when these modified "oil" droplets are dispersed in an aqueous phase, they become part of a O/W emulsion. These double emulsions are called W/O/W emulsions. Double emulsions have not yet been used in foods, and a certain technology is required to make them commercial (and affordable). They could be important because the calories from a water-filled oil droplet are much lower than those of oil droplets in a regular emulsion. The nature of the emulsified product would remain the same—it would be an emulsion of "low calorie oil droplets" in water. Be on the lookout for these low calorie emulsified sauces in the future.

2.7 CAPTURING AIR

Air is an inexpensive component in food and is not listed on food labels. *Foams* are a category of materials in which a large quantity of gas (generally air) is dispersed in the form of bubbles in a liquid, solid, or semi-solid medium. The foam in beer has small bubbles of carbon dioxide distributed in the liquid. Aerated chocolate may be regarded as a solid foam in which the air cells are surrounded by walls of fat and sugar. Marshmallows have an elastic matrix so they are more like a sponge. Gas bubbles give food a softer and lighter texture (imagine what bread would be like without them) and make whipped sauces and desserts possible. Other solid sponges like popcorn and soufflés will be discussed in Section 8.6.

Both gas and liquid must be present to form a liquid foam, but that alone is not sufficient, as we know from stirring water with a spoon. Something else has to be present at the interface between the bubbles and the liquid to stabilize the foam. It is well known that adding a drop of dishwashing liquid to water will make a rich lather. The formation of a foam is also related to the surface tension of water. The surface tension of pure water in contact with gas is so high that it is necessary to add a surfactant in order for foam to form and stabilize more easily.

There are aerated food products in confectionery, baked goods, snacks, breakfast cereals, ice creams, and beverages.[10] How much air are you buying? Air makes up 95% of popcorn, 90% of a meringue, 70% of bread, 50% of ice cream, and 40% of an aerated chocolate bar. This is why some of these foods are sold by volume (ice cream by the pint or liter, for example). Foams are generated in various ways: beating air into a liquid phase (ice cream and meringues), yeast fermentation that produces CO_2 (bread), chemical reactions from baking powder (cakes and cookies), lowering the pressure of a liquid supersaturated with gas (beer and champagne), or by expansion of a gas in a vacuum (aerated chocolate).[11]

There are three types of instability that can cause liquid foams to collapse. The first is disproportionation, in which gas under higher pressure in small bubbles diffuses to larger bubbles (where it is at lower pressure), which grow until the small bubbles disappear. For this reason there is much interest in developing technologies that can produce foams with uniformly sized bubbles to minimize this phenomenon. Liquid can also drain through the layers or thin liquid films that separate the bubbles, which can be partially prevented by increasing the viscosity of the liquid phase (by adding a polymer, for example). Last, the laminae that separate the bubbles can break, causing bubble coalescence or fusion. Surfactants can be used to add elasticity and protect the interfaces.

There are seven gases commercially approved by the European Union as food additives when used in their pure form: oxygen, hydrogen, carbon dioxide, nitrogen, nitrous oxide, helium, and argon.[12] Of these, nitrous oxide is the only one not present in significant amounts in the air that we breathe (though it's found in toxic gases produced during combustion and pollution, where we don't want it). These gases are soluble in liquids, and under pressure the amount of dissolved gas increases. This is why we don't see CO_2 bubbles in soda bottles capped under 1.2 atmospheres of pressure (20% more than atmospheric pressure) under cold conditions (to have a reference, tire pressure is almost 2 atmospheres, the equivalent of 28 to 30 pounds per square inch). Different gases have different water solubility, which influences bubble formation and the structure of the foam. You can observe this by open-ing a can of *Guinness* beer: the nitrogen (dispensed from a special recep-tacle under the lid) forms a fine, creamy foam. You may think of getting different gas tanks and experimenting in the kitchen.

Here is a little trivia about food foam technology. Egg whites, essen-tial to meringues and soufflés, are so stable because a fraction of the egg protein, including globulins, denatures when beaten and migrates to the interface of the bubbles, stabilizing and preventing them from breaking. A significant group of egg proteins, the ovalbumins (54% of egg protein), remain unchanged by the mechanical action and bring a higher viscosity to the liquid inside the walls separating bubbles, pre-venting drainage. The ovalbumin denatures during cooking and turns the structure rigid. But there's more. When egg whites are beaten in a copper bowl, a complex forms between the copper metal ions and another egg protein, conalbumin, which makes the sponge more sta-ble.[13] Though it is said that the presence of yolk and oil prevent the egg whites from forming a meringue, because both compete with the pro-tein at the liquid-air interface of the bubbles, some sponge interfaces are stabilized exclusively with lipids. Such is the case with whipped cream, where mechanical action breaks the membranes surrounding the fat globules in the cream (Section 2.11), allowing the released liquid fat to act as a glue between the globules positioned at the interface of the bubbles. Chilling cream before whipping is recommended because the cold reduces the proportion of liquid fat inside the globules (the fat changes to liquid as the temperature rises, and completely melts at 32°C). When more fat globules (cream is 30% lipid) are present at the bubble interfaces, as shown in Figure 2.4, the resulting foam is more rigid, which makes the whipped cream more stable.[14]

2.8 TO GEL OR NOT TO GEL

Jellyfish are among the most curious of living creatures. Their apparent transparency comes from lacking a skeleton and being made almost entirely of an aqueous solution with only 1% organic material. Jellyfish are considered a delicacy in Asia.[15] The cytoplasm (or interior) of our cells has pretty much the same structure as these gelatinous fish. The

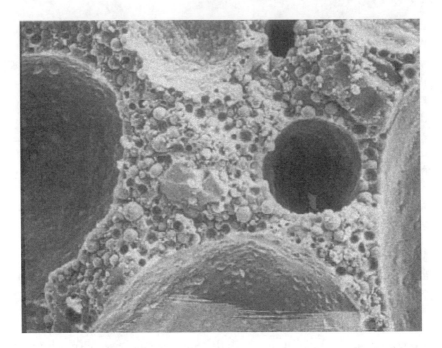

Figure 2.4   The microstructure of whipped cream as viewed with an electron microscope under frozen conditions (cryomicroscopy). Note the depth of field, which allows you to see the inside of the air bubbles. You can see the fat globules between the bubbles, and some which appear around the inside of the bubbles, which are sealed with liquid fat.

water exhibits a semi-solid behavior because it's "held" inside a three-dimensional polymer matrix that's capable of "dissolving" or swelling in the aqueous medium. This matrix is known as a gel. A *gel* is the closest water can get to being solid at room temperature, as these soft and self-supporting structures can be 98% liquid material and only 2% solid. The process of *gelation* or gelification is similar to solidification, in that the phase change occurs from a solution called *sol* to the gel state. Gels are important in the kitchen for making quasi-solid structures that are delicate and transparent, as well as for retaining water and trapping exudates.

The gel matrix is a network made of polymer chains (collagen in gelatin, alginate, etc.) or chains of aggregated proteins that join together like a pearl necklace (gels of casein, egg white albumin, or whey). Water or

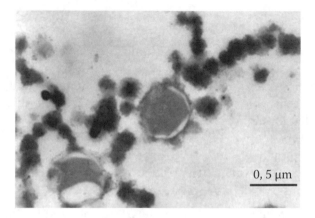

FIGURE 2.5   MICROSTRUCTURE OF A YOGURT-TYPE LACTIC GEL VIEWED UNDER TRANSMIS-
SION ELECTRON MICROSCOPE. THE DARK ROUND OBJECTS ARE CASEIN MICELLES THAT ARE
JOINED LIKE A "STRING OF PEARLS" TO FORM THE GEL NETWORK. YOU CAN ALSO SEE A PAIR
OF FAT GLOBULES. THE GRAY AREA REPRESENTS THE AQUEOUS SOLUTION TRAPPED INSIDE THE
PROTEIN NETWORK.

the solution is then trapped inside this network (Figure 2.5). These large polymer chains or threads of aggregated proteins unite in certain points or areas of cross-linking that restrict local movement and give stability to the structure. Alginate polymers form areas of cross-linking with calcium ions (Ca^{+2}) that act like bridges between adjacent polymer chains, while some carrageenans do the same in the presence of potassium ions (K^+). In a protein gel, the basic linking mechanism is through hydrophobic attractions (Section 2.2). Both the ingredients that form gels and the gelification process (that is, the transition from sol to gel) are extremely varied, and it's necessary to consult expert sources when making them.[16] There are gels that form after cooling a hot dispersion, like gelatin and κ-carrageenan (kappa-carrageenan) (see Section 11.2). Globular proteins such as those in egg whites, egg yolks, soy, whey, and so forth, generally form gels upon heating which are not reversible (like hard-boiled eggs). The proteins must unfold or denature first, forming small aggregates less than 1 micron in diameter which later interact and form chains. The pH and the ionic strength of the medium (determined by the concentration of dissolved salts) play a fundamental role in the consistency and transparency (or opacity) of these gels. In the laboratory it's possible to make a transparent gel from egg whites.[17]

Yogurt is a gel that is formed by the action of two acid-producing beneficial microorganisms on milk: *Lactobacillus bulgaricus* and *Streptococcus thermophilus*. The milk must be heated to 85°C for several minutes in order to denature the whey proteins prior to inoculation with the bacteria. The denatured proteins interact with a fraction called κ-casein which is found on the surface of casein micelles, and the complex formed contributes to the creamy texture of yogurt. As the pH lowers gradually to 4.6 from the production of acid by bacteria, a soft gel that we know as yogurt forms. Under an electron microscope, yogurt looks like a network of casein aggregates that hold the aqueous phase inside, as you can see in Figure 2.5.

Fun tricks can be performed with gels. The "hot and iced tea" developed at the famous British restaurant *Fat Duck* is prepared by adding a gelling agent to ordinary tea to form a soft gel. The gel is then finely ground into a fluid and divided into two parts, one of which is heated. If a temporary divider is placed in the glass, you can pour hot fluid on one side and the cold fluid on the other side without them mixing. At first glance it appears to be a glass filled with a single liquid which must be served and enjoyed quickly.

Aerogels and collapsible gels (also called *intelligent gels*) are not far off on the gourmet horizon. Aerogels are obtained by carefully removing the liquid from a gel without collapsing the network. The result is a solid foam that is very light and extremely porous. This technology, which is far from straightforward, is already used to make thermal insulation and glass protectors. The formation of collapsible gels exploits the process of gelation as a phase transition (e.g., going from liquid to gas), in which a small temperature variation causes an impressive change in volume. In the case of water in its liquid phase at 99°C and under atmospheric pressure, an increase in temperature of just a couple degrees causes the molecules to violently disperse as water vapor (boiling) with a thousand-fold increase in volume. The opposite happens if the process is reversed and water is condensed from vapor. In certain gels, a small change in pH or temperature causes the collapse or the swelling of the structure, which may be applicable in making artificial muscles or smart devices. It would certainly be remarkable if a dessert had a gelled pill at the bottom of a liquid that could instantly swell into an exquisite *mousse* with the application of some lemon or a flame. Science will never stop "feeding" magic to chefs.

2.9 BREAD: FROM MOLECULES TO STRUCTURES

The importance of bread in Western civilization is obvious from the many sayings that relate this precious food to our lives: "give us this day our daily bread," "earn your daily bread by the sweat of your brows," "man cannot live by bread alone," "bread is the staff of life," and so on. Leavened bread has accompanied humans since the beginning of civilization, from the time Egyptians mixed wheat flour and yeast around 3,000 BC. Presently, it is estimated that in many countries there are several hundred types of bread. Germans appear to lead in its consumption per capita: 90 kg per year.

In the context of this book, bread is a notable example of how the presence of a peculiar class of molecules conditions the type of structures that can be formed (dairy products are another example, see Section 2.12). Cereal flours derived from wheat are unique in that they are capable of forming an elastic dough when mixed with water and kneaded. This occurs because the proteins in wheat turn into *gluten*, a complex viscoelastic material. This characteristic of wheat products is encoded at the molecular level, in the form of two kinds of protein called *glutenins* and *gliadins*. These proteins make 80% to 90% of the protein in wheat but only 10% of the flour content. Glutenins are very large polymers formed of many subunits linked by disulfide bridges (a covalent bond of the type -S-S- joining two amino acids in different parts of a protein chain). Gliadins, in turn, are monomeric or small single protein units.

The elasticity of gluten, so important for holding the expanding bubbles and giving a porous structure to baked products, results from two mechanisms operating at different levels. At the molecular level, some parts of the glutenin molecule behave as "springs" that can be stretched as needed. At the dough level, small gliadin molecules act as "bearings" permitting the extended networks of large glutenin molecules to slide

and thus "plastisize" the dough. In fact, these types of molecular structures and interactions give gluten its unique properties. The possibility
of developing new strains of wheat with higher amounts of glutenins
(which are responsible for over half of the variation in bread-making
performance) through breeding or gene technology is just around the
corner, because the genes encoding for these proteins have already
been identified.

How does the final structure of bread come into being? We have to
start by examining the microstructure of the wheat dough. The dough
develops into an interconnected gluten network having the starch granules embedded throughout (Figure 2.6). Three major events must take
place in the oven at just the right moment. First, air introduced during kneading, the gases produced during fermentation or generated by
leavening agents (even ethanol may evaporate), and water vapor must
start to form bubbles, which are accommodated as they grow by the
elastic dough. Then, as the temperature increases, the starch gelatinizes
at around 65°C and the wheat proteins start to coagulate, forming an
elastic crumb. Last, a network of interconnected gas cells develops, the
final structure is consolidated, and with further baking the outer layer
dehydrates to form a dark brown crust, thanks to the Maillard reaction.[18] Control of the final structure depends not only on the ingredients

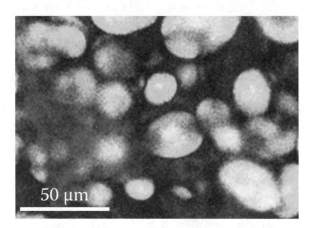

FIGURE 2.6   MICROSTRUCTURE OF A BREAD DOUGH. THE PROTEIN MATRIX FORMED BY GLU-
TEN (DARK BACKGROUND) IS HIGHLIGHTED USING A FLUOROCHROME. STARCH GRANULES (LIGHT
OVALS) ARE DISTRIBUTED WITHIN THIS MATRIX.

(e.g., lipids that give the fine layered dough structure in croissants) but also on processing factors such as oven temperature (which may vary between 180 and 300°C), as well as the position in the bread loaf pan.[19]

We have demonstrated that in a presliced loaf of bread the air cells at the end of the loaf are larger than those in the central slices. Bread slices are easy to image on both sides using a simple photocopying machine. Then all that is needed is to develop a software that will identify air cells in digital images and then to size them by counting pixels inside each of them (Section 5.8).[20]

2.10 CHANGING STRUCTURES

Standardization of raw materials is a basic requirement for commerce because it allows products to maintain the same identity and quality. Few industrial activities involve raw materials that change overnight, like the food industry. We hope that every package of breakfast cereal or jar of jam will be identical to the one we enjoyed before. But biological structures are the sources of our food, and they can change with the climate, the type of storage and transport, and, in general, over time. McDonald's claims that you can eat the same hamburger at any of its locations, whether you're in Alaska or in Tel Aviv or Nairobi. This is surprising because their ingredients come from diverse sources, travel through varied weather conditions, and are susceptible to important changes right up until the consumer takes his or her first bite.

It's difficult for two apples harvested from the same orchard to be exactly equal from a chemical point of view. They don't begin to grow at the same time, and they are not exposed to the sun or the cold in the same way. The flavor of meat, for example, depends on what the animal is fed, and its texture is affected by the animal's condition at the moment it's sacrificed. This environmental influence is well exploited by vintners, who search for perfect soil and climate conditions (the *terroir*) to produce wine with unique aromas and flavors from the same grape strains.[21]

Excluding the loss of quality due to microorganisms, there is a list of reasons why raw materials change over time. Some foods are still living or at least continuing their metabolism during storage, right up to the point of consumption. In fact, if we add lemon to oysters before eating them and they don't shrink as they do when they are still alive, this makes us suspicious. Fresh fruits and vegetables are the most important food structures in which respiration continues until they are consumed. Dry grains like legumes also keep their basic metabolism. One popular school experiment is to germinate beans on moistened cotton, where they will produce roots and a stem. Germination, which transforms barley into malt and soybeans into sprouts, is an example of the capacity to resume important biochemical activities that are latent in these and other seeds.

Fruit and vegetable respiration basically involves the consumption of oxygen and the liberation of CO_2, generating heat and water vapor. With respiration, complex molecules like starch, sugars, and organic acids are converted to simple carbon dioxide and water molecules, generating energy. Fruit ripening involves important changes in the chemical characteristics of the fruit, such as the appearance of volatile aromatic components, flavor alterations from conversion of starch into sugar, and changes in physical properties like texture and color. In one important group of fruits (e.g., apples, apricots, avocados, peaches), CO_2 production increases to a maximum during maturation and is accompanied by the production of ethylene (also a gas) and other hormones. In some cases the signs of ripeness are obvious, like bananas, which are "green" when sold but turn yellow with brown spots as they ripen. As an apple ripens, the pectins in the cell walls solubilize and absorb more water, softening the cells and making them separate. You can appreciate this when you bite into an over-ripe apple, because there's no noise as you chew, no juice comes out, and the separated cells give the apple a rough, sandy texture.

Once a fruit is harvested, respiration proceeds differently depending on the type of fruit, making it difficult to make general recommendations about storage and handling. Postharvest handling aims to find the right conditions of temperature, relative humidity, and atmosphere around the fruit to maximize its quality and value. The rate of respiration decreases with temperature, which is why some fruits are stored in the refrigerator. Bananas and avocados, however, ripen best at room temperature and can be damaged if refrigerated. Storing apples and stone fruits (peaches, plums) at low temperatures causes metabolic disorders that result in damaged and mealy interiors. The composition of gases in the atmosphere can affect the shelf life of fruits and vegetables, so gases are added and removed to adjust atmospheric conditions in the storage yards and shipping containers. The term *controlled atmosphere* refers to a precise manipulation of the gases (generally O_2 and CO_2) throughout the entire time of storage, while the term *modified atmosphere* normally indicates that the food (e.g., precut produce often found in supermarkets) was packaged under a certain gas composition or the atmosphere inside a package was created through product respiration.

In the case of a slaughtered animal or fish, there are many catabolic processes (chemical breakdown of certain molecules) that influence the structure of the muscles. The stiffness of a cadaver, or *rigor mortis*, that lasts for several hours after death is caused by the irreversible binding of actin and myosin (Section 2.1), so that the muscle fibers contract and produce stiffness and rigidity of the muscles. These changes depend greatly on the physiological state of the animal or fish at the moment of death and later on the storage temperature. It takes weeks for rigor mortis to disappear from beef that is stored at 0°C and only a few days for fish. As meat ages, it slowly softens as enzymes called *cathepsins* act on the muscle filaments, and other enzymes act on proteins and fats, producing certain desirable flavors, all of which make the muscle tissues more palatable for consumption.

The variability of ingredients and reactivity of food is something that food technologists and chefs have to assume. That's why it is so important to start with the best quality ingredients available, and once they're in your hands, to store them optimally, as will be discussed in Section 8.1. Producing consistent products or dishes is a challenge for chefs, especially as they gain a reputation and the demand for them increases. Never forget that most foods are living structures.

2.11 DAIRY NANOTECHNOLOGY

Nanotechnology is the new hope for deriving technologic solutions to many real-life problems. *Nanotechnology* is the manipulation of matter at a size never before accessible to humans, in between the molecular level where chemistry operates, and the cellular level, which is already manipulated through physiology and biotechnology. The definition of nanotechnology is "the creation of products, equipment and systems manipulating materials on a scale from 1 to 100 nanometers"—that is, dimensions smaller than one thousandth of a hair.

It is obvious that there is nanotechnology in nature, as we've seen how nature starts with simple molecules and creates living structures from them at multiple levels. These structures then break back down into molecules by digestion, metabolism, or degradation. This cycle occurs, forward and back, throughout the range of nanotechnology. The most amazing food nanotechnology can be found inside a milk carton. *Milk* is the fluid that mammals feed their young for development and growth, and the udder or breast is the "nanofactory." Milk contains three main elements necessary for the construction of the structures in dairy products: fat globules, casein micelles, and whey proteins. The molecules in these structures and their assembly process take place inside the mammary cells in the udder of the cow (Figure 2.7).

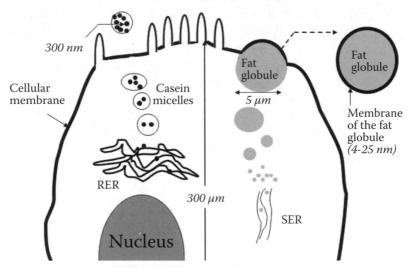

FIGURE 2.7   CELL FROM A COW UDDER, SHOWING THE SYNTHESIS AND ASSEMBLY OF THE CASEIN MICELLES (LEFT) AND THE FORMATION OF FAT GLOBULES (RIGHT). BOTH STRUCTURES ARE DISCHARGED TO THE AQUEOUS PHASE OUTSIDE OF THE CELL, BECOMING PART OF THE MILK. ABOVE RIGHT, THE STRUCTURE OF A FAT GLOBULE.

The most abundant proteins in milk (caseins, beta-lactoglobulin, and alpha-lactalbumin) are synthesized from amino acids in the molecular factories of the rough endoplasmic reticulum (RER). The casein molecules are grouped into micelles of about 200 to 400 nanometers (in the *nano* range) with the help of calcium and phosphorus and are transported outside the cell, where a solution of lactose and mineral salts waits for them. The triglycerides in milk fat are synthesized in another cellular compartment called the smooth endoplasmic reticulum (SER) and come together in tiny droplets that fuse into larger droplets as they move toward the cell membrane. To leave the cell, the fat droplets must be drawn into the cell membrane, so that each globule of milk fat is covered by a biological membrane: these membranes around fat globules have a thickness that varies from 4 to 25 nm, precisely in the nano range (Figure 2.7). Thousands of these cells empty their contents into alveoli from where they eventually flow into the reservoir that stores the milk and feeds the nipple.

Although the bovine mammary gland cell is an amazing nano-apparatus that produces milk "from the bottom up" with great precision, its product does not meet 100% of our present needs: fat separates in the bottle (creaming) and there is too much of it. For this reason we have to "redesign" cow's milk using human technology, operating "from the top down." Anyone over 50 years old will remember that bottled milk used to have a layer of the less dense milk fat that rose to the top. Today there is *homogenized milk*, in which fat globules are reduced in size by a physical process called *homogenization*, so that they remain in suspension much longer (Section 5.2). A second drawback of cow's milk was its natural fat content (about 3.5%), which provided an undesirable excess of calories. Centrifugation is a process that spins a volume of milk at high speed, so that the fat globules quickly separate into cream (30% fat) and skim milk (almost 0% fat).[22] This separation is possible only because the fat is in the form of globules between 0.1 and 10 microns in size and is not distributed at the molecular level (which would make separation more difficult). Once this partition occurs, milk with varying fat contents can be produced by remixing the separated fractions in the right proportion. In the supermarket one can find reduced-fat milk (2% fat), part-skim milk (1.5% fat), and low-fat milk (1% fat), all of which contain less fat than the original milk but still contain all the other components. For many people, part-skim milk tastes as good as whole milk, yet it has ¾ the amount of calories. Have you ever wondered why these lower-fat milks cost more than whole milk although the dairyman gets to keep the removed fat or cream? It's the cost of processing.

Let's return to nanotechnology. A nanoparticle of silver, which is smaller than a virus, presents a very large surface area per unit of volume, implying that a high proportion of silver atoms occupy the outer part of the silver nanoparticle. This feature gives nano-silver certain properties that are very different from an ingot of silver in a bank vault. There is much hope that nanotechnology can change lives by providing durable, lightweight materials, nano-robots that can repair cells, catalysts that improve energy efficiency, and so forth. This remains to be seen. The underlying concern is that the nanoparticles or "nanothings" being created have never existed before. Some experts warn that the risk of introducing them into the environment is that they may end up in our bodies, and we don't know exactly what effects that may have. Experiments have shown that the very small size of some nanoparticles enables them to enter human cells and even the cell nucleus.[23]

Intentionally adding nanoparticles to food can only be justified if the benefits were extraordinary and unmatched by other technologies, and if the risks involved were tolerable. For now the applications of nanotechnology with regard to food are limited to the food environment (packaging and external sensors) and agriculture. The fact that the word *nanotechnology* does not appear in a published text or Web page of any major food company confirms that the future of this technology is still uncertain. Certainly the concepts, techniques, and tools developed by nanosciences—that is, the basic scientific knowledge of the phenomena that occur at the nano level—will be of great utility for examining the inside of our food and understanding the food structures that form and break at the nanoscale level. It's very possible that some future food production processes will copy this "bottom up" model (see Section 1.2), so as to design structures as nature does, by starting with the correct molecules and assembling them into more complex structures.

2.12 THE OTHER MILKY WAY

The Milky Way is the galaxy where our planet Earth resides. The galaxy owes its name to its milky appearance in the sky. There is a group of "star foods" that are derived from the fluid that mammals feed their young, hence the title of this section. This "galaxy" of dairy products is clearly visible at the supermarket and includes a wide range of food structures, deserving our special attention.

From the point of view of an expert in soft materials, dairy products are admirable structures. First, they are constructed from only three of the constituents of milk: fat globules, casein micelles, and whey proteins. Second, the manner in which these components interact and combine on a scale less than 1 micron is a remarkable example of molecular self-assembly and microtechnology, which is not appreciated by material scientists (Section 2.11). Finally, the structures that are formed cover a wide range of materials from liquid (milk), soft and hard solids (cheeses), spreadable plastic materials (butter) and solid particles (powdered milk), to emulsions (cream), foams (whipped cream), and gels (yogurt), as shown in Figure 2.8.

Cheese making is considered an art, but science and technology are also involved. There are hundreds of types of cheese, and just as many books on cheese making. For specific details about making different cheeses these books are helpful, but the basic science is common among all of them.[24] The manufacture of cheese begins with the origin of the milk and depends on the type of animal (including breed), the animal's feed, milking period, and so forth. Cheese structure starts with the cheese curds, which are gels (Section 2.8) that form from the joining of casein micelles that have been destabilized by the acid produced by microorganisms or by the enzyme rennin (rennet) that cleaves the long peptide ("hair") that sticks out from the surface of the micelles (see Figure 2.8). The formation of the curd is also influenced by the heat treatment of the milk, the amount of fat, whether or not the milk is homogenized, and so on. It's easy to imagine the almost endless varieties of cheese that are possible. The other 20% of the milk proteins that don't form into the gel remain in the aqueous whey (noncasein fraction)

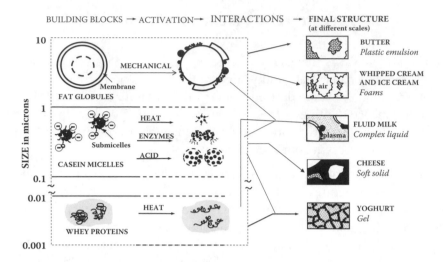

FIGURE 2.8 DEVELOPMENT OF MICROSTRUCTURES IN CERTAIN DAIRY PRODUCTS. EVERYTHING STARTS WITH JUST THREE BASIC UNITS: FAT GLOBULES, CASEIN MICELLES, AND WHEY PROTEINS IN MILK. THE ACTION OF VARIOUS AGENTS (MECHANICAL ENERGY, HEAT, ENZYMES, ETC.) ON THESE BUILDING BLOCKS PRODUCES ACTIVE INTERMEDIATES, WHICH ARE NOW ABLE TO INTER-ACT AND BUILD THE DIFFERENT STRUCTURES OF THE FOOD PRODUCTS.

and are not part of the curd. These soluble proteins are called *whey proteins*. The main whey proteins are beta-lactoglobulin (~65% of total protein in the serum) and alpha-lactalbumin (~25%). Another soluble fraction of milk protein that remains in the whey is the peptide cut off by hydrolysis. This protein "hair" is known as casein-macropeptide and has been shown to have antimicrobial and probiotic properties as well as immunologic effect.

To make fresh cheese, the curds are cut into small cubes for easy removal of water and later treated with salt and pressed. At this point the mass can also be stretched in hot water to transform the protein network into thick elastic fibers, which is how a *Mozzarella* cheese is made. But it's the subtle structural details and especially the flavor that develop during the maturation process. Each type of cheese requires certain optimal humidity and temperature conditions. The aromas associated with cheese are primarily derived from the enzymatic hydrolysis of lipids (lipolysis) and proteins (proteolysis) produced by microorganisms. The structure and creaminess of cheeses like *Camembert* and blue cheeses like Roquefort are due to the action of molds that grow on the surface of the cheese in the first case as well as in the holes within the cheese, in the latter. These fungi secrete powerful enzymes whose action on different substrates provides the valued smooth and creamy texture and tastes. As a result of proteolysis the amino acid tyrosine accumulates in *Parmigiano Reggiano* cheese and after 30 months of storage it crystallizes into small grains that can be tasted on the tongue. Far from being a defect, this graininess means the cheese is sufficiently aged (several years).

It's no wonder that cheese is expensive. Only a fraction of the protein in milk is used in the process, so that 100 liters of milk only makes about 10 kilos of cheese (the exact amount depends on the moisture content and the type of cheese). For example, a thousand liters of milk is required to make two 35-kilogram *Parmigiano Reggiano* cheeses. The dairy industry is an example of a traditional industry adapted to make great improvements in sustainability. Current technology allows for the processing of whey, which used to be discarded directly into the environment. The whey is fractioned into beta-lactoglobulin and alpha-lactalbumin that are then dried, generating powdered protein ingredients high in functionality and commercial value (Section 8.4).

2.13 YOUNG AND VARIED STRUCTURES

For millions of years our food supply consisted of the food structures provided by nature and in their natural state. Then, changes in structure came from solar drying and the application of heat. Good microorganisms came into play later on, and fermented foods, with their special textures and flavors, arrived on our menu. Some of these fermented foods, such as yogurt, have been enjoyed for millennia, but widespread consumption and popularity of yogurt did not occur until the mid-twentieth century, when yogurt gained a reputation for being healthy, and sweetened, commercially flavored yogurts with fruit became available.

As shown in Table 2.1, some of the most popular processed foods are made of easily identifiable structures that have only recently (in the long history of food) become dietary mainstays in their commercially

TABLE 2.1

Young and Famous Food Structures, Together with Some of Their Inventors

Food	Type of Structure	Origin and Approximate Date
Mayonnaise	Emulsion	End of the 1700s
Whipped cream	Liquid foam	Nineteenth century
Milk chocolate	Particulate solid	Around 1818
Ice cream	Frozen aerated emulsion	Around 1832
Ketchup	Structured fluid	H.J. Heinz (1876)
Breakfast cereals	Porous, hard solids	J.H. Kellogg (1884)
Cotton candy	Filament	Around 1900
French fries	Rigid, filled beam	Post World War I
Potato and corn chips	Brittle solids	Around 1930
Instant coffee	Porous, soft solid	Nestlé (1938)
Flavored yogurt	Gel	Dannon (around 1950)
Puffed snacks	Solid foams	Around 1950

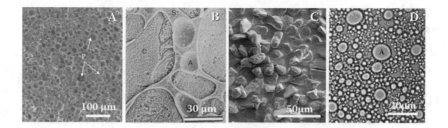

FIGURE 2.9   EXAMPLES OF THE STRUCTURES OF SOME OF THE FOODS LISTED IN TABLE 2.1.
(A) INSTANT COFFEE (*P* = PORES); (B) ICE CREAM (*C* = ICE CRYSTAL, *A* = AIR, *S* = SOLUTION);
(C) MILK CHOCOLATE (DEMONSTRATING COCOA PARTICLES, POWDERED MILK, AND SUGAR)
(COURTESY OF P. BRAUN, BUHLER AG); AND (D) MAYONNAISE (*A* = DROP OF OIL).

prepared form. The microstructure of several of them is shown in Figure 2.9.

Several of these products are new forms of known materials, produced by twentieth century technologies that contribute to a greater variety of textures and flavors in food. These new foods were developed for diverse reasons. Some come from a nutritional fundamentalism, like the breakfast cereals created by the Kellogg brothers. Their intent was to replace the traditional high-fat breakfast of greasy sausage, bacon, scrambled eggs, and omelets with healthy cereal flakes. In many ways milk chocolate was the undertaking of M.S. Hershey, who after a couple of failures, in 1903 built a town in Pennsylvania dedicated to chocolate. There are innovators like H.J. Heinz, who turned a humble raw material like tomato paste into a seasoned condiment—ketchup—that is now added to many dishes. These and other names became companies and brands that are now global, such as Nestlé (valued at around $80 billion), McDonald's, Lindt, Cadbury, Barilla (Italian pasta), Guinness and Carlsberg (beer), and so forth.[25] Other products had to wait for the necessary technology to achieve mass consumption, such as ice cream (ice machines are mid-nineteenth century), puffed snacks, and some extruded breakfast cereals (Section 8.4).

From a food history point of view, the food structures presented in Table 2.1 and Figure 2.9 are all very young. The oldest have only been around for a couple of centuries. The obvious question is: Are there other food structures that we haven't yet discovered or rediscovered?

The same question can be extended to manufacturing technologies. The extrusion process that is used to make some breakfast cereals and snacks, for example, has been used for less than 60 years and was copied from the plastics industry. One might wonder if the microtechnologies currently being developed which can manipulate molecules and fluids in tiny quantities will someday be available to dispense the right nutrients within the correct structures to produce better and affordable processed foods.

2.14 MEASURING WITH INSTRUMENTS

Because foods are materials, food engineers try to quantify their properties in a similar way as they do with other engineering materials. In fact, the adjectives used in materials science are also used to describe the behavior of certain foods during chewing: tough meat, viscous cream, and so on. Food materials laboratories have a number of instruments for measuring important properties like deformation after applying forces of all kinds, the viscosity of liquids and pastes, the phase transitions (melting and softening) induced by heat effect, optical characteristics like color and transparency, the noise emitted during fracture, and so forth, in an accurate and reproducible way. The challenge is to find or design engineering instruments whose results are related to the desired perceptions that have been determined by a sensory panel or consumer groups.

Mechanical testing of foods is one of the important physical measurements and generally attempts to simulate what happens in the mouth because foods have to break during chewing under the mechanical action produced by the jaws. The mechanical properties are evaluated in a testing machine that applies a deformation at a controlled rate and measures the force used in each moment until the sample is destroyed. It is similar to breaking a peanut shell between your fingers, but the instrument will determine the newtons of force that were required to break it and the millimeters of deformation that occurred before it broke.[26]

It is important to have good communication between chefs and engineers so that the terms used in these trials are understood in the same

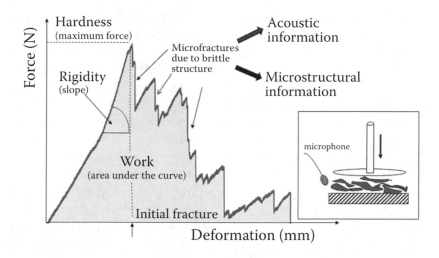

FIGURE 2.10   MECHANICAL COMPRESSION TEST (CRUSHING) OF POTATO CHIPS IS SHOWN IN
THE INSERT IN THE RIGHT. THE RESULTING DIAGRAM SHOWS THAT THE COMPRESSIVE FORCE
REACHES A MAXIMUM VALUE AT THE MOMENT FRACTURE BEGINS. AFTERWARDS LESS AND LESS
FORCE IS NEEDED TO TRIGGER A SERIES OF MINOR FRACTURES THAT GIVE RISE TO ACOUSTIC
PHENOMENA (PERCEIVED AS NOISE) AND TEXTURAL SENSATIONS FROM THE MICROSTRUCTURE.

way. A material is "rigid" when it doesn't deform after applying force,
and a material is "hard" when it requires a lot of force to fracture it. Thus,
hard candy is both rigid and hard, but peanut shells are rigid but soft
(you can break them easily with your fingers, without prior deformation).

The diagram obtained during a mechanical test, in which a group
of potato chips were slowly compressed with a plunger, relates the
applied force at each moment to the resulting deformation, as shown in
Figure 2.10. Sometimes a tiny microphone is incorporated to record the
acoustic signal emitted during the test, as the sound of breaking potato
chips is also important. This mechanical test provides information
about the rigidity and strength (or hardness) at the time of breakage,
and then shows a series of microfractures that continue to occur until
the potato chips are reduced to almost a powder. The breaks in the
curve provide microstructural and acoustic information (e.g., crunchiness) and are equivalent to a fingerprint or "signature" for the product,
which can then be used to develop similar foods, evaluate new formulations, or study the food's behavior during chewing.[27]

Commercial gelatin is obtained from the bones and hides of pigs and cattle and is available in translucent sheets or in a powder form. Because the raw material is highly variable, so is the consistency of the gel that forms (and its taste), something cooks know. Gelatin producers indicate the Bloom value in their specifications, which represents the resistance of a pure gelatin gel to penetration with a punch. However, supermarket jelly consists basically of sugar, commercial gelatin, flavoring, and coloring, with the latter two in very small proportion to the first two. One of the projects that the students in my Food Materials Science course did at the end of the semester was to buy different food gelatins, prepared them according to manufacturer's directions, and then they measured the strength of the gels, using a similar mechanical compression test to the one shown in Figure 2.10. After all, what one is buying is gel strength. The test basically consists of slowly lowering a metal disk about 2 cm in diameter until it compresses the gelatin, and then recording the force that opposes the gel until fracture occurs. Dividing the fracture strength by the unit cost of the product (in dollars [$] per gram) determines the cost per unit of "gel strength," which is what is really of value in this kind of product. For an engineer, this is enough information for now—the problems of flavor and taste, although very important, will remain.

A calorimeter is an instrument that measures *thermal properties* of foods such as the melting point and the calories needed to heat a given amount. The differential scanning calorimeter (DSC), which is used to study thermal properties of food, is a sophisticated and expensive instrument. (I tell my students that it costs the same as the latest BMW 500 series, so that they take good care of it.) The heart of the apparatus consists of a tiny "furnace" where a sealed metal capsule that holds less than one gram of the sample is introduced. This small quantity ensures that the entire volume of the material quickly reaches a homogeneous temperature. The sample is heated or cooled gradually at a precisely controlled rate (°C per min) and within a preset range of temperatures (hence the name scanning). The instrument measures changes in the heat input (gained by the sample) or heat loss from it at each moment. The increase in temperature of the food from the heating effect is related to the specific heat (the amount of heat per unit mass required to raise the temperature by 1°C) which is almost constant. Any major change in heat flow on top of that of the specific heat, like the denaturation of a protein, for example, an egg white's transition from liquid to solid, the gelatinization of starch (paste formation), the freezing of water, or the melting of a fat (when cocoa butter becomes soft) appears as a peak in the "thermogram" (readout), whose area is proportional to the heat absorbed or released by the sample. A DSC test can also determine the glass transition temperature Tg, or that temperature above which a glassy, brittle material softens (Section 2.3).

2.15 MEASURING WITH THE SENSES

Instrumental measurements provide information on the physical behavior of a food product, which may be important if the product must flow through a pipe or be heated for sterilization, for example, or to design containers that provide mechanical protection to them. Instrumental measurements are limited, however, in predicting the sensory quality of a product, or how people perceive it through their senses (e.g., its texture). Mastication involves many types of forces, but more important, sensory characteristics are multidimensional. There is a branch of food science known as *sensory evaluation*, which uses a group of panelists, or people who are trained to describe the textural, visual, odor, and taste properties perceived with the senses, also called the organoleptic properties of a food. The sensory organs and the capacity of the brain to interpret the properties become "the instrument." Sensory evaluation is the gold standard against which any chemical or physical property of a food should be compared, even before it enters the mouth. An apple can contain all the desirable nutrients that we expect and be perfectly ripe, but if our vision detects a mark on the skin, it won't make it to the shopping bag. There is no equipment that can replace human tasters for determining the color, aroma, and taste characteristics of beer and wine.[28]

The static methods of sensory evaluation have been in use for a long time. They reflect the integrated set of sensations that are perceived by the panelist from the moment a product enters his or her mouth until it is swallowed. These methods are used to compare reformulated products with traditional ones and to make profiles of the various characteristics of a food. Lately more emphasis has been placed on the variation in time or the dynamics of the sensory perception during chewing. In the time-intensity analysis, the panelist will note how the release of flavors and texture change during mastication, thereby generating a profile in time. In the case of aromas, this process can be complemented with direct sampling at selected intervals, using tubes inserted in the nostrils, so that volatile compounds that are coming to the nose can be subsequently analyzed by chromatography and mass spectroscopy (Section 7.3). This way subjective or sensory perceptions can be compared to the chemistry of the molecules involved.

There are certain limitations to using people for the characterization of food, including problems with availability, the unreliability of our senses, the interference of environmental factors, health, and so on. Another limitation is the panelist's capacity to describe his or her perception of textures and flavors in a uniform and consistent way. Judges and panelists practice with standardized products or products that represent certain textures and flavors and develop lexicons or even dictionaries based on many products in the same category, so that they will have a standard, shared nomenclature. Sensory evaluation is an essential tool for product development, quality control, and assessment of acceptability by consumers.

2.16 THAT'S THE WAY I SEE IT

People may see different things in foods. Painters become fascinated with their colors and shapes (as in the realism of still life); poets reminisce about their hidden meanings; chemists value the elements they contain; nutritionists may see foods as a route to better health, and so on. Engineers look at foods as they flow through processing lines and become marketable objects. But considering foods as soft and tasty structures may seem strange, more so because the details of these structures cannot be seen with our eyes. The fact is that we eat structures, not nutrients or chemical elements, contrary to what nutritionists and food chemists may say. If we consider structure to be the main value of foods, this must change the perspective of food technologists,

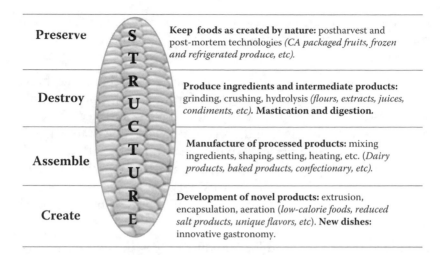

Preserve	**S**	**Keep foods as created by nature:** postharvest and post-mortem technologies *(CA packaged fruits, frozen and refrigerated produce, etc).*
Destroy	**T R U**	**Produce ingredients and intermediate products:** grinding, crushing, hydrolysis *(flours, extracts, juices, condiments, etc).* **Mastication and digestion.**
Assemble	**C T U**	**Manufacture of processed products:** mixing ingredients, shaping, setting, heating, etc. *(Dairy products, baked products, confectionary, etc).*
Create	**R E**	**Development of novel products:** extrusion, encapsulation, aeration *(low-calorie foods, reduced salt products, unique flavors, etc).* **New dishes:** innovative gastronomy.

FIGURE 2.11   MAKING FOODS IS A DEDICATED EFFORT THAT INVOLVES PRESERVING, TRANS-
FORMING, ASSEMBLING, CREATING, AND DESTROYING FOOD STRUCTURES. WHEN WE EAT FOODS,
WE ARE ENJOYING HOW THESE STRUCTURES BREAK DOWN IN OUR MOUTHS AND LATER, ALMOST
UNCONSCIOUSLY, ARE REDUCED TO MOLECULES IN OUR DIGESTIVE TRACT.

nutritionists, chefs, and even the consumer, as I hope will be demonstrated in the pages that follow (Figure 2.11).

To begin we are reminded that in order to preserve natural food structures, careful control must be placed over the postmortem events that occur in meat and fish as well as what happens to fruits and vegetables after they are harvested (postharvest). The value of these foods is proportional to their freshness, so many technologies have been developed to delay unavoidable decay, including refrigeration, fast freezing, and controlled storage and packaging. Dry legumes and grains, staple foods in most of the world, have low moisture content and therefore only require cool, dry, and hermetic storage.

Some structures produced by nature must be destroyed so that basic intermediate materials such as wheat and corn flours, starch, fats, and sugars can be released and extracted, becoming products in their own right. Gums and essential oils need to be isolated from their natural sources. Grinding, scraping, and pressing obliterate the matrices that contain these valuable components and permit their extraction and refinement. Structures are also broken down to extract juices from fruits and vegetables, and to derive the substrates for fermented beverages and spirits.

The enormous processed foods industry is assembling the previous intermediate structures and transforming them into recognizable classes of finished products. That's how pasta, baked and dairy products, snacks, candies, and processed meats come into being, as well as sauces and beverages. Mixing, heat transfer, and shaping are some of the major operations performed in large processing plants, artisanal shops, and kitchens for this purpose. We expect these formulated and converted structures to be consistent, stable, and microbiologically safe.

Hundreds of new or modified products show up on supermarket shelves each year, and restaurants are expected to change their menus at least once a year. One of the biggest challenges for food technology experts and chefs alike is the creation of new food structures. The wide assortment of textures and flavors offered today arose from a mixture of intuition, hard work, and chance. In the future, creativity, refined ingredients, and improved structuring operations such as foaming, gelling, emulsification, and other techniques will bring multiple opportunities for food processors and cooks alike, as they will continue to be the main providers of what we eat. Hopefully, the future development and manufacture of new food structures as well as the creation of new dishes will provide a greater variety of enjoyable foods from which we can derive a better nutrition and a healthier life.

NOTES

1. McGee, H. 2004. *On Food and Cooking: The Science and Lore of the Kitchen.* Scribner, New York.
2. Apparently this comes from Goethe and his "Theory of Human Chemistry," which relates the affinity between people to reactions between molecules. There is a more recent book, Thims, L. 2007. *Human Chemistry*, volumes 1 and 2, LuLu, Morrisville, NC, that also tries to explain the analogy between humans and chemistry.
3. Those interested in the subject may consult the book Stead, J.W., and Atwood, J.L. 2009. *Supramolecular Chemistry*, 2nd ed., Wiley, Chichester.

4. The ultimate reference on the subject of thermodynamic separation of polymers and associated complex molecular structures in foods is Russian scientist Vladimir Tolstoguzov. He is the former director of the famous Institute of Organo-Element Compounds of the USSR Academy of Sciences. He relocated to the West in 1992 and wrote many papers on the subject, including Tolstoguzov, V. 2005. Some thermodynamic considerations in food formulation. *Food Hydrocolloids* 17, 1–23.

5. In terms of the physics of polymers, the partition of polymers into two immiscible phases, each enriched with a specific polymer, is called *thermodynamic incompatibility*. Associative separation or *complex coacervation* is the formation of complexes between two polymers in solution which separate in concentrated form (both polymers mixed) from the solvent.

6. The fundamental work of the scientists from Nabisco, Louise Slade and Harry Levine, is in the book Slade, L., and Levine, H. 1991. *Water Relationships in Foods*. Springer, New York.

7. It is said that the glass in ancient cathedrals is thicker at the bottom due to the slow downward flow of this "supercooled liquid" caused by gravity. According to Zanotto, E. 1998. Do cathedral glasses flow? *American Journal of Physics* 66, 392–396, any observed thickening is most likely due to imperfections in glass manufacturing from those times and could not have been caused by flow. According to Zanotto it would take millions of years to produce a very small change in thickness, given the high viscosity of the glass.

8. Wheat gluten gives elasticity to bread dough which is developed during kneading when wheat proteins become hydrated with water. Wheat gluten is associated with celiac disease, a disorder of the small intestine caused by a complex immune response. It should not be confused with corn gluten, which is a protein by-product of wet corn milling and does not develop elasticity.

9. Belitz, H.-D., Grosch, W., and Schieberle, P. 2004. *Food Chemistry*, 3rd revised ed., Springer, New York, pp. 268–288.

10. A recently published book that covers diverse topics related to culinary foams is Campbell, G.M., Scanlon, M.G., and Pyle, D.L. 2008. *Bubbles in Foods 2: Novelty, Health and Luxury*. Eagan Press, St. Paul, MN.

11. A complete and updated review on foods containing bubbles can be found at Niranjan, K. 2008. Bubble-containing foods. In *Food Materials Science: Principles and Applications* (J.M. Aguilera and P. Lillford, eds.), Springer, New York, pp. 281–303.

12. European Community, Directive No. 95/2/EC from February 20, 1995.

13. Sagis, L.M.C., de Groot-Mostert, A.E.A., Prins, A., and van der Linden, E. 2001. Effect of copper ions on the drainage stability of foams prepared

from egg white. *Colloids and Surfaces A: Physicochemical and Engineering Aspects* 180, 163–172. The authors show that adding copper ions directly into the egg white will slow production of the foam, but the resulting foam is more stable (independent of the container in which the egg whites are beaten). This article is one example among many of how scientific literature contains relevant information for cooks.

14. For a more complete explanation of the mechanism for stabilizing whipped cream and the difference between UHT homogenized cream and nonhomogenized, see Kulozik, U. 2008. Structure dairy products by means of processing and matrix design. In *Food Materials Science: Principles and Applications* (J.M. Aguilera and P. Lillford, eds.), Springer, New York, pp. 439–474.

15. As I once observed at a banquet in Shanghai, the Chinese are fond of eating jellied seafood products. See also: Jellyfish—Food of the future, *New Scientist* 2698, 2009, which suggests that new chefs could begin to transform algae and jellyfish into exquisite dishes.

16. A good general reference is Harris, P. 1990. *Food Gels*. Elsevier, London. Surprisingly, to my knowledge this is the only text that covers all types of food gels.

17. Kitabatake, N., Shimizu, A., and Doi, E. 1988. Preparation of transparent egg white gel with salt by two-step heating method, *Journal of Food Science* 53, 735–738.

18. An x-ray image of a slice of bread showing the continuous protein-starch matrix holding air cells is shown in Figure 3.2.

19. More on wheat proteins and bread as a structured product can be found in Dobraszczyk, D.J. 2008. Structured cereal products. In *Food Materials Science: Principles and Applications* (J.M. Aguilera and P. Lillford, eds.), Springer, New York, pp. 474–500.

20. Actual data showing that the distribution of air cell sizes along slices of a bread loaf varies are presented in Ramírez, C., and Aguilera, J.M. 2011. Determination of a representative area element (RAE) based on nonparametric statistics in bread. *Journal of Food Engineering* 102, 197–201.

21. Agronomists distinguish between *genotype*, which is the particular set of genes of a plant, and *phenotype*, which is the group of characteristics that are expressed by the interaction of the genome with the environment.

22. The terminal velocity at which a body moves within a fluid is directly proportional to the square of its size and to the prevailing acceleration (see Section 5.2). On Earth the gravitational acceleration is constant ($g = 9.8$ m²/s), but in a centrifugal field (e.g., when the trajectory is curved) the acceleration is given as $\omega^2 r$ and depends therefore on the distance from the center to where the body is rotating (r), and the rotational angular

velocity (ω). In a lab centrifuge ω can be changed within an ample range (e.g., 1,000 to 15,000 rpm), so an object may move (decant) thousands of times faster than under gravity.

23. More about nanotechnology and foods can be obtained from a report by the Institute of Medicine in 2009 entitled *Nanotechnology in Food Products*, The National Academies Press, Washington, DC.

24. I highly recommend this classic book on cheese and fermented milks written by my professor at Cornell University, who first introduced me to this fascinating, delicious, and nutritious subject: Kosikowski, F.V. 1977. *Cheese and Fermented Milk Foods*, 2nd edition. Edward Brothers, Ann Arbor, MI. It describes in detail the procedures for preparing different types of classic cheeses. He also wrote the article Kosikowski, F.V. 1985. Cheese. *Scientific American* 252(5), 88–99.

25. The market value of some of the leading commercial brands can be viewed at Clark, N. 2009. Biggest brands: Top 100 global brands by value, 2009. *Marketing*. www.marketingmagazine.co.uk/news/wide/901385/ (accessed August 12, 2009).

26. One newton (N) is the force needed to provide an acceleration of 1 m/s^2 to an object whose mass is 1 kg. For example, 1 N is equal to the force with which gravity pulls a small apple (or in other words, the apple's weight).

27. Chewing is actually a very complex process involving deformations produced by various types of forces (in addition to compression) and cycles of breaking and wetting the particles with saliva. The artificial mouths that have been developed so far are unable to completely simulate the behavior of a material in the oral cavity.

28. There are several books available on sensory evaluation of foods, but this book is especially noteworthy: Lawless, H.T., and Heymann, H. 2010. *Sensory Evaluation of Food: Principles and Practices*, 2nd ed. Springer, New York.

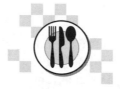

CHAPTER 3

Journey to the Center of Our Food

We eat food, not molecules. But during production, processing, and cooking, the molecules gradually become food structures that are familiar and appealing to us. It's a shame that we can't visually perceive the elements and organization of these structures. Fortunately, there are many techniques to help us get inside of the food and display at different scales its astonishingly complex microstructure. Despite their intrinsic beauty—at least in the eyes of food microscopists—the challenge ahead is to relate the observed (and now quantified and measured) structures with desirable properties such as texture, flavor, and nutritional effects.

3.1 FLAVORFUL STRUCTURES[1]

Of all the structures that we create, food must be the most complex. A loaf of bread seems rather simple: just crust and crumb. But the crumb contains air cells held between solid walls, and these walls in turn contain starch that is trapped in a protein matrix lubricated by fat. The matrix isn't made of just any protein. Wheat gluten is made of two types of special macromolecules that give dough its elasticity, which is unique among all cereals. Thus, we have dropped by nearly seven orders of magnitude from the length of a slice of bread to the size of these molecules (20 to 50 nm) (Figure 3.1). But that's not all. The amount and distribution of starch, gluten proteins, and fats and how they interact with one another result in the hundreds of different types of bread, even though the basic raw material remains the same (wheat flour). Moreover, these structures are different from others we encounter in our daily life because they exchange moisture with the environment, many are alive or vary over time (e.g., they "age" or ripen), suffer attacks from microorganisms, and eventually disappear from the face of the Earth. Last, they have to break down in the mouth and be tasty.

We have discussed food structures without explaining exactly what the term means. For our purposes, we understand the word *structure* to mean the distribution elements that make up a whole and their inter-relationships. Note that we speak of "elements," from which it follows

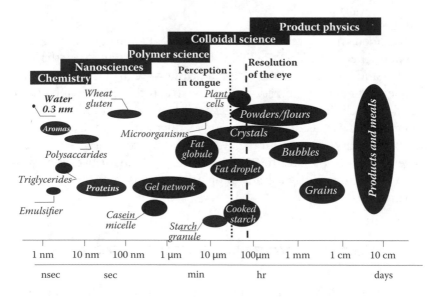

FIGURE 3.1 IMPORTANT FOOD COMPONENTS AND THEIR APPROXIMATE SIZES. LISTED AT THE TOP ARE SOME OF THE MOST IMPORTANT SCIENTIFIC DISCIPLINES INVOLVED IN THE STUDY OF FOODS AT THE DIFFERENT SPACE AND TIME SCALES INDICATED ON THE BOTTOM AXIS.

that one can distinguish classes of objects that are different from each other. In engineering, the structure of a building or bridge is critical because its properties depend on the materials used in its construction and how they are assembled together. An anti-seismic building can withstand an earthquake without major damage because its structure has been designed to dissipate the energy that is transferred during the telluric event. Structure is also synonymous with organization, and so we hear about social structure, mental structure, and so on. In food science, *microstructure* refers to the arrangement of elements on a scale that is smaller than the thickness of a hair (<80 microns). This concept is relatively new and appeared in early 1970 with the widespread use of electron microscopes. Techniques that allow scientists to peer inside foods and unlock the secrets found in their microstructures are now used regularly in both academia and industry (Section 3.3).

The microstructure of a food is central to many of its properties, including texture, flow, chemical stability, nutritional value, and even color. For example, when we say that the meat is tough, that the mayonnaise curdled, or that an apple is mealy, one might think that we're talking about changes in chemical composition. But these conditions are almost always the result of a reorganization or interaction at the microstructural level of the original chemical components. Returning to the original example of bread, it's not an issue of chemical composition that makes fresh bread taste differently from stale bread. A chemical analysis would show that the main components of both breads are present in almost exactly the same amounts. What happens when bread ages is that some of the molecules in the starch (mainly amylopectin) become ordered into crystal structures, which gives us a different perception when we chew the bread (Section 3.5). With respect to color, smooth surfaces appear "lighter" than those with micropores because the light fails to penetrate and illuminate the interior (so the pores look dark), a phenomenon used to make instant coffee with identical composition but different color intensities (see Figure 2.9A).[2]

The analysis of the food microstructures and their relation to the properties of foods is an area of great activity in food science.[3] It has been mentioned that over the past 10 years the number of publications related to food microstructure has tripled. There is much progress being made toward the quantification and characterization of structural elements using computer software. The ultimate goal is to relate the objective aspects of the microstructure to the relevant properties of food in order to improve the chemical and microbiological stability during food storage, substitute possible undesirable ingredients, lower the caloric density and increase the satiety effects of some foods, develop new culinary creations, enhance texture perception and flavor release in the mouth, and favor an easy digestion with increased absorption of nutrients, among other things.

3.2 WE CAN'T SEE THE BEST PART

Unfortunately food technologists and chefs are unable to see the most intimate details that make such a difference in their creations. It's as if an architect was unable to appreciate how the building materials were assembled during construction, could not go inside once the building was finished, and could not see details such as the veneer on the doors or the designs on the bathroom tiles, but was only allowed to observe the exterior of the building.

A micron or micrometer (μm) is one thousandth of a millimeter (1 mm = 0.001 microns) or one millionth of a meter (10^{-6} m), which corresponds to 1,000 nanometers (nm). For reference, the average thickness of a hair is about 80 microns. Our vision is limited and we only see one single object when there are actually two objects, if they are separated by less than about 60 to 80 microns. This is called the limit of *resolution* of our vision (Figure 3.1). Another important sensory limitation in food science is the minimum size of a particle that can be perceived by the tongue. If an ice crystal in ice cream or particle of mustard in mayonnaise is less than about 40 microns in size, it will not be sensed in our mouths and both products will taste creamy, smooth, and delicate.

The naked eye cannot appreciate colloidal systems, which are composed of small clusters of molecules or very fine particles less than about 0.2 microns in size. These clusters are dispersed in water and move erratically, as their small size causes them to collide constantly with molecules of the solvent.[4] We can't see the cells of fruits and vegetables that contribute to their texture, because some of these cells measure on the order of 80 to 100 microns; we also can't see the starch granules (between 5 and 50 microns) that we add to thicken sauces, or the oil droplets (about 10 to 40 microns) that are dispersed in a mayonnaise. We definitely cannot see bacteria that may be contaminating our food (which measure 1 micron in size). Still less can we appreciate the casein macromolecules (0.4 microns to 400 nm) that give structure to cheese. Fortunately, we aren't able to see the particulate matter that pollutes our air which has an average size of 10 microns (known as PM_{10}), or the more obnoxious material that is of 2.5 microns ($PM_{2.5}$) that goes deep into our lungs, because it would depress us with every breath. Figure 3.1 shows several important structural elements in food and their approximate size. In the microworld, size advances in multiples of 10. An atom is 10 times more minuscule than a small molecule, which in turn is 10 times smaller than a protein, which is 10 times smaller than a virus, until another jump of 10 leads to a micron, the size of a bacterium. Because one must refer to many dimensional scales in a single graph, the axis of Figure 3.1 progresses from 10 by 10s (logarithmic scale).

Among the instruments used to look at the food, the magnifying glass is a converging lens placed between the eye and the object, which allows amplification of surface details up to about 60 times their size (60×). When the lens is mounted on a base to control the distance to the object and to focus the lens, it is called a *stereomicroscope*. Inexpensive versions of pedestal magnifiers adapted with a digital camera or camcorder for capturing images are widely available.

The *compound microscope* (so named because it has several lenses), also known as the optical or light microscope (LM), was invented around 1600, after the telescope. Basically a transmitted light microscope consists of a visible light source that is focused with a condenser lens onto a "transparent" sample placed on a slide. The light that passes through the sample and "carries" the image goes into a tube containing two more lenses. The objective lens close to the sample magnifies the image up to 40 times (in multiples of 10×). Then the image is further magnified about 10 to 20 times in the ocular lens located at the top of the tube, which is close to the eye, or a mounted digital photo or video camera. The light microscope was used in the nineteenth century to detect adulteration of foods, particularly spices. At that time, microscopic observations were reported as exquisite hand-made drawings, because photomicroscopy (pictures taken from the microscope) began after 1850. Today different types of light microscopes have many routine applications in microbiology and food science as well as in research. With special stains it is possible to improve the contrast between different tissues and even discriminate between proteins, fats, and starches (Figure 3.6). More sophisticated microscopes use beams of light at a specific wavelength for *fluorescence microscopy* (Figure 2.6), or may be attached to various types of spectrographs[5] so that specific molecules can be located *in situ*. The optical microscope has a resolution limit of about 200 nm (0.2 microns) which is determined by the wavelength of visible light (0.4 to 0.7 microns).

Since 1980, the *confocal laser scanning microscope* (CLSM) has made possible the observation of biologically active samples such as cells and tissues, in a direct and nondestructive way. Thanks to the penetrating power of its laser beam, the microscope can scan a specimen at different depths, acquiring only the information that is in that plane. These two-dimensional images or "optical sections" are taken successively at increasing depths and are later reconstructed into three dimensions with computer software. Another microscopy technique borrowed from biology allows the localization of specific molecules in food by making them react with "tagged" antibodies, which are then visible under the microscope lens. This technique has made it possible to see where whey proteins are located in the microstructure of a pâté or to understand the specific role of alginates in stabilizing salad dressings.[6]

3.3 EYES WIDE OPEN

If visible light imposes a limit on the size of what we can see with a microscope, the logical next step is to change the source of illumination. In the last century it was discovered that if electrons were used to "illuminate" an object (e.g., by impinging over it), the magnification of the object could be increased many times. This discovery led to the birth of *electron microscopy*, and the first instrument of its kind was developed by Canadian James Hillier in 1937. This type of microscope was able to amplify objects by more than five thousand times, meaning that an ant would appear as if it were standing right in front of your eyes and measured 10 meters long. Today, electron microscopes are essential tools for food research, and the information they provide is not only useful but also aesthetically impressive.

In an electron microscope, electrons are generated in a heated filament (usually made of platinum) and are directed toward the sample with magnetic fields (replacing the glass lenses of a light microscope). With *transmission electron microscopy* (TEM), the electrons are focused on very thin sections of a sample (less than 1 micron thick) and by passing through the electrons generate a flat image like that from a transmitted light microscope (see Figure 2.5). Sample preparation for TEM is complex, requiring specialized equipment and instrumentation and above all lots of experience, but when it's done professionally TEM provides invaluable information.[7] With *scanning electron microscopy* (SEM), the beam of electrons sweeps or scans the surface of the sample, generating a three-dimensional view of the surface, like as seen with a magnifying glass (see Figure 2.4). Moreover, the impact of electrons on the sample generates new electrons and x-rays whose analysis provides information about the atomic composition of the surface being analyzed. Electron microscopes require a strong vacuum inside, so the samples must remain dehydrated to avoid the presence of water vapor. This is a significant problem for most foods, which tend to have high moisture and when dehydrated experience considerable shrinkage, making the observed structure differ from the original.[8] Electron *cryomicroscopy* uses special equipment that can observe samples under frozen conditions with liquid nitrogen (Figure 2.4). At these very low cryogenic conditions (e.g., −196°C) water is frozen into ice, so for practical purposes it doesn't evaporate. Fast freezing is much gentler on a structure than dehydration.

But electron microscopes are not sufficient for viewing things on an atomic scale. In the 1980s two remarkable discoveries were made at the IBM research and development center in Rüschlikon, near Zurich: the scanning tunneling microscope, which can "see" at the atomic level, and a ceramic material that conducted electricity without any resistance at temperatures higher than ever before (which is known as "superconductivity"). Each of these discoveries won the Nobel Prize for Physics in consecutive years, first in 1986 (G. Binnig and H. Rohrer with E. Ruska) and then in 1987 (J.G. Bednorz and K.A. Müller), which was a stunning achievement in basic research performed at a private company, one that also happened to be associated with computing. The *atomic force microscope* (AFM), which looks much less impressive than an electron microscope, operates on a principle similar to the old turntable. A sharp point travels across the sample's surface, and the interactions between the tip of the point and the outer layer of electrons from the sample are measured. The deflections of the flexible bar (cantilever) that holds the sharp point are translated into force and distance (at nanometer level) for each point on the surface. Computer software is responsible for transforming these signals into three-dimensional images (see Figure 1.2).

The availability of microscopic techniques for studies in foods depends on the development of hardware for biology and material sciences research. Most industrial and academic labs that perform advanced research in food materials science own or have access to a battery of microscopy equipment. As a consequence, the number of scientific articles published on the microstructure of food has increased fourfold over the past 15 years, and in 2009 exceeded 320 in 1 year.

3.4 FOOD UNDER THE SCANNER

The ability to scrutinize the inside of certain foods to check for defects that might be invisible from the outside without "invading" or destroying the food is very useful. That is exactly what doctors do when they send their patients for a magnetic resonance imaging (MRI) scan or for a CT (x-ray computed tomography) scan: they observe organs in place, and noninvasively (the organs are not changed by the examination). Why not use these same diagnostic techniques for food?

Magnetic resonance imaging (MRI) is based on the principle that nuclei that carry charges, like the hydrogen atom (^1H) in the water molecule, are capable of interacting with the equipment's external magnetic field. The result of this interaction is unique for each of the various tissues and organs and can be translated into signals of different intensity that are then converted into images that show good contrast between the different tissues. When an apple falls onto the ground, the immediate

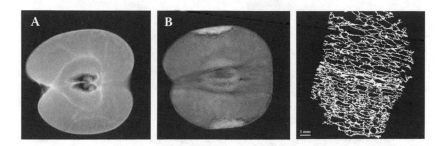

FIGURE 3.2   LEFT: IMAGE OBTAINED BY MAGNETIC RESONANCE IMAGING (MRI) OF AN
APPLE THAT HAD BEEN HIT WITH A HAMMER. (A) IMMEDIATELY AFTER THE HIT. (B) WITHIN
5 DAYS. RIGHT: X-RAY EXAMINATION OF A SLICE OF BREAD. (WITH PERMISSION OF *JOURNAL OF
FOOD SCIENCE*.)

effect on the flesh may not be visible. It can be detected by MRI, however, and the consequences of the fall on the internal tissues (bruise)
become evident after a time (Figure 3.2). The MRI scan is neither inva-
sive nor destructive (it does not alter the state of the tissue), and it does
not generate radioactivity. There are multiple applications for MRI in
food science research such as in the study of fat and ice crystallization (freezing and thawing), moisture migration in products, gelation,
encapsulation, and temperature mapping during processing.

X-ray imaging works by exposing objects to short wavelength radiation that can penetrate an object. The contrast shown in the resulting image reflects the relative densities through which the radiation
traveled. The denser portions of the sample are less "transparent" to
x-rays and appear more prominently in the picture. More dense items
like pieces of bone in packaged meat or metal debris contaminating
jarred or canned food can be easily detected by x-rays, in the same way
that airport scanners find hidden food. For research, the x-ray microscope works just like the hospital x-ray machines, but with a resolution
of about 10 microns. This is sufficient for distinguishing the internal
structure of many foods without having to destroy the food. The fine
protein-starch matrix in bread (Section 2.9) is visibly highlighted by
this analysis (Figure 3.2).

Swiss cheese is an emblematic case for the desire to inspect the inside
of a food without destroying it. A wheel of *Emmental* cheese can measure up to 90 cm in diameter, have a thickness of about 20 cm, and

weigh over 100 kilos. The quality of the cheese depends in great part on the size, distribution, and smoothness of the holes hiding inside.[9] These holes are produced by carbon dioxide (CO_2) that is generated by a special type of bacteria. The CO_2 accumulates in the form of bubbles during the ripening process. Scientists at the University of California–Davis showed that it is possible to use magnetic resonance imaging to sample virtual slices from a wheel of cheese, and use that information to make decisions about value and destination.[10] The maximum resolution of MRI is about 30 microns, which is enough for medical studies but not high enough for certain food applications. Nondestructive food inspection has many promising applications in quality assurance and traceability. It is now possible to image animals that are being fattened for meat production using a portable ultrasound scanner in order to monitor the proportion of meat and fat accumulation. Perhaps some day the inside of all packaged fresh fruits will be rapidly checked using MRI (leaving no visible trace on the fruit), and the hidden spines in salmon fillets will be detected by x-ray imaging and subsequently removed, ensuring a safer product.

As we've seen, thanks to advances in other scientific disciplines, there is now an extensive battery of instruments available for visualizing the microstructures of food, in all the necessary range of scales, by both destructive and nondestructive methods. The nondestructive techniques are the most fascinating because they allow scientists to track changes over time, like what happens to the bruised apple in Figure 3.2 or a french fry as it cooks, without stopping or intervening in the event. This prevents the use of different samples that can introduce variability and hinder the analysis. Although one might think those powerful microscopes and other inspection techniques are enough to learn more about the role of microstructure in food, this is not true. What really matters is to be able to relate the objective characteristics of the microstructure with the desirable properties of the products.

3.5 COOKING UNDER THE MICROSCOPE

Unfortunately many of the significant changes in food structure that occur during preparation and cooking cannot be seen. In our laboratory we have created ovens, dryers, freezers, stoves, and fryers that can be placed under the lens of a microscope and observed in real time (with a digital video camera attached to the microscope—standard equipment nowadays) the changes that occur in a small sample of a food. For this we used miniaturized devices that allowed us to directly heat or cool the small sample, to simulate what happens in a home oven or commercial freezer.

On average, a grain of uncooked rice consists of about 70% starch, but as it cooks the grain absorbs a large amount of water and swells (most cooking instructions call for 2 cups of water per cup of rice), and the starch content in cooked grain falls to about 10% of the total weight. We can simulate what happens inside a grain of rice during cooking by heating a granule of starch in lots of water. Although the gelatinization of starch is described in Section 2.4, "a picture is worth a thousand words," as the saying goes. Figure 3.3 presents a sequence of four photomicrographs that show the starch granule swelling and disintegrating when heated in water at 75°C on a microscopy hot-stage. The gelatinized granule is soft, and its disintegrated structure allows digestive enzymes (amylases) to have access to the amylose and amylopectin molecules and transform them into glucose (Section 7.7). Starch gelatinization occurs during the cooking or baking of any product that contains both starch and water, helping to make the food more palatable and digestible. Simple experiments like this, performed with a basic light microscope equipped with a hot-stage, a video camera, and connected to a monitor, could be very enlightening for school-age students.

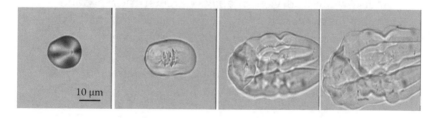

FIGURE 3.3   GALLERY OF IMAGES TAKEN FROM A VIDEO SHOWING THE GELATINIZATION OF A STARCH GRANULE OVER TIME AS IT COOKS IN WATER. THE GRANULE SWELLS BY ABSORBING WATER AND EVENTUALLY RELEASES ITS AMYLOSE AND AMYLOPECTIN MOLECULES INTO THE MEDIUM (RIGHT). NOTICE THE HUGE EXPANSION OF THE GRANULE AS IT IMBIBES WATER.

But this is not the end of the story. Once released from the granule, the amylose and especially the amylopectin molecules tend to crystallize, or arrange themselves orderly into a compact form, a phenomenon known as starch *retrogradation*. This process is responsible for the aging of bread and occurs at a maximum rate at 4°C, which is why bread should not be stored in the refrigerator. Starch retrogradation is partly reversible with heat as you notice when bread is reheated.

3.6 FRYING IN LILLIPUT

Forty percent of the potato production in the United States ends as french fries after a process that even the most recalcitrant critics of "junk food" would admit is nearly flawless. The following is a "collage" of phrases from the book *Fast Food Nation: The Dark Side of the All-American Meal,* by Eric Schlosser (one of those critics). Schlosser is describing his impressions after visiting a U.S. factory that makes frozen french fries:[11]

> The plant is a low building, clean and tidy. Operates 24 hours a day, 310 days a year, making french fries. Inside the building, a maze of conveyor belts crisscross between machines that wash, sort, peel, slice, blanch, dry, fry and rapidly freeze potatoes. Workers in white suits and hardhats keep everything under control, examining the french fries for defects. In the laboratory, white-clad women analyze french fries day and night, as every half hour a sample arrives for analysis. They pass me a plate full of fries, extra-long Premium quality—the kind that go to McDonald's—salt and ketchup. The fries were delicious, crispy and golden. I finish them and ask for more.

Frying causes significant changes in the texture and taste of food, changes that make fried products very appealing (see Section 8.7). The problem is that fried foods absorb some of the hot oil in which they are cooked, becoming quite high in calories (and until recently, unhealthy types of fats). The percentage of oil in some fried foods like potato chips can reach 35%.[12] One in three potato chips is pure oil. During the last 10 years, scientists have intensified their efforts to understand how oil is introduced into fried products and possibly control the amount. A brief inspection of a french fry (and our fingers) reveals that the crisp, dry crust, less than a millimeter thick, contains nearly all of the oil, while the interior of the fry is cooked, moist, and oil free.

In Jonathan Swift's *Gulliver's Travels*, the shipwrecked hero lands on a beach in the kingdom of Lilliput, which is populated by beings less than 15 cm in height. Presumably, the cooking utensils of the Lilliputians were proportional to their size, and their potato chips measured around 5 mm. Our laboratory has designed the world's smallest "micro-skillet" in order to study the process of deep frying, consisting of a micro-pan that fits under the lens of a light microscope. An attached video camera can observe the cell changes in a single potato cell (~100 microns) as it cooks in hot oil at 180°C.[13] Figure 3.4 contains a gallery of selected images from the video showing that the cell surrounded by its cell wall is initially a "bag" of water (say, 85% by weight) holding many starch granules (image A). At less than 7 seconds elapsed, the temperature of "water" reaches about 65°C and the granules begin to gelatinize (see Section 2.4), absorbing water and swelling rapidly until they occupy the entire interior of the cell (image D). When the cell temperature reaches about 100°C, it begins to dehydrate (image F) and then turns golden (images G to I).

This "micro-skillet" has allowed us to confirm that even at the high temperatures of frying, the potato cells are not destroyed and oil does not enter the interior of the cell. Only the external parts of the cell are "wet" with oil. Consequently, if slicing the potatoes caused only minimal damage to the cells below the cut surface, it would be possible to reduce the oil that accumulates in the pores of the crust after frying. If you could remove the oil from the surface by some means, it would lower the oil content even further. This is what happens when pan fried potatoes are quickly transferred to a piece of absorbent paper, but unfortunately we remove only about one tenth of the oil that way (though that's better than nothing).

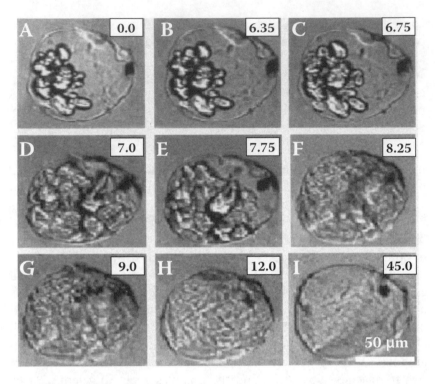

FIGURE 3.4 GALLERY OF IMAGES OBTAINED WITH A LIGHT MICROSCOPE OF A POTATO CELL IN THE "MICRO-SKILLET" FRYING IN HOT OIL AT 180°C. THE BRIGHT OVAL BODIES IN IMAGES (A) THROUGH (C) ARE STARCH GRANULES. THE FRYING TIME IN SECONDS IS SHOWN IN THE UPPER-RIGHT CORNER OF EACH IMAGE.

It's said that for every $100 of french fries sold, fast food chains earn $80, making fries the most lucrative food in the world. North Americans eat about 12 kg annually of fries *per capita*, 90% of which are purchased in restaurants and fast food outlets. This is a great incentive for companies to improve and to sell more. There are many recent innovations for making crisper fries with less oil (*light* fries), such as cutting the potatoes with precise "water knives" that cause less damage to the cells, superficial heat treatment of the cut potatoes before frying, coating potatoes with starch and other hydrocolloids so that they absorb less oil, to name a few. However, consumers still prefer conventional french fries, as *Burger King* well knows, after their experiment 10 years ago with coated french fries was a complete failure.[14] In spite of the adverse nutritional evidence, the fried food business is still going strong. There is more about fried foods in Section 8.7.

3.7 COOKING PASTA

Pasta has a widely disputed origin, which has even been reached by the field of archeology. A group of scientists recently discovered long thin strips made of a grain (not wheat) in a 4000-year-old settlement in northwestern China, which could be the ancestors of modern *spaghetti*.[15]

Commercial noodles are produced by forcing dough of semolina (durum wheat flour with larger particles than normal wheat) and water through a perforated plate. Dozens of dough strips emerge from each press cycle, which then undergo a long 8-hour drying process of hanging on a rack like neckties in a closet. Traditionally the holes in the plate are drilled with a bronze bit, so that the surface of the holes has ridges that give the pasta a rough surface. This helps the sauce adhere to the pasta as it's lifted with a fork, so that we taste the right sauce-to-pasta ratio in our mouths. Production engineers discovered that if holes in the plates were covered with a smooth surface like Teflon® (see Section 8.3), the pasta dough slid through much faster, increasing the productivity of the machinery significantly. Scientists from the University of Milan used a scanning electron microscope to study the effect of the new material on the surface of spaghetti.[16] Unfortunately, the pasta pushed through the Teflon holes had such a smooth surface that the sauces slipped right off of the fork before reaching the mouth. What a task for the chefs, who had to increase the viscosity of their sauces so they would adhere to the new pasta.

Dry pasta has a structure that is a compact matrix in which starch granules (~70% of total) are trapped in a network of protein (12% to 15%). During cooking, water should gelatinize the starch (Section 3.5) and the protein should coagulate, which means that water must migrate to the interior and the temperature must exceed 70°C. The cooking progress can be observed with the naked eye (but even better with a magnifying glass). The hard white center gradually disappears

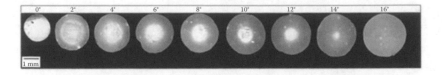

FIGURE 3.5   CHANGES IN A CROSS SECTION OF SPAGHETTI WHILE IN BOILING WATER (99°C)
FOR 16 MINUTES. THE WHITE CENTER IS THE UNCOOKED PORTION, WHILE THE DARK OUTER
RING SHOWS THE COOKED PORTION. IT TAKES AROUND 15 MINUTES TO COOK A NOODLE "AL
DENTE." NOTICE HOW THE SPAGHETTI SWELLS AS IT IMBIBES WATER AND HOW STARCHES IN THE
OUTER PORTIONS GET PROGRESSIVELY GELATINIZED.

as the outside cooks. When the noodle is cooked to *al dente*, the white center is just about to disappear (Figure 3.5). For many people pasta in this state still seems somewhat raw and hard.

Interestingly, the degree to which starch is cooked has a significant effect on its degradation in the digestive tract (Section 7.7). Some studies suggest that when pasta is cooked to the *al dente* state, a portion of the starch does not convert to sugar (and provides no calories). Urgent studies are being conducted to verify this hypothesis, which would allow us to eat pasta *al dente* with less guilt.

3.8 MICROSCOPY IN FOOD GERONTOLOGY AND ARCHEOLOGY

Gerontologists study the aging process in humans, which in its external form is expressed through various physical and structural changes. Senescence in plants covers the processes that occur once they have been harvested and are past their optimum maturity. These physical losses that occur postharvest are substantial worldwide. It's estimated that between 10% and 40% of certain raw materials from agriculture and fishing never reach direct human consumption. There are multiple causes for this, which depend on the type of food. Fruits, vegetables, and seafood undergo rapid biochemical and microbiological deterioration, while cereals and legumes are very susceptible to insects and rodents.

Dry legumes such as beans, chickpeas, and lentils (and other legumes from Africa) will suffer a loss of quality if stored in hot and humid conditions. This damage is not apparent physically and is only noticed when the beans do not soften during the normal cooking time and remain tough and unappetizing. These beans will sometimes become tender with prolonged cooking times, but at higher energy costs. Some very "old" legumes will not soften no matter how long they are cooked. This phenomenon has to do with microstructure and has been called the "hard-to-cook" condition. For the beans to soften, the cement between the cell walls must dissolve (Figure 3.6). There are two important mechanisms that hold neighboring plant cells together at their cell walls. The first involves the bonding of pectin molecules in both cell walls by Ca^{+2} ions, which act like bridges between the

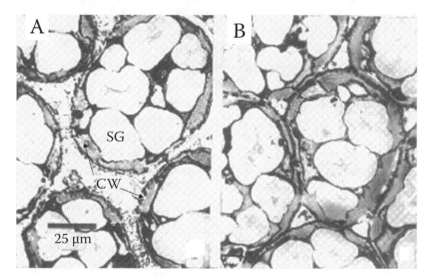

FIGURE 3.6   PHOTOMICROGRAPHS SHOWING THE INSIDE OF A COOKED BEAN, STAINED WITH TOLUIDINE BLUE. (A) SOFT BEAN. NOTE THAT THE CELL WALLS (CW) ARE NOT UNITED AS THE MIDDLE LAMELLA HAS DISSOLVED DURING COOKING AND THE CELLS ARE SEPARATED. SG IS A GELATINIZED STARCH GRANULE. (B, RIGHT) THE MICROSTRUCTURE OF A BEAN THAT WAS COOKED FOR THE SAME AMOUNT OF TIME BUT REMAINED TOUGH. THE CELL WALLS DID NOT SEPARATE. (FROM STANLEY, D.W., AND AGUILERA, J.M. 1985. A REVIEW OF TEXTURAL DEFECTS IN COOKED RECONSTITUTED LEGUMES. THE INFLUENCE OF STRUCTURE AND COMPOSITION. *JOURNAL OF FOOD BIOCHEMISTRY* 9, 277–323. WITH PERMISSION.)

negatively charged groups in the polymer. In grains that have not been damaged during storage, these bonds can be reversed during cooking. The second mechanism is simply a false senescence that occurs in grains that are exposed to high temperature and high relative humidity during storage, which results in lignification (lignin accumulation) of the middle lamella that separates the cells. This process is irreversible because lignin forms a three-dimensional, insoluble network infiltrating the outer walls of the adjacent cells. The structure of plant cells is discussed in Section 2.1.

The relationship between the microstructure of a bean and its texture can be explained by an analogy with the structure of a wall. If the bricks are stacked on top of one another without anything holding them together, the wall would come down with only a push. If the bricks are set in mortar, however, the wall is strong and may even withstand an earthquake. During mastication, the cells of a tender cooked bean will slide relative to one other, because the cement holding them together has been dissolved (Figure 3.6A). An older, tougher bean is harder to chew because the cell walls must be broken apart with our teeth. Adding baking soda (sodium bicarbonate) to the cooking water makes the pH more alkaline, which improves softening by replacing the divalent Ca^{+2} ions (that bind the negatively charged groups of pectin molecules together in cell walls) with Na^+ ions. The Na^+ ions are unable to bind to two negative charges at the same time, so they disrupt the bonds between the cell walls.[17] But although this method is often used in home cooking to soften beans, their taste and texture are different from soft beans that are cooked in water.

Some foods "die" structurally, in the sense that they become unattractive or inedible: stale bread, melted ice cream, limp french fries, collapsed soufflés, and so on. The death of a powder by caking, for example, occurs after the originally dry particles are exposed to high humidity and absorb water. Their surfaces become rubbery (soft and wet) so the particles stick together forming compact clumps. The air in a half-empty jar of instant coffee powder that is opened and closed many times in a humid environment (near the ocean, for example), renews and brings more water vapor into the head-space inside of the jar. This humidification "glues" the particles together and causes later a solidification of the material as water gets redistributed in the whole mass. This is not necessarily a problem, unless it forms such a compact solid that the powder cannot be removed with a spoon (more on this in Section 8.1). Anticaking substances that can trap the excess moisture are dispersed between the particles to prevent them from sticking together. Silicon dioxide and various silicates are among the anticaking agents approved for use in foods.

Interestingly, food microscopy has been used not only as a forensic technique but also in archaeological applications. Food archeologists face the disadvantage that organic matter decomposes rapidly and generally leaves no traces. Archaeological food remains are preserved only if they survive insect attack and microorganisms by being somehow frozen or dehydrated in their environment. Seeds, grains, and pollen are particularly resistant to the passage of time and are favorite materials for the archaeologists who study diet during human evolution. Electron and light microscopy have directly shown (not through pictorial traces) that the ancient Egyptians sprouted grain to make bread and beer.[18]

Indirect evidence about ancient foods can be obtained from plant remains through phytoliths, or mineralized copies of plants that have developed when silica dissolved in water was deposited on the specimen. Later the silicate dried and formed a sort of replica. The use of microscopy by archaeologists has been an important source of information about what our ancestors ate. One approach has been the microscopic study of the teeth found with fossil remains. The wear of the teeth is associated with the hardness of food. Other anthropologists have used light microscopy to study the effect of different cooking methods on the starch structure of various botanical sources, and thus document the diets of prehistoric human groups by examining meal leftovers.[19]

3.9 CHOCOLATE "BLOOM"

Xocoatl is a special spiced cocoa beverage used by the Maya in religious ceremonies. The cocoa produced by the tree *Theobroma cacao*, which means "food of the gods" (from the Greek theos = god and broma =

food) was brought from Mexico to Spain around 1520 by a Cistercian monk who accompanied Hernán Cortés. The monks of the Monasterio de Piedra, south of Zaragoza, were the first to prepare the chocolate in Europe, although milk chocolate has been consumed on a regular basis only since the nineteenth century.[20] Cocoa is rich in polyphenols, especially catechins and procyanidins, that act as antioxidants and may even help brain function. We cannot see the microstructure of chocolate, but our palate can certainly detect it. Milk chocolate contains cocoa, sugar, and milk powder in the form of minute particles ground to less than 40 microns in size (so that they feel smooth to our tongue and palate), drenched in cocoa butter, a quasi-solid fat whose last solid fraction melts at 36.2°C, just below body temperature (Figure 2.9C).[21]

Unfortunately it is not uncommon to encounter chocolates and sweets whose surfaces have lost their luster and appear whitish and opaque. There is nothing really wrong with chocolate in this state—it has been wounded but is not dead. There aren't any microorganisms or toxic substances involved, but all the effort on the part of the chocolatier to produce glossy, shiny chocolates is for naught. Part of the cocoa butter migrated to the surface and recrystallized or solidified into a different crystal structure, forming needles that look like a lacy white covering (Figure 3.7). This phenomenon is called *chocolate bloom*.

It is not easy to create shiny chocolates that have a nice snap as you bite into them. Extensive research conducted since 1930 had given chocolatiers the scientific know-how to build an industry with annual sales of about $70 billion. When the triglycerides in liquid cocoa butter are cooled, they crystallize into various forms, a phenomenon known as polymorphism. Cocoa butter can derive different molecular arrangements and structures from the same chemical composition. One of the six possible crystal forms, called form V, produces the best shine and snap in a bar of chocolate. Tempering chocolate is an important part of the manufacturing process and consists of subjecting the hot chocolate solids and liquids (above 50°C) to a controlled cooling process in order to form tiny particles or "nuclei" of type V crystals. Any subsequent crystallization grows from these good nuclei and not others (see Section 2.3). Subjecting chocolate to uncontrolled temperature changes, like temperatures greater than 33.8°C, for example, increases the proportion of liquid fat that can migrate to the surface and produces

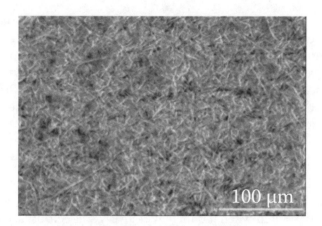

FIGURE 3.7 PHOTOMICROGRAPH OF THE SURFACE OF A CHOCOLATE WITH "BLOOM." THE NEEDLES THAT PROTRUDE FROM THE SURFACE ARE COCOA BUTTER CRYSTALS THAT MIGRATED FROM THE INSIDE AND RECRYSTALLIZED. THE MARKER IS EQUAL TO 100 MICRONS. (COURTESY OF D. ROUSSEAU, RYERSON UNIVERSITY, CANADA.)

bloom, while favoring the formation of the undesirable crystals, which are curiously more stable (melt at a higher temperature).

The bloom that occurs in chocolates that are filled with almond cream has another origin. In this case it is the oils in the nuts or creamy centers that migrate to the surface and crystallize.

Chocolate bloom has been a complicated problem for scientists. The rigorous standards that govern what can be labeled as "chocolate" limit the use of additives that might ameliorate the problem. A good way to avoid bloom is to store chocolate in a cool place (about 10°C), or even better, eat it quickly after purchase.

3.10 REINFORCED TEXTURES

Often a valuable material is suitable in many ways but lacks a key desirable property. Think of natural rubber, a superb elastic material but so soft that it is used as an eraser to remove the marks left by lead pencils. That is why automobile tires are not made of rubber only. There are also small particles made from a special carbon (which is why they are black) dispersed uniformly throughout the rubber to give tires more tensile strength and better wear resistance. Moreover, the sidewalls are reinforced with steel cords that provide extra strength. Reinforced concrete contains iron mesh or bars for greater strength, similar to the function of the cellulose fibers in plant cell walls (Section 2.1). Reinforced materials exist in nature (e.g., wood) and engineers also use them when a certain mechanical property needs to be accompanied by other characteristics like weight reduction, abrasion resistance, or lower cost.

In Japan there is a gel called surimi (Section 4.8), which is made by heating a fish paste called *kamaboko* in the presence of small amounts of raw starch (potato or cornstarch)—just a little bit of starch, not much. Why add the starch when it only makes a very soft gel? In fact, the goal is to have a firm texture similar to that of shrimp. The principal reason is cost. Fish protein starts to gel at 70 to 75°C and starch gelatinizes or swells with water starting at 65 to 70°C (Section 2.4). If about 5% by weight of potato starch is added to the kamaboko, and the mixture is heated, the first thing that happens is that the starch begins to swell at 65°C, and acts as a sponge, absorbing water. When the protein begins to gel at 70°C, it is therefore more concentrated (water was removed as the starch hydrated) so the gel that forms around the swollen starch granules is stronger. In fact, the strength of a gel varies approximately with the square of the concentration of the gelling agent (fish protein in this case). The gelled protein network becomes the beams and pillars of the reinforced masonry and the starch becomes the weaker internal walls. If you add too much starch, the swollen granules completely surround the small hard particles of gelled protein, weakening the structural support of the gel and making it soft.[22] The texture depends on the continuous phase: high if the continuous phase is protein, low if it's starch. This is another example of foods with similar chemical composition having very different properties, thanks to their underlying structure.

Meringues can also be reinforced with a little bit of starch. The albumen in the egg whites coagulates at 80°C, a higher temperature than the gelatinization of starch. Some commercial preparations of egg for meringues and icings already have some incorporated starch.[23] The surimi technique has been used to develop meringues with less egg white and some potato starch, with good results at lower cost. The key is to add native starch to the beaten egg whites, because in this state it will swell with water to gelatinize. Oat and rye starches have the lowest temperature for onset of gelatinization (about 50°C), but are not widely used in pure form. Potato starch begins to swell at around 56°C, six degrees before cornstarch.[24] Armed with this information you may try adding a little starch to avoid the leakage of liquid (weeping) from the bottom of soft meringues, as well as heating them to around 65 to 70°C so that the starch granules get soaked with the extra water.

3.11 ALL IN DUE TIME

Don't leave this chapter with the idea that given certain ingredients the formation of food microstructures or key elements (e.g., droplets, crystals, bubbles, etc.) will occur regardless of how you proceed. In addition to size, timing is an important factor. The molecules need time for the different components to settle into their proper and most convenient places, and to react with other molecules (the kinetics of chemical changes, Section 5.4). Both the sequence in which you add or mix ingredients in a recipe, and the rate at which energy is applied to mixing them, play a role in the outcome. You have to wait for leaf (or sheet) gelatin to fully hydrate. Hot sugar syrup must be added slowly to the egg whites when making an Italian meringue.

Building engineers know how to coordinate the many tasks that must be completed in a certain order when building a home. The tasks are described through diagrams filled with rectangles and arrows that indicate the sequence of events (the Gantt chart). This tangible graph shows the critical path, or the steps that must be completed before progress can continue. Doors and windows can't go in without walls. Foods are not necessarily constructed this way. Many foods assemble more like a tent. First a few of the parts are set up, and then the rest self-assembles with the "pull of a cord" during cooking.

A time-length diagram showing some of the important events that occur during food processing can be useful for understanding what happens inside food structures on both the micro and macro levels. Figure 3.8 shows the diagram for the production of edible foams (see Section 2.7). To make a foam, the surfactant molecules must rapidly

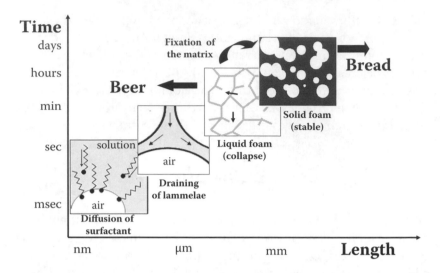

FIGURE 3.8   TIME-DISTANCE DIAGRAM FOR THE FORMATION OF A FOAM SHOWING THE
SEQUENCE OF EVENTS THAT HAVE TO DO WITH THE BIRTH AND DEATH OF THE BUBBLES. THE
PERSISTENCE OF THE FOAM OVER TIME (VERTICAL AXIS IN LOGARITHMIC SCALE) DEPENDS ON
HOW STABLE THE WALLS ARE, WHICH IS WHY THE BEER FOAM IS MUCH MORE PERISHABLE THAN
THAT IN BREAD (SECTION 2.9).

reach the interface of the bubble and stay there as air is introduced.
These molecules are many times smaller (measuring a few nanometers)
than a bubble and migrate to the liquid-gas interface relatively quickly
(on the order of seconds or less), because the distances involved are
also small. If this does not occur and the molecules prefer to associate with each other or the medium is so viscous that they cannot rush
to interface, there won't be any foam. Once the foam is stabilized, the
liquid between the bubbles (distributed in thin films called lamellae)
tends to drain under the effects of gravity and differences in pressure,
which also cannot be seen (see Section 2.7). The consequences can
be observed after a few minutes, however: the lamellae break and the
bubbles begin to join together and collapse, just like what happens to
beer foam after 10 minutes or so. To stabilize a foam for longer periods
of time the walls must be stiffened in order to obtain a thick matrix like
in milkshakes, a semisolid like marshmallows, or a true porous solid
like meringues or bread.

The practical methods of making foams and emulsions (that is, dispersing one phase into another) have been around for centuries (Sections 2.2 and 2.7). These methods have little control over the scarce and usually expensive molecules that need to be located at the interfaces. A "normal" mayonnaise has one yolk emulsified into about 180 cc of oil. Given the amount of phospholipid molecules (surfactants) that are in one yolk, careful kitchen experimentation reveals that it is possible to transform more than 20 gallons of oil into mayonnaise using a single egg. This assumes that all of the surfactant molecules manage to reach their place in the oil-water interface at the appropriate time and the fat globules do not "crowd," for which you must continually add water.[25]

3.12 FOOD STRUCTURE DESIGN

To design something is to create, fashion, execute, or construct it according to a plan. Most products in our daily life have been designed to fulfill specific needs: houses, cars, computers, cell phones, and our clothes. Even the cover and the interior pages of the book containing this manuscript will have to be designed. But processed foods are unique among the products we consume in that their structures have never been designed. Although the origin of sweetened whipped cream can be traced back to the inspiration of a French cook named Francoise Vatel in the mid 1600s, it was not "designed," and it is still prepared in the kitchen much in the same way as it was in the time of Louis XIV.[26]

The obesity problem (largely a result of eating too much and not having enough physical activity) is an opportunity for restructuring foods. One potential solution is to introduce imperceptible air bubbles, microgels or microdroplets of water, and tasteless tiny particles of fiber to reduce the caloric density, while keeping portion sizes the same. A sophisticated approach to redesigning some troublesome products or designing new ones must take into account the limitations of food products compared to other industrial products (Table 3.1).

Several things are needed in order to design and construct processed foods from the bottom up like a building, so that they will be able to

TABLE 3.1

Comparison between Products "Designed" for Daily Life and Foods "Processed" to Be Eaten

Designed Products	Processed Foods
Based on exact blueprints	Based on vague recipes
Use almost unlimited types of materials	Use only food-grade ingredients
Structural elements mounted sequentially	Structure develops during processing
Equipment is of the size of the elements created	Equipment is much larger than elements formed
Events occur at macroscale	Changes take place at microscale
Structures designed not to fail	Food structures must disintegrate
Properties are well determined (e.g., measured with instruments)	Properties are elusive (e.g., measured sensorially)
Good body of science	Science is emerging

meet the needs of the future. First, the science of soft materials and the formation of food structures need to be better understood. We need more information about how given structures relate to specific food properties, particularly those related to our senses. We need new building blocks, for which some ingredients will have to be modified or analogs created, and these new molecules must also be safe. Food processing equipment must be able to manipulate smaller amounts of key components and locate them sparingly and precisely (i.e., at the microscale), as the cow does in making milk (Section 2.11).

Let's engage in some "food science fiction" based on what is currently done in laboratories. For example, we could shape droplets of oil of almost any size in a microchannel (smaller than a needle of a syringe) and cover them with the exact amount of surfactant using a "molecular dispenser." These identical droplets could then be dispersed individually into the continuous phase of a product adding to stability and reducing the amount of surfactant used. Similarly, gel particles of different sizes and shapes may be produced by deforming the droplets of polymer solutions by shear and elongational stresses prior to gelation. It may soon be possible to locate salt microcrystals only in the parts of a food that come in contact with taste receptors for salt during the mastication time, therefore avoiding superfluous salt content. Bleached microparticles of fiber could imperceptibly replace "white" flour particles in wheat flour by increasing proportions, in much the same way that milk has different fat content (Section 4.13). Precise amounts of fat-soluble vitamins could be dispersed into microscopic oil droplets and then covered with a hydrophilic surfactant so they could be introduced almost unnoticeably in aqueous foods. It would even be possible to make very small ice crystals and of different shapes, which could be added to ice cream mixtures, rather than producing them in an uncontrolled fashion as the whole mass freezes in a large heat exchanger. Several nutrients and beneficial molecules could be microencapsulated and protected inside food matrices, so they reach target zones in our digestive system almost unaffected.

To do all of this and more we need the ability to manipulate components on a microscopic level and control the sequence of the different stages of structure formation. The food industry still hasn't scaled up to production level the techniques available in the world of microtechnology and microprocessing. When these capacities become available to the industry (cost being one limiting factor), technologists will imitate the way in which the cell from the udder of a cow makes milk, the most ideal food (Section 2.11).

Those who are apprehensive about too much intervention and "processing" of some of our foods—the ones that need redesigning—should know that industry has already been doing some of this in an uncontrolled way (sounds like the case of accidental gene exchange in nature and controlled manipulation through biotechnology). Homogenization

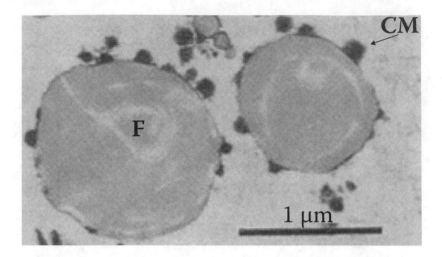

FIGURE 3.9 A HOMOGENIZED DAIRY EMULSION OBSERVED BY TRANSMISSION ELECTRON MICROSCOPY (**F** = FAT GLOBULE; **CM** = CASEIN MICELLE). NOTE THAT CASEIN MICELLES BECAME ADSORBED ON THE SURFACE OF FAT GLOBULES AS A CONSEQUENCE OF HOMOGENIZATION. SOME REMNANTS OF THE ORIGINAL FAT GLOBULE MEMBRANE PROBABLY STILL COVER THE INTERFACE OF THE HOMOGENIZED FAT GLOBULES BUT CANNOT BE SEEN AT THIS RESOLUTION.

of milk fat is the rupture of the original fat globules in milk to produce smaller ones, so that creaming can be delayed. As a consequence there is an increase in the total surface area of the population of fat droplets, so that portions of their surfaces can no longer be covered by the original fat globule membrane (i.e., there is not enough). Immediately after breakage, milk proteins like caseins and whey proteins adsorb randomly onto the nude interfaces and give new (and different) functional and nutritional properties to the homogenized fat globules (Figure 3.9).[27] Breakage of fat droplets occurs in the channels of a homogenizer that are 100 times larger than the size of the fat globules. (It's like crushing a grape with a bulldozer.)

NOTES

1. The most loyal and dedicated readers are encouraged to review the book by Aguilera, J.M., and Stanley, D.W. 1999. *Microstructural Principles of Food Processing and Engineering*, 2nd ed. Aspen, Gaithersburg, MD.

2. In the article by Aguilera, J.M. 2005. Why food microstructure? *Journal of Food Engineering* 67, 3–11, several examples of how microstructure affects different properties of food are presented in more detail.
3. Foods under the microscope (www.magma.ca/~scimat/) is a Web site with many images of the microstructures of various foods and associated information and is well worth review.
4. The previously mentioned term *hydrocolloid* is derived from this phenomenon. It refers to systems in which the aqueous suspension has particles that are larger than the solvent molecules but less than 1 micron in size. These colloidal suspensions have unique properties. Understanding the chemistry of colloids is fundamental to comprehend the formation and behavior of emulsions, foams, and gels.
5. *Spectroscopy* is the analytical technique used to identify and quantify molecules based on the vibration of certain chemical groups within the molecules which occurs when they are excited by electromagnetic waves (energy). For more information visit Helmenstine, A.M. About. com. Spectroscopy Introduction. http://chemistry.about.com/od/analyticalchemistry/a/spectroscopy.htm.
6. Kalab, M., Allan-Wotjas, P., and Shea Miller, S. 1995. Microscopy and other imaging techniques in food structure analysis. *Trends in Food Science and Technology* 6, 177–185. This article remains an excellent presentation on microscopic imaging techniques applied to the analysis of food structures.
7. I have always counted microscopists as some of my best friends. Any technician can produce an image under a microscope, but getting an accurate picture of a product is a work of art that only experienced microscopists can produce. All the bottles of wine that I have given as presents to microscopists over the years have been amply repaid by the work they have done helping me to see the microworld of food.
8. Currently there are "environmental" SEMs that operate under low vacuum (almost atmospheric pressure) and do not require sample dehydration. However, operating these microscopes requires great expertise.
9. According to U.S. Department of Agriculture (USDA) regulations, the quality standards for Grade A Swiss cheese state that "the cheese shall be properly set and shall possess well-developed round or slightly oval-shaped eyes which are relatively uniform in size and distribution. The majority of the eyes shall be 3/8 to 3/16 inch in diameter."
10. Rosenberg, M., McCarthy, M.J., and Kauten, R. 1991. Magnetic resonance imaging of cheese structure. *Food Structure* 10, 185–192.
11. Schlosser, E. 2005. *Fast Food Nation: The Dark Side of the All-American Meal*. Harper Perennial, New York.

12. The approximate oil content (in percentage) of some other foods is as follows: french fries (8 to 16), fried chicken (28), fish croquettes (22 to 34), fried fish (7 to 18), donuts (9 to 31), and corn tortillas (23 to 34).

13. Aguilera, J.M., Cadoche, L., and López, C. 2001. A microscopy study of potato cells and starch granules heated in oil. *Food Research International* 34, 939–947.

14. In 1997 Burger King introduced fries coated with a crunchy layer of starch that absorbed less oil and remained rigid for longer periods. In 2001 the company recognized that the fries had been a failure because they tasted terrible and were not appetizing. To learn more see: How Burger King got burned in quest to make the perfect fry. *Wall Street Journal*, January 16, 2001.

15. Lu, H., Yang, X., Ye, K.B., Liu, Z., Xia, X., Ren, L., Cai, N., Wu, N.Y., and Liu, T.S. 2005. Culinary archeology: millet noodles in late Neolithic China. *Nature* 437, 967–968.

16. Lucisano, M., Pagani, M.A, Mariotti, M., and Locatelli, D.P. 2008. Influence of die material on pasta characteristics. *Food Research International* 41, 646–652.

17. This phenomenon is similar to the ion exchange process that is used to soften water. When water contains a significant amount of calcium and magnesium, it's known as "hard" water. Hard water clogs piping and prevents detergents from dissolving. Ion exchangers replace calcium and magnesium ions with other ions like sodium and potassium.

18. Samuel, D. 1996. Investigation of ancient Egyptian baking and brewing methods by correlative microscopy. *Science* 273, 488–490.

19. See Henry, A.G., Hudson, H.F., and Piperno, D.R. 2009. Changes in starch grain morphologies from cooking. *Journal of Archaeological Science* 36, 915–922, for a gallery of light microscopy images of different starches obtained from 10 domesticated plant species and subjected to various types of cooking and fermentation.

20. Castells, P. 2009. The chocolate. *Investigación y Ciencia* 390, 45.

21. The classic book on the science and technology of chocolate is Beckett, S.T. 2008. *The Science of Chocolate*, 2nd edition. Royal Society of Chemistry, London.

22. The experimental proof that heat-induced food protein gels (see Section 2.7) can be reinforced with the addition of small amounts of native starch is in the article (written with an undergraduate student) Aguilera, J.M., and Baffico, P. 1997. Structure-mechanical property relationships in thermally induced whey protein/cassava starch gels. *Journal of Food Science* 62, 1048–1053.

23. Buckman, J., and Viney, C. 2002. The effect of a commercial extended egg albumin on the microstructure of icing. *Food Science and Technology International* 8, 109–115.

24. The gelatinization temperatures of pure starches from different origins depend on how the temperatures of starches are determined, the size of the granules, moisture content, and so forth. Therefore these temperatures differ greatly from one source to another. Keep in mind that the onset and the end of gelatinization spans a temperature range of approximately 10°C (e.g., between 60–70°C).

25. This mayonnaise experiment and the calculations behind it are described in McGee, H. 1999. *The Curious Cook*. McMillan, New York, pp. 116–133.

26. In fact, this may not be true but a legend around Vatel has been based on his suicide after the fish failed to arrive in time for a banquet at a Chateau de Chantilly honoring Louis the XIV (an event which may also be false). Vatel was immortalized in a film starring Gérard Depardieu and Uma Thurman.

27. Aiqian Ye, A., Cui, J., and Singh, H. 2010. Effect of the fat globule membrane on in vitro digestion of milk fat globules with pancreatic lipase. *International Dairy Journal* 20, 822–829. Michalski, M.-C., and Januel, C. 2006. Does homogenization affect the human health properties of cow's milk? *Trends in Food Science and Technology* 17, 423–437.

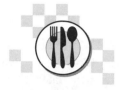

CHAPTER 4

From Farm to Cells and Back

It is time to enter the real world and see from where and how we get our food. The long journey through the food chain that starts at the farm and ends in our mouth requires a lot of science and technology nowadays, including some surprises. In the future, this ancestral axis will intersect with a new axis connecting our brain, gut, and cells. The journey from the farm to our cells will become more complex as it will have to respond to various stringent and proactive consumer demands. The cells in our bodies (particularly those in our brains) will send signals to the farm and the whole food chain about what is desirable.

4.1 FROM FARM TO FORK

Once upon a time human beings stopped "eating to survive," and began to have some control over the availability of food. The beginnings of agriculture started around 10,000 to 12,000 years ago. The first cities appeared in Mesopotamia between 4000 BC and 3000 BC, and settlements like Ur of the Chaldeans soon grew to about 20,000 inhabitants crowded into an area less than 100 hectares. Cities in Egypt, India, and China and what is now Europe were built around irrigated and highly productive places where fishing and agriculture developed quickly. It is estimated that at least half a million people lived in Rome by mid-second century BC, and the food supply was already a problem, one that may have played a part in the later fall of the Empire. By the early nineteenth century millions of people were living in cities. Nine cities already had more than one million inhabitants in 1900. It is estimated that by 2020 about half of the world's population will live in urban centers, and in places like Latin America the estimate approaches 80%. This phenomenon of urbanization and the recent emergence of megacities are possible largely because of technological improvements in conservation and transformation of food, as well as advances in transport logistics, warehousing, distribution, and sales.

This is the origin of the food chain, or the sequence of events that move foods from agricultural and aquaculture production, passing through the process of transforming of raw materials into products, and then the packaging and distribution of the products to consumers (Figure 4.1). The flow of food and nutrients from their source to our plates is euphemistically called "from farm to fork," reflecting their ancestral path from land and sea to the table.

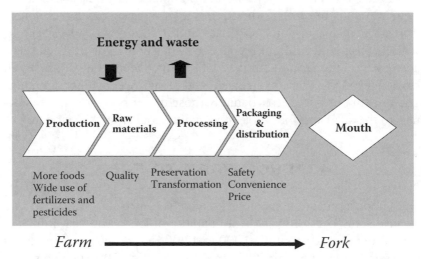

FIGURE 4.1   THE CONCEPT OF THE "FARM TO FORK" FOOD CHAIN AT THE END OF THE TWENTIETH CENTURY. NOTE THAT THE BOTTOM ARROW POINTS FROM LEFT TO RIGHT, INDICATING THAT THE CONSUMER HAS LITTLE INPUT IN WHAT KIND OF FOOD IS PRODUCED OR HOW IT OCCURS.

Presently there are various food chains that move products from their origins, through processing, conversion into packaged foods, marketing, and distribution. First, there is an industry that handles large volumes of a few raw materials and produces ingredient commodities such as flour, starch, fats and oils in bulk, and refined sugar. This industry extracts and purifies the proteins, carbohydrates, and lipids that are dispersed in natural matrices and transforms them into stable, nearly pure ingredients. Other important food chains, such as the postharvest management of fruits and vegetables and the handling of meat and fish, make every effort to preserve natural structures for as long as possible (Section 2.16).

The main supply chains are associated with the processed food industry, where raw materials undergo major changes that result in more appetizing and varied foods that are easy to eat and preserve. One method is to mix ingredients (flour, oil, refined sugar) and transform them into breads, cakes, candies, sauces, and dairy products of various kinds, using energy-consuming equipment. Another branch of the processing industry turns the same raw materials into more convenient forms, such as powdered milk and instant coffee, canned foods, frozen prepared foods, and so on. There are also food chains for using surplus or lower quality ingredients (which are inevitable in crop and livestock production) to produce dried fruits, juices and fruit concentrates, jams, sausages, frankfurters, deli meats, and so forth. The last part of the food chain (also requiring energy) is the packaging, storage, distribution, and wholesale or retail sale. Some of the processed food chains make extensive use of water resources and generate waste that ends up in the environment. For these reasons, food chains will be under fierce scrutiny in years to come.

4.2 WHY MALTHUS WAS WRONG

The unfulfilled prophecy of the English economist Thomas Robert Malthus (1766–1834) established that the natural tendency of a population was to grow faster than its resources could sustain. In mathematical terms, the Malthus theory stated that populations tend to grow geometrically (i.e.,

2, 4, 8, 16), but that food resources only grow at linear rates. He believed this would lead to terrible famines and increasingly poor quality of life.[1] In fact, the world's population grew exponentially during the twentieth century, without producing worldwide hunger, though isolated episodes of famine did occur that had nothing to do with Malthus' theory (but with civil wars, droughts, etc.). Malthus was mistaken because he underestimated the human capacity to mobilize knowledge through technological advances, innovation, and entrepreneurship.[2]

In 1968 the biologist Paul Ehrlich took a turn, predicting in his book *The Population Bomb* that within a few years hundreds of millions of people would be starving because of the inexorable growth of the population. This neo-Malthusian prophecy failed to come true because in the 1960s scientists created new high-yield cereal varieties using traditional plant breeding. During the 40 years of the Green Revolution (see Section 1.9) the grain production of farmers in India increased 2.4 times. There is so much food around today that Americans have the luxury of feeding enough grains to their livestock (for meat production) to satisfy the nutritional needs of 850 million people.

In 2000, less than 1% of Americans were directly engaged in agriculture production, yet they produced almost one and a half times the daily requirement of nutrients for the entire U.S. population (although subsidies discouraged the production of certain crops) and exported nearly 15% of production. Today 40% of our food grows on irrigated land and almost 50% of our fish is produced through aquaculture. Don't be too hard on Malthus and Ehrlich, however, because it is difficult to predict what the impact of new technologies on productivity will be. They could not have foreseen the conditions that encouraged entrepreneurship either. Global population growth is expected to stabilize at around 9 billion people by 2050 (the population was estimated at 7 billion in 2011).[3] Modern efficient irrigation systems, hydroponics (less land use), agricultural biotechnology, and industrial-scale cell culture have done their part, and the scientific discoveries of today will be in their production stage tomorrow. The big question now is what effect climate change will have on food production.

Malthus could have proposed that the only way to feed an exponentially growing population was to have a parallel increase in energy consumption, which has been proven to be true since the 1950s. Even though agricultural technology has allowed farmers to achieve high yields, it now takes almost twice as much energy to produce one unit of food than it did 50 years ago. The manufacture of fertilizers and pesticides and consumption of fossil fuels are responsible for approximately 60% of the energy input into intensive agriculture.[4] The nearly 3,800 kcal per capita of food available to Americans require about seven times that amount of energy to be produced. We need to ask ourselves if this scenario is compatible with feeding over 9 billion people in the future.

Advances in agricultural and aquaculture production are supplemented by technological advances in the development of more convenient and secure products. If you drive for 15 minutes on the windy road from the Lausanne train station to the hills overlooking Lake Leman, you arrive at the Nestlé Research Center, the research laboratory of the largest multinational food company in the world. Over 120 scientists with doctoral degrees in disciplines as diverse as engineering, physics, chemistry, microbiology, medicine, nutrition, and psychology together with a technical and support staff form a team of approximately 600 people. This group is the apex of a research and development pyramid that transfers knowledge to the company's various businesses in 160 countries by way of 17 product development centers spread all over the world. Founded by Henri Nestlé in 1857, *Nestlé* has annual sales of $85 billion and each year invests about $1.2 billion in research, development, and innovation (R&D+i), which far exceeds the GDP of many countries. Other major food companies such as Unilever, Kraft-General Foods, and Danone spend a similar proportion of their sales on R&D+i.[5] In this era of abundance, these companies want to be regarded as more than giant food factories—they want to be regarded as promoters of improved nutrition, health, and welfare for their consumers in the coming decades.[6]

In addition to this effort on the part of industry, there are thousands of scientists in universities and government institutes around the world who are dedicated to research in the areas of food, agriculture, and food biotechnology. The European Union has invested nearly 2 billion euros in the Seventh Framework Programme for 2007–2013, promoting collaborative research in these areas. This money comes from the national budgets for R&D+i of the member countries. The proposed 2011 budget of the U.S. Food and Drug Administration (FDA) (which regulates food safety in the United States) is about $1.4 billion. In Malthus' time it was difficult to foresee the significant impact that scientific and technological advances would have on the food chain (see Figure 4.4 in Section 4.9).

4.3 THE ROUTES THAT
LEAD TO OUR MOUTHS

Figure 4.1 shows the food chain as a series of black boxes that move molecules and structures toward the mouth. In order to get an idea of the technologies involved in the production of the processed food we consume each day, we must now examine what happens inside the black box labeled "processing." It normally requires a couple of university-level courses to cover the topic of food processing, which is examined in detail in many texts if the reader is interested in delving further into the subject.[7]

To appreciate all of the technologies involved in food processing and preservation, it's helpful to visualize the shelves of a modern super-market, noting where and how different products are located within the store. Figure 4.2 summarizes the main processing paths that raw materials take on their way to the final consumer.

Some of the major food processing technologies are briefly described below. Though some of the terms and concepts are not explained due to space constraints, there are sufficient search terms included, in case the reader would like to go to the Internet for further information. Food that has been subject to one or more of the technologies presented below is what people usually refer to as *processed food*.

- *Management of moisture*: The reduction of moisture and the addition of solutes have been widely used to stabilize raw materials and processed products that are stored at room temperature. Dehydrated products (dried fruits, pasta, rice and beans, etc.), baked products (bread and cookies), snacks (fried and baked), instant products (coffee, soups, and instant potatoes), and all types of spices are stored at moisture contents lower than 0.5 g

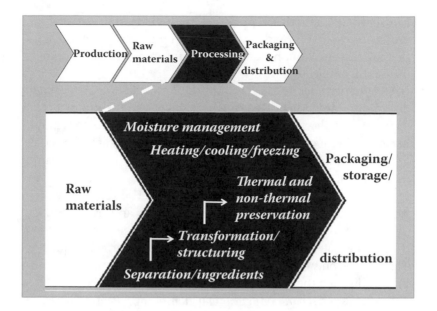

FIGURE 4.2   THE VARIOUS FOOD PROCESSING TECHNOLOGIES ARE GROUPED ACCORDING TO
THEIR PRIMARY IMPACT ON THE FOOD CHAIN. SOME FOODS, ESPECIALLY FOODS GROWN FOR
SELF-CONSUMPTION IN THIRD-WORLD COUNTRIES, AND OTHERS LIKE NUTS AND FRESH FRUITS
AND VEGETABLES, GO ALMOST STRAIGHT TO THE MOUTHS OF CONSUMERS.

water/g of product (Section 8.1). Intermediate-moisture foods can
be stored at higher humidity without microbiological risk using
added solutes (sugar or salt), pH adjustment (acid), and added preservatives (Section 2.2). These products include jams, tenderized
fruit, salami, jerky, and pickles, among others. All these products
are moist but stable at room temperature and can be found on the
shelves at the supermarket.

• *Thermal and nonthermal preservation technologies*: Food that contains enough water to promote the growth of microorganisms
must be heat-treated in its packaging (canned foods) or beforehand (ultra high temperature [UHT] milk) but then packaged
under controlled conditions (aseptic packaging) in order to be
of high quality and microbiologically safe. Canned foods have
an excellent record as cheap, convenient, and safe food. UHT
products (milk, juices, soups) are filled in an aseptic environment into presterilized laminated cardboard boxes (Section 5.5).

Nonthermal methods of preservation include the use of high pressure, irradiation, and various other industrial technologies that are less used but have interesting future potential as there is no significant heating involved.

- *Heating/refrigeration/freezing*: Heating technologies are increasingly directed toward either delivering heat directly to the product (like in microwave heating), or applying heat in small doses without harming the quality of the food (e.g., aseptic packaging, Section 5.5). The ability to rapidly remove heat and turn liquid water into ice has given rise to the category of frozen products that are widely recognized as healthy, safe, and convenient. The removal of sensible heat (cooling) from pasteurized products and fresh produce (fruits and vegetables, meats and fish) is widely used (Section 8.1). A new category of chilled prepared foods is growing quickly. These foods only require refrigeration and are challenging the frozen products in the market.

- *Technologies for separation and production of ingredients*: There are several processes used to free up valuable compounds from the raw materials where they are contained, separating them out with solvents and concentrating them into liquid or powder products. Carbon dioxide at high pressures is a safe and flexible new method for obtaining different high-quality fractions from the same extract and is already used to decaffeinate coffee and tea, and to extract hops for beer (Section 8.4). Technologies using porous membranes, which act as sieves on a scale less than 100 microns (micro-, ultra-, and nanofiltration), are already established in many food industries. The separations occur at room temperature and the membranes are increasingly selective, resistant, easy to clean, and cost effective.

- *Technologies for transformation and structuring of foods*: Industrial food processing involves mixing, transforming, and giving structure to raw ingredients. Dairy products, breads, confectionery products, desserts, snacks and baked goods, processed meats, sauces and salad dressings, noodles and pasta, juices and beverages, among others, all fall into this category. The most frequently used technologies such as emulsification, gelification, extrusion, fermentation, and frying are discussed in other parts of this book.

- *Packaging/storage/distribution technologies*: Packaging technologies provide protection, convenience for purchasing and use of food, and information to consumers. Containers made of glass, rigid and flexible plastic, paper and cardboard, aluminum and tin cans, and even laminate multimaterials such as UHT milk cartons can all be found at the supermarket. Some packages have a gas atmosphere surrounding the product (e.g., nitrogen in the case of cheese, fried snacks) or raw materials (fruits and vegetables) to extend their shelf life. Future technology will allow the packaging, product, and environment to interact in ways that extend the shelf life, provide information on nutrition and quality, and even facilitate the use of food at home (active and intelligent packaging). Packaging materials will also become more environmentally friendly. The migration of chemical substances from packaging into foods continues to be of concern.

4.4 THE WORLD'S LARGEST INDUSTRY

This is the title of an article published by *Forbes* magazine about the food processing industry, which is the largest industrial sector worldwide with annual sales (turnover) exceeding \$3.5 trillion.[8] In the United States alone, consumers spent \$1.17 trillion on food in 2008, of which 51.5% (\$600 billion) accounted for meals at home and 48.5% (\$565 billion) on food consumed outside of the home. Of this last total, 74% (about \$420 billion) is related to consumption in restaurants of various kinds, 6% is spent on school meals, and 4% is direct sales in stores and vending machines.[9] In 2010, the expected annual sales for full-service restaurants were about \$184 billion and for fast food restaurants they were on the order of \$164 billion.[10] The above figures suggest two important conclusions about our "modern diet": that in the United States, food consumed away from home is becoming as important as food eaten at home, and that we spend as much on fast food as we do at more formal restaurants. We must keep these trends in mind as we analyze food habits in other parts of the world, especially in emerging countries with large urban populations.

However, the 10 largest food companies in the world generate less than 10% of total food sales worldwide, close to $300 billion in 2005.[11] In other words, the food industry is mostly composed of small and medium enterprises (SMEs), which are an important source of jobs and family income. In Europe over 95% of processed food companies have fewer than 50 employees. In Italy there are over 400 small companies that only produce salami and other processed meat products. Each of these products is recognized and preferred by its unique traditional, regional, and gourmet characteristics.[12]

In many countries the food industry is the first or second largest employer (after the government). For example, the 858,000 industry businesses that sell food in the United States (including restaurants, fast food chains, cafeterias, etc.) are the largest source of private employment in the country.[13] The food industry also contributes to the economies of rural and coastal regions, and the decentralization of economic activity, as many raw materials must be processed rapidly near their source (e.g., dairy, fish, fruits, and vegetables).

Since its inception at the end of the late nineteenth century, the modern food industry has been tremendously successful in transforming artisanal food preparation into large-scale production processes, thus providing people with a wide variety of popular products that are convenient, stable, and safe. Most households purchase 70% of their food from supermarkets, which offer between 8,000 and 10,000 different products with average life cycles of 2 to 3 years, on average. Food production can now be characterized as a high-volume industry producing multiple products at low unit prices, with reduced margins. At the same time, the food service industry has developed to meet the growing market for prepared meals consumed outside of the home.

Before the emergence of the modern processed food industry, people (mainly women) had to spend several hours out in the field and in the kitchen to produce and prepare food. The fact that women now have many alternatives for easily and safely feeding their families is one of the factors that has allowed them to incorporate fully into economic, social, and political life outside of the home, one of the great achievements of the last century. More than two thirds of women with young children today are able to work and generate their own income, an achievement that has been somewhat disregarded by the critics of the massification and industrialization of foods. The generation of people who are around 50 years old today can remember how much time their mothers spent buying food and preparing three meals a day, every day of the year. It has been estimated that nonworking women in the United States now spend just over 70 minutes per day preparing food, whereas women who work full time spend 38 to 46 minutes per day.[14] One might say that a store-bought cake is not the same as their mother's homemade one (and that's true), but many mothers do not stay home all day every day of the week. Nowadays dads and young cooks get their turn in the kitchen.

One great challenge for multinational food companies operating around the world is to offer cheaper products for poor consumers. Over 1.4 billion of these people demand better nutrition but have food budgets that are less than $1.25 per day.[15] The company *Danone* predicts it will have one billion monthly customers by 2013 for its liquid yogurt product that costs 10 cents/unit.[16]

4.5 EATING ON EARTH

The way foods are presented to the modern consumer has undergone considerable changes over the past couple of decades. Today's hectic lifestyles leave little space for elaborate family meals that now have to compete with various forms of manufactured foods and prepared meals that are regarded as more convenient and tasty.

Some advocates of healthy eating say the first dilemma for the consumer is whether he or she wants to eat processed foods or "natural" foods (often called "whole" foods), a simplistic distinction between modern industrial foods and older kinds.[17] This alternative presupposes that there is a clear line between the two and apparently does not give room for mixed choices. Reputed food scientists have recently addressed this issue in a very comprehensive way.[18]

A second issue deals with the formats in which foods and meals are usually presented before we put them in our mouths. Table 4.1 was created solely for the purpose of developing an arbitrary classification

TABLE 4.1
Nomenclature Used in This Book for Some of the Main Formats in which
Prepared Food Alternatives Are Presented to the Modern Consumer

Food Type	Some Characteristics	Associated Concept
Fast food	Standard menu meals placed on trays and consumed in dining areas (e.g., institutional cafeterias, food courts). May include calorie-dense meals (see below)	Self-service
Snacks	Any portion of shelf-stable, packaged food, smaller than that of a regular meal that is generally eaten between meals	Portability
Calorie-dense meals	Low-cost food, such as hamburgers, pizzas, fried chicken, and sugary beverages and desserts, with lots of calories per portion; generally contains high levels of fat, salt, and sugar	Standardization, advertisement
Takeout meals	Time-honored practice that ranges from street food to refrigerated and frozen prepared meals that are intended to be eaten off of the premises	Convenience

TABLE 4.1 (*Continued*)
Nomenclature Used in This Book for Some of the Main Formats in which
Prepared Food Alternatives Are Presented to the Modern Consumer

Food Type	Some Characteristics	Associated Concept
Typical cuisine	Well-known meals usually associated with regions, which were eaten already by forefathers; emphasis on local raw materials; includes most meals prepared at home ("home cooking")	Tradition, local tastes
Fine cuisine	Elegant and sophisticated cooking with established rules for the preparation. Includes classic recipes and ethnic cuisines; consumed at recognized restaurants	Gourmet, specialization
New cuisine	Combines high-quality raw materials and new ingredients shaped into novel meal structures; emphasis on sensorial experiences	Creativity, art, and science

of the main alternatives that modern consumers face in their daily food
consumption and a nomenclature that would facilitate the reading of
the following sections. Of course there is some overlap between the
different forms of delivering foods and gradations within each of them.
I have taken the liberty of using the expression "junk food" because
the term is by now used colloquially to describe a range of menu items
such as sandwiches, pitas, hamburgers, fried chicken, french fries,

chicken nuggets, tacos, pizza, and hot dogs. Although it is generally assumed that junk food is bad, *per se*, their nutritional profile may be similar to that of traditional or "natural" foods. Take a chunk of blue cheese, one of many items adorning the cheese table at a cocktail party or in a fancy restaurant, for example. A 20-gram portion of blue cheese has approximately 60 kcal, 3.2 grams of saturated fat, and 240 mg of sodium. The same 20 grams of a cheeseburger ("junk food") contains 50 kcal, 1 gram of saturated fat, and 117 mg of sodium.[19] At the end, it is a matter of how much we eat of these foods and how often.

It is possible to measure the impact of street food and calorie-dense food on current eating habits (Section 4.4). Because of its low cost and convenience, it is estimated that street food (which is not necessarily synonymous with "junk food") is consumed daily by about 2.5 billion people worldwide. In Latin America, street food purchases account for up to 30% of urban household spending.[20] Lack of hygiene during preparation continues to be a main concern with this type of food. On the other hand, the market for "junk food" is estimated to exceed $100 billion in annual sales. McDonald's alone serves some 40 million people daily through approximately 32,000 stores located in over 120 countries around the world (figures from 2009).[21] The worldwide snack market, where consumption is based on its convenience and "portability," could reach between $70 billion and $300 billion a year (depending on how snacks are defined). Pressures are building on these segments of the food industry to offer healthier products, opening exciting opportunities for innovation.[22] In contrast, the global market for organic foods was estimated at about $60 billion per year in 2010.[23] In 2010 the value of the organic market in the United States was around $27 billion and was growing at a rate of nearly 8%. Europe remains the biggest market for organic products.[24]

The right column of Table 4.1 contains some associated concepts that distinguish each type of food based on how it's produced or delivered. Obviously there is a clear tendency toward industrialization, mass production, and standardization of products and services. Some differentiation is based on the formulation of product lines within each category that are higher quality (*premiumization*) or more sophisticated ("*gourmetization*"). It is unlikely that the above trends can be reversed in the short term, given prevailing lifestyles, so for the short term, efforts should focus on developing healthier versions of these foods.

4.6 EATING IN SPACE

The ability to feed human beings here on Earth is fairly established, but providing meals for undertaking space travel goes beyond mere technology challenges.[25] You don't want to add the psychological burden of monotonous, tasteless food to the already inherent stress produced by the conditions and the complexity of the trip. The National Aeronautics and Space Administration's (NASA) manned space expeditions during the second half of the last century, during which astronauts needed meals for several days and even weeks, resulted in major advances in food technology. There was also a unique opportunity to design food for specific purposes using cutting-edge science and technology. One early challenge was to minimize the weight of the food, as every kilo of cargo on the spaceship cost about $10,000. The next challenge was to design food that would occupy the least possible volume.

The first NASA astronauts complained that food was unappetizing, the portions were only bite-size, creams came out from aluminum tubes, and there was only cold water to hydrate the lyophilized powders. In addition, the astronauts had to eat very carefully to prevent detached crumbs from contaminating the spacecraft instruments. Their protests were noted and the Gemini missions (1964 to 1966) did not include any tubes. Food portions were coated with gelatin to prevent particles from dislodging and floating around in the zero gravity chamber. Shrimp cocktail appeared. Skylab astronauts had a refrigerator and a freezer as well as a table where they could "sit" to eat, choosing from a menu of 72 dishes, thus becoming the first "*Gastronauts*." On today's space shuttle missions, astronauts can choose from a wide variety of foods, many of which could have come from a supermarket. An intense food exchange has occurred between American astronauts and Russian cosmonauts on the International Space Station, which is stocked with over 250 items.

Thus, the conquest of space has led to some ostensible advances in the technology of food. One of these is the process of freeze-drying, which removes water from food while it is frozen, a method that preserves color, flavor, nutrients, and textures much better than any other method of dehydration. Innovations in packaging and convenience of use came about because of the space missions. Unsurprisingly, land conquests have also contributed to the development of new foods. Margarine (Section 4.8) and canned foods are some of the ready-to-eat (RTE) foods that were originally developed as military rations. These technological innovations in food preservation and distribution are in widespread use today.

NASA announced a manned mission to Mars that is planned for mid 2030, a journey that would last about 30 months.[26] Naturally we wonder what the astronauts will eat during that time, and what the consequences will be. There is not much discussion in the press about this, and there are no details to be found on NASA's Web site. It's hard to believe that the astronauts will be reduced to eating only the sterile packaged foods that can be loaded onto the spacecraft, especially considering that the cost of transporting a kilo of weight into space is now around $22,000. The trip to Mars will last several months, and they may stay on the red planet for several years. Will these astronauts have the same nutritional needs as they do here on Earth, or will they need to eat special foods? A 4-month experiment is going on right now at NASA on space cuisine to understand menu fatigue—a typical complaint of astronauts. The NASA project will consider building modular equipment for processing tomatoes that are grown hydroponically (without soil) in space, for example, so as to obtain tomato slices and juice, ketchup, and salsa. They also hope to use the same methods to cultivate other plants like potatoes, soybeans, rice, peanuts, and mushrooms.[27] One thing is clear about this trip: they won't be bringing anything back to Earth for us to put into our pots and frying pans.

4.7 LESS POSITIVE OUTLOOKS

Some of today's criticisms toward the food industry deal with the same concerns that Upton Sinclair addressed in his 1906 novel *The Jungle*, which denounced the poor working and health conditions in the Chicago slaughterhouses and meatpacking industries of the time.

The novel precipitated the enactment of legislation that improved the working conditions in the U.S. food industry. Today the food industry faces similar charges about the use of child labor for the harvesting of coffee and cocoa in Africa, poor working conditions and hygiene in fast food chains, as well as alarm over recent incidents involving contaminated food.

In the foreword of the book *The Chemical Feast*, Ralph Nader justified his criticism of the food industry that appears throughout the book with a provocative phrase: "food is the most intimate consumer product."[28] Food enters our body daily and becomes a part of it. For this reason, consumers are more intensely concerned about their food than they might be about other products, and the same can be said about the technologies involved in their production.

But critics also point to a certain "superficiality" on the part of corporations with regard to their social responsibility to address public health problems. The food industry has been compared to the tobacco industry, which used advertising to foster unhealthy, addictive habits.[29] The food industry is accused of loading processed foods with excessive fat, sugar, and salt, while the fast food business lures consumers with super-sized portions and all-you-can-eat meals for only a marginal added cost.[30] The inquiry focuses mainly on how these companies advertise to children. Television is the preferred medium because it can reach a larger audience who doesn't need to know how to read and establishes a brand identity. A U.S. study showed that 70% to 80% of the food advertisements during the TV programming for children and adolescents were for "junk food" products, while only a tiny percentage of ads had to do with fruits or vegetables. Foes contend that industry does not seem to have better nutrition in mind when, for example, it removes the more nutritious outer layers from cereals in order to make products that are more "white" and therefore more appealing.

It is suggested that corporate greed may be what motivates the industry's excessive use of food additives, antibiotics, and hormones (all of which end up in our bodies) that help to mask bad practices and maximize profits. The antibiotics that are given to the animals and fish raised for food eventually result in fewer treatment options for some human diseases, because the microorganisms involved are able to develop antibiotic resistance. In the case of genetically modified or transgenic crops (Section 1.9), it is argued that economic greed has introduced potentially harmful genes into the environment, while the potential benefits of the modified crops have not reached the neediest populations in the world.

Some people accuse the food businesses and trade associations for the use of lobbying and public relations campaigns (and even donations to academic research programs) to try to influence legislators and the government agencies that regulate them. In practice, one might argue that the big companies determine most of what we eat and are therefore responsible for our health. Companies contend that there are no good or bad foods, but that all foods can be part of a healthy diet if properly consumed. They also argue that some results of nutrition research are not always conclusive enough to be relevant, and that consumers are free to make choices and are responsible for their own personal nutrition. The vice president for nutrition of a large food company once told me that most consumers say that they want to eat healthily, but when faced with healthy products in the supermarket they don't buy them. This reality has also been documented by data collected in interviews with consumers which reveal discrepancies between their ideas about a proper meal and what they actually consume. The net result of all of this is that people eat more food, and obesity is rampant.[31]

4.8 PIG IN A POKE?

The human palate decided that some harvested fruits, some of the fish caught in the net, and some parts of an animal were not suitable for direct consumption. Economic pressures and the desire to maximize the utilization of raw materials led to the production of diverse "second grade" products such as jams, fish sauce (such as *garum*, a fermented fish condiment used by the Romans), *surimi*, pâté and sausages, as well as ingredients like pectin and gelatin.

War prompted the development of replacements or supplements for foods that were scarce or expensive. The most notable case is the invention of margarine for the French navy in 1870 by Hippolytus

Mège-Mouriés, at the request of Napoleon III. The original product was an emulsion of animal fat with bits of cow udder for flavor, very different from today's margarine. That was probably the origin of analogous foods or substitutes, and also the beginning of lobbying on the part of the food industry (in this case by butter producers who did not want competition).

Well into the twentieth century, with a greater understanding of the properties of food molecules and food structures, scientists began to develop lower-cost analog food products to replace natural foods, taking advantage of newly available ingredients. Soy meat or *textured vegetable protein* (TVP) is an inexpensive product made from defatted soy flour (50% protein). The soy flour is passed through an extruder, a fast-turning Archimedean screw, acquiring a fibrous texture like meat with a neutral taste (Section 8.4). As the soy passes through the extruder, its globular proteins (which were originally rolled up like a ball of yarn) denature at high temperatures (approximately 90 to 120°C) and stretch with the rotation of the screw, then group together in fiber bundles during a final alignment and heating. The process of transforming the amorphous powder into fiber takes only a couple of minutes. TVP is sold in dry pellet form and must be hydrated in water before mixing it with ground beef (which is why it is also called a meat extender). The combination of meat and TVP is rarely detected by consumers, and the TVP improves retention of juices when hamburger patties are fried. If you have ever eaten in a cafeteria, cheap restaurant, or hamburger joint, it's likely that you have tasted soy meat. The first patent on textured soy proteins dates back to the 1950s, and since then much research has been done with other vegetable protein sources. Chromatography or electrophoresis analyses, which are performed in many chemical laboratories, can determine whether a "meat" product contains vegetable proteins. These techniques separate the multiple protein subunits according to size and charge, generating a kind of "fingerprint" that can be compared to the pattern obtained from pure beef. These tests (and forms of DNA analysis) can be used to determine the species of animal from which a meat product came. Thanks to science you can no longer be sold "a pig in a poke."

Around 1970 a similar process to the one used to make rayon fibers was applied to the production of spun soy protein, using a purified soy protein or soy isolate (90% protein). Many spun protein filaments were bound with egg protein and cut into pieces that gave them the appearance of chunks of poultry. The idea was to make products using vegetables that could simulate the texture of meat for those who could not eat meat for religious reasons. Using vegetable proteins to produce textures similar to animal meat is also attractive from an energy standpoint, because it takes 10 times more energy to produce a kilo of beef protein compared to a kilo of vegetable protein.

There are other substitutes or well-known imitators. *Surimi* is a very inefficient but practical way to introduce fish protein with low commercial value into the human food chain. In fact, the surimi is fish that has been washed and turned into a protein gel, but the fake shrimp or crab that we normally eat is called *kamaboko*. There are also substitutes for cocoa butter made with less expensive fats that can replace all or part of this expensive raw material in manufactured chocolates. Anyone who has bought very inexpensive chocolates has eaten these substitutes, which are recognizable by their waxy mouthfeel.

The cost reduction of using substitutes depends on how similar the sensory properties of the substitutes are to those of the original product. This challenge has provided an opportunity for creating innovative formulations and has sometimes even resulted in the development of healthier products. Analogs of pizza cheese (i.e., substitutes of mozzarella cheese) are made from casein or caseinate milk derivatives and other sources of protein, vegetable oils and fats, additives to provide stability, and natural flavorings. With these substitutes, it is possible to reduce the amount of fat or cholesterol, as well as the proportion of saturated fat. To make these cheese analogs, protein and emulsified fats are heated to form a homogeneous matrix, which is subjected to a process of mechanical stretching to develop the fibrous and elastic characteristics of melted cheese. These products are not to be confused with processed cheese, which is usually sold in supermarkets in a layered form. Processed cheese is prepared by blending batches of different cheeses that are molten at high temperatures. The molten material is mixed with water, salt, colorings, and emulsifying salts (phosphate compounds that prevent fat separation), and the homogeneous mass is molded and heat packaged.

Nature is an inexhaustible source of inspiration for cooks and scientists, but it sometimes happens that their attempts to mimic natural products do not lead to the most appropriate solution, as in the case of butter. Butter is an emulsion of water that is dispersed as fine droplets in a lot of fat (80%), and its plasticity and spreadability come from the "stickiness" between the many fat globules and their physical state (the ratio of liquid fat to solid fat at a certain temperature). Margarine, the substitute made from vegetable oils that are partially hydrogenated for a more solid consistency (see Section 1.2), has no fat globules. Instead, margarine's structure consists of an interconnected network of fat crystals, which are responsible for its spreadability (Figure 4.3). Some low calorie spreadable margarine products (spreads) that have been developed recently are made with monoglycerides (glycerol molecule having only one fatty acid attached to it; Section 1.2), gelatin, and water. Thus, they are "zero fat" but not zero lipid. The trick is to structure monoglyceride molecules into fine bilayers that occlude part of the water inside the two layers. These extended monoglyceride-water sandwiches are converted into layers of fat crystals (lamellae) that form a network, giving the product texture and plasticity. The remaining liquid, which contains flavoring and coloring agents, is immobilized as gelatin microgels and dispersed in the lipid network. The result is a type of very low calorie "margarine" or spreadable product, which has

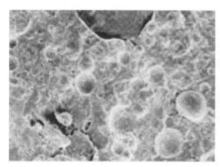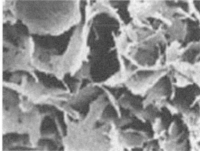

FIGURE 4.3   MICROSTRUCTURE OF BUTTER (LEFT) AND A DIET MARGARINE (RIGHT). THE FAT GLOBULES FROM CREAM ARE CLEARLY DISTINGUISHABLE IN THE BUTTER. ON THE RIGHT YOU CAN APPRECIATE THE LAYERS OF FAT CRYSTALS (LAMELLAE) THAT FORM A NETWORK. (THE PHOTOMICROGRAPH OF MARGARINE IS COURTESY OF DR. I. HEERTJE, UNILEVER.)

been controversial for its laxative effect in some people. Moreover, as it's almost pure water, it can't be used for frying.

You can't claim to feel cheated if you buy a "Rolex" on the street for a few dollars. Many substitute foods are cheaper than the originals, provide nutritional alternatives, can offer similar textures to natural foods using different raw materials, have their own composition standards, and are duly authorized. To find out what you are eating you must read labels and learn how these products are manufactured. These foods are legitimate substitutes, and the manufacturers are not attempting to trick consumers (i.e., they are not selling a "pig in a poke").

4.9 FROM CELL TO FARM

By the turn of the twentieth century, there was a change at the end of the food chain. Consumers were not simply satisfied with variety, convenience, and low prices, but also demanded better health, well-being, and adherence to ethical principles. This paradigmatic shift reversed the direction of the food chain, which now points from demand back toward supply. Modern food chains must pay attention to a new axis that is centered on the consumer, and runs from the brain cells. Now producers must respond to their motivations, emotions, tastes, and concerns about healthy lifestyles and a clean environment (Figure 4.4). With the advent of this axis that connects the mouth, the brain, and the cells, the stages of our current food chains have become more complex. Food production must now comply with increasingly demanding requirements from external sources (environmental impact, efficient use of resources, etc.) as well as new deliverables ("complete" safety, total value, gratification, weight control, etc.).

This new "empowered" consumer of the twenty-first century has not only reversed the direction of the food chain which formerly pointed "from the farm to the fork" but also extended its reach and now must point "from the cell to the farm," as shown in Figure 4.4. Today the consumer determines what, how, when, where, and how much is eaten. The consequences of this change are beyond pure semantics; they have to do with a reduction in the scale of the intervention (e.g.,

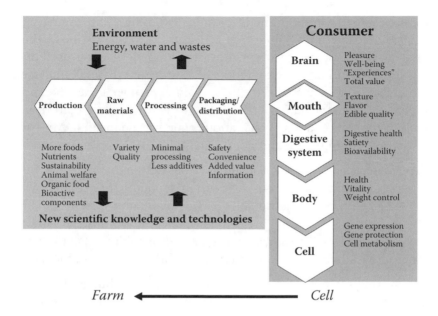

FIGURE 4.4   THE TWO FOOD AXES OF THE EARLY TWENTY-FIRST CENTURY. FOOD CHAINS ARE MORE COMPLEX AND HAVE A CLOSER RELATIONSHIP WITH THE ENVIRONMENT AND WITH SCIENTIFIC-TECHNOLOGICAL KNOWLEDGE (LEFT). THE NEW CONSUMER-ORIENTED AXIS (RIGHT) IS BASED ON DEMANDS TO DERIVE CERTAIN BENEFITS FROM FOOD. THE BOTTOM ARROW NOW POINTS FROM THE CELL TO THE FARM.

from products to structures, molecules, and genes) and the emergence of psychological and physiological wants to satisfy.

How has this come to be? Largely because a significant segment of societies in First-World countries have more than met their basic food needs. Increases in per capita disposable income in these countries have led to a demand for higher-quality, healthier foods, with more variety and more exotic menus.[32] The United States, the European Union, and Japan have a growing proportion of people who have higher education, smaller family size, and are living longer. Consumers (especially in Europe) are demanding more organically farmed products and have concerns about the welfare of farm animals as they are raised, transported, and slaughtered. This is causing a radical change in agricultural production methods. Farmers are raising more animals that are grass fed, and are moving away from feedlots (which confine animals for quick fattening). These same consumers are now much more aware of the carbon footprint of their food, as well as its water footprint, or the amount of water used during production and transportation of raw materials and processed foods. Nothing better reflects the shift in consumer focus shown in Figure 4.4, than the name of the ministry in charge of agriculture and food in the Netherlands, which at one time was changed to Ministry of Nature, Environment and Food Quality.

The emergence of this new consumer "axis" means that industry must place a greater emphasis on engineering products that comply with the expected benefits (deliverables), while maintaining the traditional objectives of higher output, better quality, and cheaper costs. It is much more complex to sell health, wellness, and sustainability than to simply reproduce traditional food production on a large scale, as in the past.

Discovering the route that a food follows inside the human body has become an exciting challenge for scientists. Obviously, the scale of analysis is now reduced from the large processing equipment and products (measurable in feet and inches) down to the microscale and molecular level. The new areas of research include the microstructures formed in the digestive system, the molecules that are released, and their interaction at the cellular level with molecular receptors, and eventually the genes. Moreover, this kind of research requires more sophisticated and specialized analytical tools, as well as greater interaction between food science and food technology, and other disciplines such as material science, medicine, neurobiology, psychology, and molecular genetics.

4.10 FOOD EVERYWHERE

In the second millennium BC, Greek historians described caravans laden with spices from India that reached the ports of southern Arabia and made their way slowly to Egypt. Starting in the sixteenth century, crops from the Americas made transoceanic trips to Europe, and Europeans discovered corn, potatoes, peanuts, tomatoes, chocolate, chili peppers, and sweet potatoes. By the late nineteenth century, steam-powered ships brought the wheat produced in the United States, India, Australia, and Argentina to the European markets, initiating the internationalization of grain trade. In 1877, frozen mutton was shipped from Argentina to France for the first time, and in 1882 New Zealand began exporting frozen meat to Great Britain. But it was not until the 1960s that the international food trade became massive and global. Over the next 40 years the value of exported foods tripled and their volume quadrupled.

Fruits and vegetables that were once seasonal in many northern countries are now available nearly year round thanks to the opposite season production in the southern hemisphere. Technology has made it possible for fruit to be transported under controlled temperatures and controlled atmospheres long enough to be shipped overseas, while the more perishable foods like fresh fish and berries travel by air. Fruits that were virtually unknown in most markets 40 years ago, such as the kiwi, are now available in their "2.0 versions" (e.g., the golden kiwi), and there is great demand for tropical and exotic fruits in international markets. This is a manifestation of the "experience economy," where consumption is not driven solely by price, but also by the desire of consumers to experience new sensations and emotions. A fancy restaurant like El Bulli sources 70% of its products locally (fish, seafood, vegetables, fruits, meats, truffles, mushrooms, etc.) and 30% from other geographical zones, including dehydrated seaweeds from Japan, couscous from North Africa, cheeses and chocolate from France, caviar from Russia, as well as exotic ingredients like salt from the Himalayas (China), pickled daisy blossoms (North America), pumpkin seed oil (Austria), and miraculin (Australia).

The globalization of the food economy has generated a series of reactions from some consumers, from demands about the provenance of their food to protests over the disappearance of certain varieties.[33] There are worldwide movements promoting the consumption of local and artisanal foods. The high volume of the international fruit trade has led to standardizations that threaten the diversity of both imported and exported fruits. For example, the production of apples, grapes, and other fruit in England tends to be dominated by a few "commercially desirable" varieties, to the detriment of local varieties that have already disappeared or are about to disappear.

But the foods themselves are only one component of international trade. Free trade agreements, which involve a wide range of products and services, threaten local producers, and the importing countries can react with protectionism. The demands on food safety reach farther into the supply chain, and as a result involve national security concerns and the threat of food terrorism. The United States and the European Union now require foods to be "traceable"—their path from origin to final destination must be available, with each step and handler identified. To settle this point, the Codex Alimentarius Commission, which sets international food norms, is proposing a principle of equivalence, so that food safety requirements are objective, science-based, consistent, and uniform.[34] There is also talk of limiting the transportation of food over long distances, or "food miles," to decrease environmental impact. This would create disadvantages for imported products that can be replaced with local products.[35] This move is obviously supported by environmental groups, as long distance shipping requires fuel for transport and refrigeration, and creates packaging waste. One concern is that Third-World countries whose development depends on the farming and export of fresh produce, especially African countries, will compete at a disadvantage even if their production is environmentally more sustainable than that of the importing countries.[36] Proponents of this view argue that the impact of food production on the environment involves more than just "food miles," but also the use of farming machinery, fertilizers, and other advanced technological inputs, as well as the energy required to support the lifestyles of farmers from developed countries, including their transportation, housing, heating, and air conditioning.

International trade and the search for new flavors, textures, and nutrition provide an opportunity for the rediscovery of ancient food crops. Legumes such as lupins and chickpeas, South American Andean grains like amaranth, quinoa (or quinua), and cañihua are all examples. Peruvian quinoa exports have climbed in recent years and the price of quinoa has more than doubled, thanks to its nutritional value and culinary characteristics. This new global market also favors the cultivation of exotic fruits and unique spices.

But the globalization of food trade involves more than commodities like grains, meats, and fruits. It has created an industry of ready-to-eat processed foods, which can be observed in all its glory at the super-market. A symbolic product of this phenomenon might be a butterfly breaded shrimp, which is made in China, distributed by a company in Florida, and enjoyed by millions of people around the world. But that is not all. Of the ingredients listed on the frozen shrimp package, only the water is definitely of local origin. The rest of the ingredients, including the shrimp, the wheat flour, the modified corn starch, the whey, soy oil, and others are all standard ingredients that could have come from many different parts of the world. China was merely the place of assembly.

4.11 A BIT OF FUTUROLOGY

While the immediate concern may be to understand the food we eat and how it affects our lives, it never hurts to have a global perspective and to consider trends that might become important in the future. Much of futurology consists of projecting the past into the future with a certain boldness, which in most cases is like driving a car using the rearview mirror and pressing the accelerator. Changes in our lives are unpredictable, and that is what new knowledge brings us, especially science. Nobody voted to develop the ability to manipulate genes or to establish global communication through the Internet and cell phones. But now these technologies are here and they are a big part of our lives. The first synthetic bacteria were just created, and next may be computer chips inserted into our brains, the discovery of life elsewhere in the universe, and average life spans of 120 years.

A less ambitious and more limited kind of futurology can generate possible medium-term scenarios based on what drives certain global trends. In the case of the food industry, the driving forces are social, economic, environmental, political, technological, and scientific.[37]

The social driving forces arise from consumers' attitudes and beliefs about food, and their changing demographics and lifestyles. Apart from safety, consumers in First-World countries are increasingly concerned about where their food comes from, including ethical issues like animal welfare, environmental impact, organic production, and fair trade. Demographic changes such as an aging population will influence the types of food produced and sold, as well as their packaging and nutritional composition. Food will be produced and marketed in ways that contribute to healthy aging ("add years to your life").[38] One very important trend in developed countries is a slow return to home cooking, which involves using local ingredients as well as preprocessed easy-to-prepare sauces and gourmet ingredients, premium food products or sophisticated versions of current products with higher quality (*premiumization*). The mobility of ethnic groups and immigration offers opportunities for a wider range of foods to meet different cultural needs and increases the variety of products available. In underdeveloped countries, growing urbanization together with an increase in women who work outside the home will intensify the replacement of traditional dietary habits. Under these conditions, diets will increasingly become more "modern" or "Westernized" (e.g., eating out, supermarket shopping, consumption of fast food, and snacking).

There is growing concern about price inflation for basic foodstuffs and the effect this will have on food availability, especially in poorer countries. As new market sectors with higher incomes continue to grow in China and India, and overall income distribution improves worldwide, there are increasing demands for agricultural and livestock products, especially animal protein. The biofuel industry is also consuming more agricultural products, which will have a significant impact on the price of raw materials. The FAO estimates that in the next decade these new pressures could increase the price of agricultural products by 20% more than the average for the past 10 years. On the positive side, new genetically engineered crop varieties can significantly increase yields of corn and soy used in feeds, and reduce postharvest losses, including physical, nutritional, and market value losses. This would help banish world hunger, a problem that can no longer wait. In developing countries, access to credit and technological improvements (including information technologies and satellite communication) by small farmers and SMEs would generate employment, as would the creation of new, more specialized food chains.

Public policy regarding food, diet, and health will undoubtedly be a major driving force in the food industry in the future, and these policies influence the need for ad hoc technological developments. Such policies could involve changes in school meals, including the technologies involved in the preparation and distribution of food for school cafeterias. Public policy will continue to address the purported health claims of certain foods, especially products directed at children, to confirm their claims are supported with adequate scientific and medical research. Other public policy efforts affect research and development, innovation, and entrepreneurship, such as providing incentives for industry to invest in new technologies and research. Governments need to provide support for the small and medium-sized businesses that are the foundation of the food industry.

Environmental concerns will continue to place pressure on the agriculture and food industry to become more sustainable. This means optimizing the use of fertilizers, pesticides, herbicides, and fungicides, as well as the use and methods of irrigation, water recycling, and reuse in industrial processes. Waste management is another environmental consideration that affects the food industry. Packaging will need to be lighter, recyclable, or biodegradable. There will be more pressure to reduce emissions and decrease the carbon and water footprints of the different production chains. In summary, the future technologies of the food industry must contribute to the safety and quality of our food, especially with regard to nutrition and health, and must be economically, socially, and environmentally sustainable.

4.12 SUSTAINABLE FOODS

Although the issue of sustainability appears throughout this book, it is helpful to summarize some of the current concerns and try to clarify a few trendy terms related to the sustainability of food production (Box 4.1). What follows may seem a bit "light" to some, but the issue of food sustainability will be increasingly important in the twenty-first century, so it deserves a special section.

It's not easy to find a widely accepted definition for food sustainability that is also succinct. A system is sustainable if it can maintain a certain desired state over a long period of time. In general terms, sustainable development refers to the conservation of natural processes that

---

BOX 4.1   SOME TERMS RELATED TO THE SUSTAINABILITY OF FOOD PRODUCTION

Organic foods. Organic farming is a system of managed cultivation that meets specific conditions, integrating practices
that promote natural resources, ecological balance, and the
conservation of biodiversity.
Eco-foods. These are foods produced by agricultural systems
with efficient use of environmental resources.
Clean production. This is the implementation of better agricultural practices that improve the use, handling, and application of agricultural inputs, food quality, workplace safety,
and environmental protection.
Life cycle. This is an accounting method used to evaluate the
consumption of resources (such as energy and materials)
and the resulting environmental burden associated with a
product or process.
Food miles. It is a "measure" of the environmental impact of
transporting food from the location at which it is produced
to where it is consumed.
Carbon footprint. This term refers to the greenhouse gas emissions of a product across its life cycle, from raw materials to
consumer use and disposal/recycling. It includes mostly carbon dioxide (CO_2), methane (CH_4), and nitrous oxide (N_2O).
Water footprint. This is the amount of freshwater used to produce a food (e.g., including that for agricultural production,
that used along the food chains, and household water for
cooking and cleaning).

---

maintain the conditions suitable for life on this planet. According to
the FAO,

> Sustainable development is the management and con-
> servation of the natural resource base and the orien-
> tation of technological and institutional change so as
> to ensure the attainment and continued satisfaction of
> human needs for present and future generations. Such

sustainable development (in the agriculture, forestry and fisheries sectors) conserves land, water, plant and animal genetic resources, is environmentally non-degrading, technically appropriate, economically viable and socially acceptable.[39]

With regard to food, this sustainable "state" is defined by social, economic, and environmental issues, as outlined in the previous section.

Figure 4.4 showed how each stage of the food chain has an impact on the environment. Some of the environmental issues associated with food production include soil and water contamination by fertilizers and methane emissions from animal production. Biodiversity is impacted when land is converted from forests to agriculture use, and overfishing threatens the sustainability of marine ecosystems. Greenhouse gas emissions are also associated with food processing, because of the high consumption of fossil energy used during production and waste disposal. Food distribution leaves a measurable *carbon footprint* and creates more greenhouse gases (food miles). The amount of CO_2 emissions per kilometer of air transport is almost 15 times greater than transport by sea, and 10 times greater than transport by land (Figure 4.5). The type of food packaging materials, and whether or not they are recyclable or reusable, is another consideration.

But it's water security that now worries food producers, processors, and consumers around the world. The concept of *water footprint*, which is basically the total amount of freshwater needed to produce a good, has been introduced as a tool to monitor a sustainable use of water. Importing fresh foods is actually a way of importing water from abroad (also called virtual water). For a food crop the amount of water depends on location, weather, and agricultural practices. Water used for agriculture and food processing accounts for between 70% and 80% of the global freshwater consumption. Table 4.2 shows the liters of water necessary to produce one unit of different foods. When it comes to crops, rice comes out on top with 3,400 liters needed to produce 1 kilogram, while corn requires almost one fourth that quantity.

There are multiple instruments and agencies that seek to contribute to sustainable development, such as political and international legal

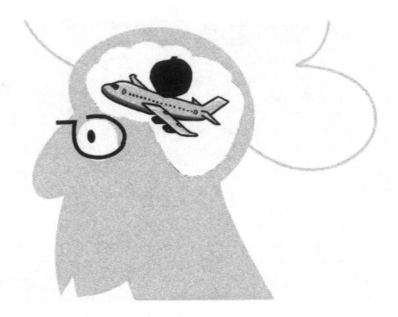

FIGURE 4.5   FOOD MILES AND WATER FOOTPRINT ARE AMONG MANY OF THE ENVIRONMENTAL
PARAMETERS THAT CONSUMERS ARE STARTING TO CONSIDER AT THE MOMENT OF PURCHASING
THEIR FOOD.

TABLE 4.2
Water Footprint of Different Foods and Beverages

Product	Liters	Product	Liters
1 glass of beer	75	1 tomato	13
1 glass of wine	120	1 slice of bread	40
1 glass of orange juice	170	1 egg	135
1 glass of apple juice	192	1 bag of potato chips	185
1 cup of coffee	140	1 hamburger	2,400

Source: FAO. Virtual Water. www.fao.org/nr/water/docs/virtual/virtual_a4.pdf

agreements, conventions, and protocols of various kinds, and global and local environmental organizations. Wealthy consumers are increasingly aware that their choices ultimately affect the sustainability of the planet, and they make this known with their dollars, euros, and yens. The question is how developing countries will grow and improve the standard of living of their inhabitants under environmental constraints that are the result of the industrial and economic development of the First-World countries.

4.13 WASTED FOOD STRUCTURES

It takes energy to make food molecules (some of it is free from the sun), but a lot of energy is also spent on processing foods into the right structures, protecting them from spoilage, and buying and cooking them. How much energy? It is estimated that food-related energy expenditure accounts for 16% of the total U.S. energy consumption.[40] We have all had to throw away rotten fruit and meal leftovers, and we've all wondered what happens to the excess food that is not sold in supermarkets and restaurants. How much of this energy converted into food structures is lost?

A recent report by FAO begins by establishing that "The results [of the study] suggest that roughly one-third of food produced for human consumption is lost or wasted globally, which amounts to about 1.3 billion tons per year."[41] In developed countries, most of the food waste occurs during the consumption stage, when the food is still good for human use. Consumers in Europe and North America throw away 95 to 115 kg of food per capita per year or approximately 300 g every day. This is equivalent to a half a cup of milk, a small apple, the edible portion of one egg, and a slice of bread. In poorer countries, food is often lost before it has a chance to be consumed. Depending on the crop, an estimated 25% to 45% of food may be lost in the field or during transport and storage. Another report estimated that 27% of food in the United States was lost by food retailers (supermarkets and other retail outlets), foodservice establishments, and consumers (e.g., during preparation and plate waste). Fresh fruits and vegetables and fluid milk accounted for two-thirds of these losses. The proportion of these daily losses that might be recoverable is not addressed, but if only 10% of them were saved it would equal one day's food supply for 8 million people.[42] UK households dispose of 8.3 million tons of food and drink waste every year, most of which could have been eaten.

Let's put these figures in perspective. The aggregate food supply in the United States provides approximately 3,800 kilocalories per person per day. Of these calories, roughly 1,100 kilocalories are lost to spoilage, processing, cooking, plate waste, and other losses, so the net average intake of kilocalories per person per day is around 2,700. This is the value that we will use later when we discuss the relationship between calories ingested and calories accumulated in our bodies. You might find it completely unrealistic to imagine that food wasted in one part of the world could help to alleviate hunger in other countries. This is true. The point is that there is much more food produced in the world than we realize; the problem is that we waste too much of it, and with that we squander energy and freshwater.

After reviewing the overall situation of wasted food, let's concentrate on the "microvision" of wasted or underutilized food components. When it comes to food structures, there's no single nutrient that fits into this category better than food fiber. This is surprising given that nutritionists say that we need to double our present average consumption of fiber to around 30 g per day with a ratio of insoluble fiber to soluble fiber of around 3:1 (see below).

In contrast with salt, sugars, and fats, people historically consumed much larger amounts of fiber (see Figure 12.1) than they do today. Fiber is mainly generated as a by-product in the processing of cereals and fruits, and finishes up as animal feed, compost, or substrate for biofuels. It is estimated that around 30% of all wheat that is milled into white flour ends up as bran and germ (containing unused B vitamins and iron) and that 45% to 60% of oranges are discarded as rind and spent pulp during juice processing, both potential sources of food fiber.

Fiber is the structural remnant of plant cells, particularly cell walls, which are not digested by humans. Soluble fiber absorbs water into a gel-like consistency and is found in cereals (oats and barley), legumes, and some fruits. It has been associated with a reduction in cholesterol levels, with binding of heavy metals, and other benefits. Its "solubility" comes from its components, mainly pectin, gums, and mucilages.

Insoluble fiber doesn't dissolve in water and comes mostly from the outer layers of roots, grains, and seeds. Its bulking effect has been related to intestinal regulation, prevention of colon cancer, and reduction in constipation. Cereals are the principal source of this type of fiber, which contains cellulose, lignin, and hemicelluloses.

Nature puts a lot of effort into creating plant cell walls, and we have not been able to develop effective processes to break them down into functional components. Fiber-rich ingredients would increase our dietary fiber content and result in products that are lower in calories, cholesterol, and fat, and that promote satiety. To exert this "dilution effect," fiber ingredients should not only act as an inert filler but also contribute to the physical and structural properties of hydration, oil holding capacity, viscosity, and texture without impairing the desirable sensorial properties and identity of existing products.

Because of fiber's alleged beneficial role in nutrition, the market is full of fiber-enriched products, and fiber has been incorporated into a variety of foods. However, the low technological functionality of these fiber ingredients (e.g., large particle size, off-white color, etc.) has frustrated the acceptance of these high-fiber foods.[43] Particles of commercial fiber not only give a darker color to the crumb of white bread, for example, but their large size (between 16 and 100 microns) also interferes with the formation of a strong gluten matrix. Microtechnology and biotechnology should be able to provide methods for improving the quality of food fiber ingredients and recuperating these natural structures in order to create better food products.

NOTES

1. "The power of population is so superior to the power in the earth to produce subsistence to man, that premature death must in some shape or other visit the human race." I found this apocalyptic quotation from Malthus' text in a footnote on page 399 of Dawkins, R. 2009. *The Greatest Show on Earth*. Free Press, New York.
2. Some authors argue that private property rights are what truly encourage and reward innovation and therefore food production. See Morton, J.S., Shaw, J.S., and Stroup, R.L. 1997. Overpopulation: Where Malthus went wrong. *Social Education* 61, 342–346.

3. This figure was established by the United Nations in a document from the Department of Economic and Social Affairs, Population Division, World Population Prospects, 2006 Revision, New York.
4. There are many studies on the use of energy for food production, and those carried out by the group of David Pimentel of Cornell University are of particular note. See Pimentel, D., and Pimentel, M.H. 2008. *Food, Energy and Society*. CRC Press, Boca Ratón, FL.
5. The interesting question is: why do thousands of the shareholders of these companies accept that more than 10% of the profits (part of their dividends) are invested in research? After all one could argue that the goal of a food company is merely to make better milk powder, ice cream, coffee, and cookies, not to develop new microchips or novel drugs to cure cancer.
6. Examples from new company logo labels: Nestlé, good food, good life!; Unilever, feel good, look good, and get more out of life; Kraft, enriches your life.
7. There are many books on food processing and food science. When I taught an introductory course I used as a textbook Potter, N.N., and Hotchkiss, J.H. 1998. *Food Science*, 5th ed., Springer, New York, which has a very readable format and introduces different subjects in simple terms.
8. The article by Sarah Murray is titled, The world's biggest industry, and it can be found at www.forbes.com/2007/11/11/growth-agriculture-business-forbeslife-food07-cx_sm_1113bigfood.html (accessed March 15, 2012).
9. Statistics on food consumption in the United States can be found on the Web site: www.ers.usda.gov/Briefing/CPIFoodAndExpenditures/ (accessed April 15, 2010).
10. Data obtained from the National Restaurant Association. 2010. Restaurant Industry Outlook Brightens in 2010 as sales, economy are expected to improve. www.restaurant.org/pressroom/pressrelease/?ID=1879 (accessed April 15, 2010).
11. Figures taken from an article in *Food Engineering and Ingredients*, 30(2), 2005.
12. Data obtained from the Italian magazine *Mercato Italia*, Rapporto sullo stato delle imprese 2008, Milán, www.agro.mercatoitalia.info (accessed April 20, 2010).
13. Based on Sloan, E. 2002. Restaurant-goers are super savvy and sophisticated. *Food Technology* 56(5), 16–17.
14. Data from the report by Mancino, L., and Newman, C. 2007. Who has time to cook? ERS/USDA. www.ers.usda.gov/publications/ERR40/err40.pdf (accessed January 27, 2012).

15. The World Bank. 2008. Poverty data. A supplement to World Development Indicators 2008. Washington, DC, p. 1.

16. Data taken from the article, Danone expande la despensa para cortejar a los pobres. *El Mercurio*, Santiago, June 29, 2010. (Danone will enter markets where people have less than $1 a day to eat.)

17. See, for instance, Polan, M. 2008. *In Defense of Food: An Eater's Manifesto*. Penguin Books, New York, p.143.

18. See McClements, D.J., Vega, C., McBride, A.E., and Decker, A. 2011. In defense of food science. *Gastronomica* 11(2), 76–84.

19. Nutritional data for both foods were taken from the same Web page, Calorie Count, http://caloriecount.about.com.

20. These data were reported by the Food and Agriculture Organization of the United Nations (FAO) in 2007. View FAO. 2007. School kids and street food. www.fao.org/AG/magazine/0702sp1.htm (accessed April 5, 2010).

21. According to a report by the Worldwatch Institute in 2008, sales of "junk food" in the United States equaled almost half of restaurant sales. See www.worldwatch.org/node/1489 (accessed April 15, 2010).

22. More details about the global market for snacks are at Bakeryandsnacks. com. 2008. Snack market set for billion dollar growth. www.bakeryand-snacks.com/The-Big-Picture/Snack-market-set-for-billion-dollar-growth (accessed April 15, 2010).

23. Willer, H., and Kilcher, L. (Eds.). 2012. *The World of Organic Agriculture— Statistics and Emerging Trends 2012*. Research Institute of Organic Agriculture (FiBL), Frick, and International Federation of Organic Agriculture Movements (IFOAM), Bonn. www.organic-world.net/fileadmin/documents/yearbook/2012/fibl-ifoam-2012-summary.pdf (accessed February 15, 2012).

24. Figure obtained from MarketResearch.com. Global market review of organic food—Forecasts to 2012. www.marketresearch.com/product/display.asp?productid=1300058 (accessed April 15, 2010).

25. Information on food and space travel up until the year 2002 can be found on NASA's Web site: NASA. 2002. Food for space flight. http://space-flight.nasa.gov/shuttle/reference/factsheets/food.html.

26. President Obama temporarily suspended Mars exploration according to the news from February 1, 2010. On April 15 the same year, the President announced that by 2030 a U.S. spaceship would be on its way to Mars.

27. This topic is discussed more fully in the article by Brody, A. 2008. Feeding astronauts. *Food Technology* 62(1), 66–68.

28. Turner, J.S. 1970. *The Chemical Feast*. Penguin Books, New York.

29. According to the Kantar Media Web site http://kantarmediana.com/intelligence/press/us-advertising-expenditures-increased-65-percent-2010 (accessed February 2, 2012), "food and candy" and "restaurants" were among the top 10 advertising categories in the United States during 2010, with expenditures of $6,672 million and $5,653 million, respectively.

30. The former FDA commissioner David A. Kessler has published a book called *The End of Overeating* (Rodale, New York, 2009), in which he accuses the food industry of creating "irresistible" foods with so much fat, sugar, and salt that they rewire our brains to overeat.

31. Nestle, M. 2003. *How the Food Industry Influences Nutrition and Health.* University of California Press, Berkeley.

32. Higher incomes have been accompanied by decreasing percentages of income spent on food. In Europe, this percentage fell by one fifth during the period from 1983 to 1993.

33. For more information read Halwell, B. 2004. *Eat Here: Reclaiming Homegrown Pleasures in a Global Supermarket.* W.W. Norton, London.

34. The Codex Alimentarius was established in 1963 by the Food and Agriculture Organization of the United Nations (FAO) and the World Health Organization (WHO) and makes recommendations related to food safety.

35. By placing "carbon labels" on packaging, for example, which could inform consumers about the amount of greenhouse gases generated during the production of the food.

36. A very enlightening article on the effect of "food miles" in certain African agricultural export economies is: From field to fork: reassessing the value of food miles. LIFT, pp. 18–24 (a publication of National Geographic). The article states that 80% of greenhouse gas emissions in developed countries occur before the agricultural products ever leave the farm, while production methods in small African farms meet sustainable practices without using fertilizers and pesticides.

37. This section is based on a paper prepared for UNIDO/FAO by Dennis, C., Aguilera, J.M., and Satin, M. 2009. Technologies shaping the future. In *Agroindustries for Development* (C.A. da Silva, D. Baker, A.W. Shepherd, C. Jenane, and S. Miranda, eds.). CABI, Oxfordshire.

38. In the early twentieth century life expectancy at birth was about 45 years. It has risen in many countries to 75 years thanks to antibiotics and public health measures that enable people to overcome infectious diseases. Future generations can expect to live past 100 years of age, depending on advances in genetic engineering and gene therapy.

39. Definition taken from FAO. Control of water pollution from agriculture. www.fao.org/docrep/W2598E/w2598e04.htm (accessed February 4, 2010).

40. A recent report on energy use in the U.S. food system is available from USDA, ERS: Canning, P., Charles, A., Huang, S., Polenske, K.R., and Waters, A. 2010. Energy use in the U.S. food system. www.ers.usda.gov/publications/err94/ (accessed February 19, 2012).

41. Gustavsson, J., Cederberg, C., Sonesson, U., van Otterdijk, R., and Maybeck, A. 2011. *Global Food Losses and Food Waste: Extent, Causes and Prevention*. Food and Agriculture Organization of the United Nations, Rome.

42. Kantor, L.S., Lipton, K., Manchester, A., and Oliveira, V. 1997. Estimating and addressing America's food losses. *Food Reviews*, January–April, pp. 2–12.

43. Rosell, C.M., Santos, E., and Collar, C. 2009. Physico-chemical properties of commercial fibres from different sources: A comparative approach. *Food Research International* 42, 176–184.

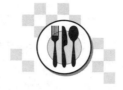

CHAPTER 5

A Pinch of Mathematics

This chapter is meant to encourage readers who fear equations and graphs. Those who skip this chapter may be reminded of it later and can return to this chapter for reference. In engineering it is essential to have mathematical expressions that relate important variables and parameters in order to describe a phenomenon. And in the experimental kitchen, it is important to be able to control, measure, and express the conditions of a process as well as keep a good record of the results through images.

5.1 HOW MATHEMATICS HELPS

A Google search conducted on August 25, 2009, yielded 7.1 million entries for the question: *Why are mathematics important in foods?* The following were some of the responses: (a) it is necessary for modeling industrial production processes; (b) it is necessary for investigating complex problems in nutrition, like energy balances; (c) math helps quantify relationships between dietary changes and their effects on nutrition and health, and (d) a very interesting one: chefs need math to deal with fractions, unit equivalents, and cost determination. The search also found the following sentence: *Mathematics is like food: you cannot live without it for more than 15 days.*[1]

These are good answers, but they are not sufficient for our purposes. Using simple engineering formulas to determine the variables that are important for improving a process or product is very useful and saves time and money. Displaying information in the form of charts or graphs allows visualization of the data and can reveal trends that are not obvious. Concluding a cooking session with a simple model that describes how the characteristics of a preparation changed over time helps us to imagine what would happen in other conditions. Understanding how digital image processing works is helpful for obtaining quantitative information about the color or defects of a pictured product. These concepts will become clear through the examples presented below.

It also helps to know a bit of math when dining out with coworkers or friends. When the bill arrives, most people only seem to know how to divide by the number of guests, regardless of what everyone eats (and drinks). This goes to show that while there is no such thing as a free lunch, those who order more expensive dishes, exotic desserts, and vintage wines get a better deal than those who go for the chef's salad, skip dessert, and drink mineral water to stay trim. You don't need an Excel spreadsheet to determine that everyone should pay for what they consumed, and not subsidize the greedy.

5.2 ENGINEERS AND THEIR FORMULAS

Engineers love to reduce phenomena down to mathematical formulas. The engineering professors at my university receive a salary that is calculated by a useful formula, but the formula cannot explain to their spouses why there is often not enough to make ends meet. There are also equations for describing the structure of certain food products. The formula combines the phases in the food (e.g., water = W; oil = O, air = G, and solid = S), with operators describing whether they are mixed (+), dispersed (/), and so on. For example, $[G + O]/W$ would be the recipe for an aerated mayonnaise.[2] The most important value of a formula is that it summarizes what is relevant and how prominent it is. Often the colloquialism "elevated to the nth degree," which assumes that n is greater than one, is used to denote something very important.

Cooks and chefs should not become frightened when looking at a mathematical formula. It is quite amazing that the most fundamental equation of our universe also has implications in the kitchen:

$$E = mc^2$$

In gastronomic terms this formula reminds us that Exquisite food is the result of outstanding raw Materials, but more importantly (and that is why the term is squared), of the Creativity of the Cook (Figure 5.1).

Formulas are developed from assumptions that outline the problem and simplify their derivation, a fact that must be kept in mind when obtaining numerical values from them. For example, under the assumption that there is no air (i.e., under vacuum), all objects would fall at the same

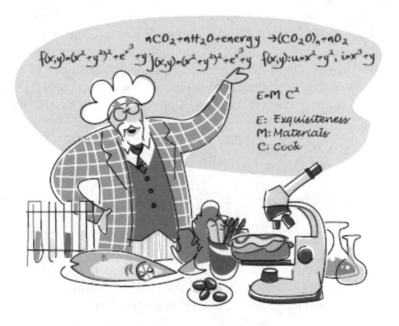

FIGURE 5.1   DO NOT BE SCARED OF MATHEMATICAL EQUATIONS. SOME FUNDAMENTAL FORMULAS CAN BE USED ADVANTAGEOUSLY IN THE KITCHEN.

speed. But this assumption neglects the fact that on our planet friction with air makes different bodies descend with different velocities.

It is important to pay attention to both the parameters and the variables of a formula. A *parameter* is a number that defines a property in the system, and a *variable* corresponds to something that can vary more or less freely (e.g., the time during which we measure something). There are also constants. If we study the heat penetration into a cylindrical jar of preserves that is heated in water at 100°C, the height-to-diameter ratio of the jar is a relevant parameter, time is the dependent variable (we chose the duration of the experiment), and temperature at the center of the jar at each time would be the response variable (what you want to determine). It is likely that the constant π appears in the final formula, which is a fixed number.

There is a basic nomenclature that helps chefs and cooks to relate to engineers, but it is not difficult to learn. In Section 2.5 reference was made to ideal liquids and solids, but this chapter will present the simple formulas that describe their behavior under the application of a force F.[3] It is obvious that when a marshmallow is pressed between the thumb and index finger it will deform, but what is less evident is the relation between the force applied and the deformation or change in distance between the fingers. For engineers, the deformation (ε) of an *ideal solid* varies linearly in direct relation (the reason for the constant k) to the applied force (F):

$$F = k\varepsilon$$

Ketchup cannot be pressed with the fingers but it can be stirred with a spoon to test thickness. The relation between force and deformation for liquids is a bit more complicated and has to do with the effort it takes to move the spoon and the intensity of stirring. The stress of an *ideal liquid*, or the force divided by the area (A), is proportional to the shear rate that is acting on the liquid ($\dot{\gamma}$). This relationship defines the viscosity (μ) of an ideal liquid, as mentioned in Section 2.5:

$$\frac{F}{A} = \mu\dot{\gamma}$$

With regard to stirring, liquids containing particles are often agitated so that particles become suspended, only to sink back to the bottom of the container a few seconds (or minutes) later after agitation is removed. Although it is sometimes mistakenly mentioned that all bodies fall at the same rate, as proposed by Galileo this only happens in a vacuum, When a small object falls through air or water (or rises up, like helium-filled balloons or bubbles), it encounters friction and after a little while it reaches a constant speed called *terminal velocity* or v_t. Although it may seem surprising, a nut falling from the top of a tree hits the ground at almost the same speed as if it had been launched from the top of the Eiffel Tower (324 meters high). In the case of the vertical motion of a rigid sphere, there is a formula for v_t. The size of the object (represented by the diameter D_p) and its density (ρ_p) both affect how rapidly it falls, as do the viscosity and density of the medium in which it moves (μ and ρ_A, respectively):

$$v_t = \frac{(\rho_p - \rho_A)D_p^2}{18\mu} g$$

The acceleration of gravity (g) is a constant in this case. The formula establishes that the velocity depends directly on the density difference between the nut and the air. v_t also varies inversely with the viscosity of the medium, which means the nut will fall much slower in water than in air (which is 100 times less viscous). The velocity also depends on the square (i.e., to the second degree, very prominent) of the diameter or overall size, which means that another nut (assuming it is a sphere) with twice the diameter will fall four times faster. One small practical problem with obtaining a value for v_t is that you have to deal with the official unit of viscosity, which is the pascal-second.[4] Resolve this minor inconvenience, and you will be able to calculate how long it takes a fat globule that is 10 microns in size to climb from the bottom of a bottle of milk to the brim. The answer: about 12 hours.

Food technologists use the above formula to make better products. Supermarket salad dressings need to appear homogenous in their glass bottles although they contain particles that like to sink and oil droplets that tend to rise. The above formula explains why salad dressings contain small solid particles and tiny globules of oil—their small size helps prevent them from falling or rising, respectively. Gums (also known as thickeners) are added to the aqueous phase in which the particles and globules are dispersed in order to increase its viscosity (according to the formula, a high μ lowers v_t), further contributing to a slow separation. Formulas can be quite useful.

5.3 WE ARE NOT ALL EQUAL

Humans exhibit a unique variability in two aspects that are important to their diet: their preferences for certain foods and the effect that some foods have on their health. In fact, we are all similar at birth, but as we grow and age our differences increase. Babies around the world eat similar foods but later some people crave caviar while others detest it. About 10% of people develop an extreme immune reaction or allergy to certain molecules present in a food, while the same molecules are absolutely neutral for the remaining 90% of the population. In other cases, individuals who consume similar diets show wide variability in certain health-related indices, like the distribution of high-density lipoprotein (HDL) blood levels, also known as "good cholesterol" (Figure 5.2).

The variability of HDL concentrations in a certain population can be examined through a distribution graph. The vertical axis (or y axis) represents the proportion of individuals (often in percentage) who have a certain HDL value, which is indicated on the horizontal axis (or x axis). In Figure 5.2, each bar represents the proportion of individuals who have an HDL value that falls within the range of HDL values indicated on the x axis. Taking into account the information in Figure 5.2, we can draw some conclusions. Based on what we learned in Section 1.8 about functional foods, it seems likely that the beneficial effect of these foods (such as increasing good cholesterol in the blood) may be higher for people who are located on the left side of the graph than for those on the right side. What the chart does not tell us is that it is likely that some of the individuals whose HDL level puts them on the risky left side of the graph will not develop cardiovascular disease, because they may have some genetic protection or by some other reason yet to

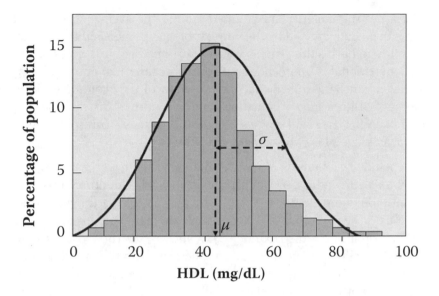

FIGURE 5.2 DISTRIBUTION OF THE CONCENTRATION OF HDL ("GOOD CHOLESTEROL") IN THE BLOOD OF A POPULATION OF ABOUT 18,000 INDIVIDUALS. THE CURVE IS A NORMAL DISTRIBUTION CURVE ADJUSTED FOR THE DATA.

be found. Discovering the complex associations between the genome and certain diseases is becoming increasingly important.

In order to get more information it is much better to fit the data (bars) of Figure 5.2 into a known curve. The normal distribution, also known as the "bell-shaped curve," or "Gauss curve," is a curve that represents a range of natural phenomena, such as the height distribution of people who are of the same gender and age, IQ values, and so forth. One benefit of the normal distribution is that the standard deviation (σ) that measures the variation of individual values from the average or mean (μ) is mathematically defined.[5] In a normal distribution, the mean corresponds to the mode (most common value in the population), and 68.2% of the population falls within two standard deviations of the mean (see Figure 5.2).

When examining the characteristics of humans, microorganisms, or particles (such as weight, heat resistance, or size, respectively) on the scale of large groups or populations, there are often many different values, but the majority are grouped around the average (the sum of values of all data divided by the number of data points) and the rest fall smoothly to both sides. This is very important when it is necessary to make nutritional recommendations for the health of an entire population. If it can be assumed that the variation of the requirement of a nutrient within a large population follows a normal distribution, the recommended dose will cover 97.5% of individuals (corresponding to the mean value plus two standard deviations).

To conclude the analysis of the normal curve, consider a case where the x axis in Figure 5.2 was the resistance of a microorganism to an antibiotic, and 99.9% of them were susceptible to the antibiotic. Obviously, the 0.1% that survived (which are many) are located to the extreme right of the distribution curve and will be the most resistant to the drug. The genetic material that helped them to survive will be transferred to their offspring. This means that when we kill off microorganisms with antibiotics, the second time it will be harder to get rid of them.

The x axis in Figure 5.2 does not have to be numerical. A food developer (or even a chef) can use a 9-point hedonic scale to measure food acceptability, by asking consumers to rate the food using terms that range from "delicious" to "extremely dislike."[6] After the taste test, the proportion of individuals in each category is then plotted on the y axis, and from there it is easy to draw conclusions. For more on the evaluation of foods by individual taste testers refer to Section 2.15.

5.4 EVERYTHING CHANGES OVER TIME

When we press on an avocado periodically to see if it is ripe, or when we open the oven door to check on a cake, we are examining how these foods vary over time. One of the best parts of cooking is tasting stews and sauces along the way and noticing how they change. In physics, chemistry, and microbiology the word *kinetics* is used to describe how the trajectories of bodies, types of molecules, or the number of microorganisms evolve over time. This concept has also been adopted by food engineers, because one characteristic common among many different foods is that their properties evolve over time (Section 1.3). For example, certain vitamins are destroyed during cooking, and bread slowly becomes stale when stored. But not every change is bad. Certain wines and cheeses improve with time, because they develop desirable aromas and textures, and eggs become edible during cooking (Figure 6.1).

Engineers like to make an abstraction from reality and derive a formula or a mathematical model that predicts when an avocado will ripen or when a cake will turn golden in the oven. It is said that all models are bad, but some are worse than others. For this reason, every model needs to be validated with good data, which is achieved by well-planned experiments and accurate measurements (see Sections 5.6 and 8.5). The two factors that most affect the kinetics of change in foods are the temperature (T) and the concentration of the compound (or other measurable property), which is called (A). It has been shown that the speed of many changes in food may during cooking take a form as simple as this:

$$\text{rate} \approx k(T) \cdot [A]^n$$

Let's interpret this equation. First, the change with time or the rate at which something happens (e.g., the loss of a vitamin, the tenderization of meat during cooking, the browning of a cookie, etc.) is proportional to a constant k. Paradoxically, k is only a constant at a fixed temperature but in general depends on the temperature. The property A, which changes over time (remember that A could be concentration, firmness, color, etc.), varies in an unpredictable way, so its value is raised to a factor n, which will be determined later when fitting the data to the equation.

Consider an application for this formula that is related to nutrition. The changes in the concentration of various metabolites in our blood during the period following the ingestion of a meal (e.g., for 2 hours), is called the *postprandial response*. The glycemic response (GR) is what you observe if you measure blood sugar levels at different time intervals after eating (the data), and the lipid response can be determined by measuring the triglycerides, and so forth. Currently it is fairly easy to determine the blood glucose levels with capillary kits, with which samples are obtained by pricking a finger. Figure 5.3 shows an idealized form of the GR after eating foods containing 50 grams of three

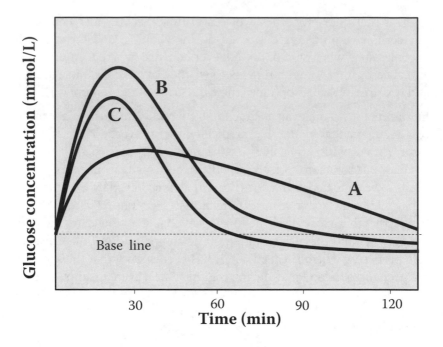

FIGURE 5.3   SKETCH OF THE KINETICS OF CHANGE IN THE CONCENTRATION OF BLOOD
SUGAR AFTER EATING STARCHY FOODS. POSTPRANDIAL GLYCEMIC RESPONSE (BLOOD SUGAR
LEVELS) AFTER INGESTION OF THE SAME TOTAL AMOUNT OF THREE TYPES OF STARCH: (A)
SLOWLY DIGESTIBLE STARCH, (B) RAPIDLY DIGESTIBLE STARCH, AND (C) RAPIDLY DIGESTIBLE
STARCH THAT HAS PARTIALLY RECRYSTALLIZED (AS IN A STALE BREAD). THE BASELINE IS THE
"NORMAL" BLOOD SUGAR LEVEL.

different types of starch: slowly digestible (A), rapidly digestible (B),
and another type equal to (B), but in which part of the starch has ret-
rograded (crystallized) and is indigestible (C). The glycemic index (GI)
of a food is defined as the area under the curve over 120 minutes multiplied by 100, divided by the area for glucose or white bread. Starch
digestion is discussed in Section 7.7, but the curves in Figure 5.3 show
that consumption of the same total amount of starch (50 g) affects
blood glucose differently depending on the type of starch, which is of
great nutritional importance.[7]

In at least two related cases, modeling of the changes in foods over
time is very important. The first is the predictive microbiology, which

uses mathematical models to predict how pathogenic microorganisms if present in certain foods will proliferate over time and under certain conditions. Predictive microbiology is used to evaluate risk during processing and food distribution, and to implement microbiological control measures to help companies produce healthier foods.

A second application of kinetic models is for accelerated storage testing of products. Suppose a company wanted to launch a functional food whose shelf life was supposed to be 1 year. The company needs to know how the activity of the functional compound decreases over time when the product is stored under normal conditions (e.g., 20°C), but they do not want to wait a year for the results. From the kinetics of the reduction of activity at higher temperatures like 30, 40, and 50°C, where the process occurs faster, it is possible to calculate a parameter (the activation energy of the reaction) which allows the reverse extrapolation of the results at 20°C.[8] The implicit assumption is that the basic reaction mechanism that decreases the activity of the functional compound does not change in the temperature range between 20 and 50°C. Another example has to do with the quality of a juice. In a study of reconstituted orange juice the changes in sensory qualities after 6 months at 10°C corresponded exactly to those after 13 days at 40°C and 5 days at 50°C. Therefore, with a good kinetic model, the changes in quality that occur during 6 months of storage in a cool place (10°C) could have been predicted with an accelerated storage study over just 1 week at 50°C.[9]

5.5 HARD-TO-KILL BACTERIA

Food must be safe. Our food should not cause disease or health ailments and some microorganisms are a major source of concern. The most frequently used method for killing pathogenic bacteria, which are more resistant than yeasts and molds, is heat application. Harmful bacteria in food have two physiological states: as active *vegetative cells*, which can reproduce very quickly and cause dangerous infections or rapidly secrete toxins, or as latent inactive *spores*, which can return to a vegetative state under certain favorable conditions. Spores are much more resistant to heat and generally more resistant to most antibacterial agents than vegetative cells. Spores are the "target" at which thermal processes of preservation are directed. For example, to reduce the number of spores in a food by ten thousand times, the food must be heated for several minutes at 121°C. If the spores have "germinated" and have become vegetative cells, it only takes a few seconds at that temperature to produce the same effect. The bacterium *Clostridium botulinum* (from the Latin *botulus* = sausage) which may be present in canned vegetables, processed meats, sausages, smoked fish, and other foods, produces a powerful toxin (Botox for plastic surgeons). If administered correctly, one drop of this toxin could kill thousands of people. Spores of *C. botulinum* are the most heat resistant among those present in foods, however, its toxin is destroyed by 10 minutes of cooking at 100°C.

Salmonellosis, which is normally associated with fresh eggs, is a major public health problem. *Salmonella enteritidis* bacteria (not to be confused with *Salmonella typhi*, which causes typhus) can remain inside eggs, and if the whites or yolks of these contaminated eggs are eaten raw (in the foam of a pisco sour or homemade mayonnaise, for example), the bacteria can cause gastroenteritis. The symptoms include fever, abdominal cramps, and diarrhea that begin about 12 to 72 hours after consumption. Figure 5.4 shows the decrease in the number of vegetative cells of *S. enteritidis* (which does not form spores) over time as the liquid egg white is heated at four different temperatures between 52 and 58°C.[10] Why these temperatures? To avoid denaturation of conalbumin, one of the major egg white proteins. This protein must be in its native state when egg whites are beaten—it is deployed at the interface of the bubbles and helps to form a good lather. If the temperature goes higher than 61.5°C, the egg white starts to get cooked.

Figure 5.4 deserves some special attention, as it shows some typical results for the kinds of studies that determine the thermal death of microorganisms (and the inactivation of bacterial toxins). The first thing to notice is that initially (at time zero) there is a very high number of microorganisms per milliliter of liquid egg white (around 10^9). Each drop of egg white therefore contains more than one hundred million viable *Salmonella* cells (or CFUs as expressed in the graph). Second, the vertical axis represents the number of bacteria as a power of 10 (in logarithmic scale), because cell death is quite rapid (at 58°C the number of

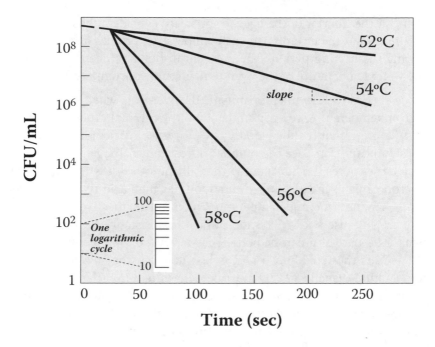

FIGURE 5.4   LABORATORY TESTS FOR THE CURVE OF THE THERMAL DEATH OF *SALMONELLA ENTERITIDIS* IN LIQUID EGG WHITE WITH RELATION TO TEMPERATURE (CFU = COLONY FORMING UNITS, A PROXY FOR THE "NUMBER OF MICROORGANISMS"). NOTE THE SIGNIFICANT EFFECT OF A FEW DEGREES INCREASE IN TEMPERATURE ON THE SLOPE OF THE LINES AND THE FINAL NUMBER OF SURVIVING MICROORGANISMS. INSET: ONE LOGARITHMIC CYCLE.

bacteria drops from 10^8 to 10^2 in less than 50 seconds). The distance between marks on this axis cover a factor of 10 (see inset left, below Figure 5.4). The most relevant information from this figure is that the data follow a straight line at a constant temperature. In other words, the bacteria die at a rate that is proportional to the number present at each moment, which is called *logarithmic death*. It is interesting to note that a few degrees change in temperature has a huge effect on the speed of bacterial death, which is indicated by the slope of the lines. Figure 5.4 also shows that heating potentially contaminated egg whites for a few minutes at 58°C significantly reduces the number of harmful bacteria, while keeping intact the proteins that form a good foam (because 61.5°C has not been exceeded). Keep in mind that this is laboratory data.[11] If we deal with whole eggs it takes some time for the temperature to start rising at the interior of the egg, so for safety considerations data from Figure 5.4 has to be combined with temperature profiles inside the egg during the heating period. The problem in home kitchens is keeping the water temperature or the oven temperature constant at 58°C.

Once you know how microorganisms die over time when subjected to a given temperature, you can understand the thermal process of sterilizing commercially canned foods. The processes are calculated in order to "significantly" reduce the number of resistant pathogens or bacteria that form spores.[12] This ensures that all the other less heat-resistant microorganisms are also killed. If a food has high acidity, or a pH less than 4.6, the time and temperature required to inactivate spores is reduced because a low pH undermines the resistance of microorganisms. The part of a can or bottle that takes the longest time to heat (known as the "cold spot") and is last to reach the selected process temperature (usually 121°C) must be determined in order to calculate the processing time. For a "solid" food like tuna, this point corresponds to the geometric center of the can. With liquid products, convection or fluid motion stirs the contents and produces a more or less homogeneous temperature throughout the container.

Considering how many millions of cans of food are produced daily, it is surprising that this commercial sterilization method has an almost impeccable safety record, especially because in theory not all of the pathogenic spores are killed. (This is what the logarithmic graph in Figure 5.4 shows, as it only decreases in fractions of 10 and never reaches zero.) In fact, in commercial sterilization of foods the probability is very small that pathogenic bacteria survive. But the use of heat does cause changes in the taste, color, and texture of canned food, so there is always a trade-off between microbiological safety and the "quality" of the food.

In the 1960s, an aseptic processing and packaging process was invented to avoid this problem of overheating viscous foods. This method involves sterilizing the food separately, then placing it into clean containers and sealing them under "aseptic" conditions. Irradiating food with powerful gamma rays is a rapid and efficient way to kill bacteria without heat, and the radioactivity is not transferred to the food. This method is increasingly finding applications in conservation, with the backing of more than 50 years of research on possible harmful effects for consumers (Section 1.12).

The structure of a food can have important effects on the growth and inactivation of microorganisms. Microorganisms like to grow where there is moisture. In the drier parts of a food, diffusion of nutrients is more limited and the microorganisms will eventually die. Something similar occurs inside the matrices of gelled foods. The microorganisms are confined to small spaces where they will grow in colonies but can't disseminate elsewhere. In a water-in-oil emulsion (water droplets dispersed in oil) microbial growth is restricted to the inside of the water droplets, and the concentrated solutes like salt, acid, and sugar inside these droplets can have an antimicrobial effect (an opportunity to redesign emulsions). The thermal properties of foods also vary with the structure. Heating a product that contains a lot of oil (or fat) is not the same as heating something that is mostly water. The thermal diffusivity (the "speed" with which heat moves in a given medium) of water is nearly twice that of oil, so in similar conditions the temperature rises faster when the continuous phase is water than when it is oil.[13]

5.6 FLAVORFUL EXPERIENCES

In a science experiment, an event takes place under a few controlled conditions. Most of the multiple extraneous effects have been eliminated or remain constant. In this way a realistic set of experimental runs can be performed and the relationships affecting the phenomenon can be interpreted, but the results are only valid under the special circumstances of the experiment. Experimentation has been fundamental to the development of science since the Middle Ages, so it seems reasonable to adopt a similar approach when testing new ideas in the kitchen. Experimentation in the kitchen can mean many things, such as substituting one recipe ingredient for another, or varying the time and temperature conditions during cooking and baking, and so forth.[14]

Let's create an experiment to determine which conditions produce a high-rising soufflé. A soufflé rises partly because of physics, when the air bubbles expand as the temperature increases, but more importantly because of thermodynamics. The amount of liquid water that evaporates increases almost exponentially with temperature, so as the soufflé heats up in the oven the bubbles become puffed up with water vapor. Simultaneously, the egg protein coagulates, so that bubbles eventually become entrapped in an elastic egg-flour matrix. More on the physics of expansion of a soufflé can be found in Section 8.6. We can only vary a few things according to our definition of an experiment, so we select three factors in the recipe to test: the amount of whole milk added to the mix, the quantity of flour, and the length of time in the oven. Everything else remains constant: the oven temperature is fixed at 190°C, the amount of beaten egg whites stays the same, and so on.

A naïve way to carry out the experiment would be to change one factor (e.g., the amount of milk) while keeping the other two factors fixed, collect the results, and then change another factor (e.g., this time the quantity of flour) while keeping the other two constant, and so forth. This method requires many experiments at a great cost of time and materials, and would not produce clear results. An *experimental design* that tested each factor at three levels (adding 7, 12, and 17 grams of flour, for example) would need $3 \times 3 \times 3$, or 27 runs in order to test all of the possibilities. If we fit the resulting data (the volume of the soufflé) onto a curve, the optimum combination of variables (if it exists) would become apparent. There are even smaller experimental designs that provide similar quality of information, and require only 15 experiments.[15] Once the results (the volume of the soufflé) of our 15 runs are obtained they can be plotted in order to determine if there is an optimal combination of the factors. Figure 5.5 shows that the maximum expansion of 32.7 cm^3 occurs at a combination of factors given by 12.6 g of flour, 63 mL of milk, and 8.7 min in the oven. Any other combination of milk and flour in the selected range produces less expansion of the soufflé. Evidently, none of our runs had that combination but now we know how to proceed optimally, and that's the beauty of using statistical designs.

Many times the only information needed is whether or not there is a relationship or linear dependence between two factors. During frying undesirable polar compounds are formed from triglycerides due to the effects of high temperature, oxygen, and moisture, and when their concentration reaches around 25% the oil must be discarded. The method to determine these compounds is based on adsorption chromatography

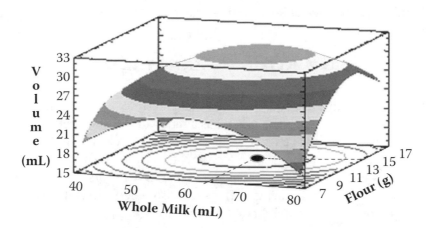

FIGURE 5.5   CONTOURS SHOWING THE VOLUME OF A SOUFFLÉ AS A FUNCTION OF WHOLE MILK AND FLOUR FOR 8.7 MIN BAKING TIME. THE GRAPH, KNOWN AS THE RESPONSE SURFACE, WAS GENERATED BY PERFORMING 15 EXPERIMENTS, AND IT SHOWS THAT THERE IS A MAXIMUM EXPANSION WHEN 63 ML OF MILK AND 12.6 G OF FLOUR ARE ADDED (BLACK DOT). (FIGURE DEVELOPED BY L. MUÑOZ.)

and it is expensive and time consuming. It is much simpler to monitor the color of the oil (this is what most cooks do) and measure it with a simple colorimeter or a digital color photo. We would like to know if color of the oil "correlates" linearly with the concentration of polar compounds. If the correlation is linear it can be determined by a correlation coefficient (symbolized by r). The values of r range from –1 (perfect negative linear correlation) to +1 (perfect positive linear correlation, meaning that as the value of one variable increases, the value of the other variable also increases). Zero indicates no linear relationship. In our example, a good positive correlation ($r > 0.95$) was found between the dark color of frying oil and the concentration of polar compounds. Interestingly, this doesn't necessarily mean that polar compounds give the dark color to the oil (causation); it's a fortuitous event that both phenomena vary with time in roughly the same way.

Statistics also teach us that experimental error exists and that we must therefore repeat the experimental trials and measure several times. It would seem that if we proceeded carefully with the methodologies and measurements, everything would resolve, but simple things like water impurities or the size of flour particles can affect the observed results.[16]

5.7 KITCHEN FRACTALS

A dish that Juan Mari Arzak and his daughter Elena offered in their restaurant in San Sebastian, which has a rating of three Michelin stars, was named "roe deer venison with fractals and black olives."[17] What flavor do fractals have and where do they source them? There is a Web site where a chef prepares fractal patterns that have flavors and textures similar to kitchen ingredients.[18] There are also "cookie fractals" whose designs correspond to well-known fractal forms.

All of this reflects the need for a "geometry" of complex structures like clouds, trees, mountains, and broccoli. Euclidean geometry can be too limiting for quantitatively describing these irregular shapes. The French mathematician Benoit Mandelbrot (1924–2010) was largely responsible for the development of fractal geometry, a term derived from the Latin *fractus* or "irregularly broken," which solves a large part of the problem.[19] A fractal object has a similar graphic aspect or pattern, independent of scale, and can be generated with a recursive algorithm. Mandelbrot showed how fractal shapes can arise anywhere in nature, even in the time series of prices of stock market shares.[20] Using the latter as an example, a graph showing how stock prices vary is similar whether you look at 1 day, 1 month, 1 year, or 40 years. A broccoli or cauliflower is made of repeating patterns (the form we see with our eyes) from a scale of 100 microns to the actual size (Figure 5.6). This means that if a tiny piece of broccoli is examined under a magnifying glass it will appear similar in form to the whole broccoli head.

What is interesting is that the fractal dimensions are noninteger numbers, different from the dimensions in Euclidean geometry in which a point equals 0, a line is 1, a surface is 2, and a volume is defined by 3 dimensions. Thus, we use "three dimensions" to describe something that occupies a volume in space (for a box we need to specify the height, length, and width). In practice, a sheet of paper obviously has a dimension of 2 because the thickness is so minuscule compared to

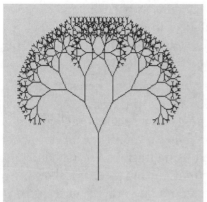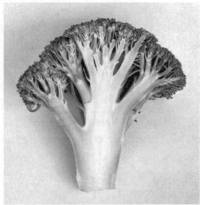

FIGURE 5.6   COMPARISON OF A COMPUTER-GENERATED FRACTAL AND A NORMAL-SIZED BROC-COLI. THE FRACTAL FIGURE IS BUILT BY THE SUCCESSIVE SUPERPOSITION OF A REDUCED SIZE Y TO THE BRANCHES OF THE LAST Y. (PHOTOGRAPH BY A. BARRIGA. A.)

length and width as to not matter. Thus, any point drawn in the plane of the sheet is represented by only two coordinates. If you then crumple the sheet with your hand, the sheet now also occupies a volume (which has a Euclidean dimension equal to 3). The more the sheet wrinkles up tightly, the closer it gets to a compact volume. With impeccable logic, fractal geometry states that the dimension of the folded and wrinkled sheet is a decimal number between 2 and 3, because it can still be considered a surface but now occupies a volume in space.

Around the year 2000, our laboratory became concerned about how to describe complex food structures using mathematical methods. Through an Internet search, one of my doctoral students found Christopher Brown, a professor at Worcester Polytechnic Institute in Massachusetts. Brown had worked for NASA, and his work involved assigning values to the roughness of the pavement where the space shuttle would land. From the point of view of the tires, the runway needed be smooth for takeoff, but rough enough to provide some friction for braking when the spacecraft landed. With sophisticated measuring devices and some software that he devised, Brown had been able to give a "fractal dimension" to the roughness of any surface that met certain conditions. Brown has been collaborating with our lab for more than 10 years now, and we have numbered the surfaces of fried foods, chocolates, and even hard candy.[21] Interestingly, the smooth and shiny surface of good chocolate becomes rough and dull as fat crystallizes in the surface (called chocolate bloom, see Section 3.9) and the extent of the phenomenon during storage (e.g., the kinetics) was quantified using fractal analysis.

This work is important because several of the mechanisms involved in the formation of food structures are the progressive assembly of microstructural elements on increasingly larger scales. Agglomeration, gelation, and possibly crystallization follow a "quasi-fractal" formation process and can therefore be studied using fractals. Fractals have also been used to interpret the fracture curves during mechanical testing of food (Section 2.14) and to characterize rough surfaces, such as those caused by cutting foods with different sharp objects.

5.8 IMAGES IN THE KITCHEN

A popular proverb states that "you eat with your eyes." The appearance of a particular food or dish is fundamental for stimulating the appetite and forms part of your appreciation of its quality. These days there are many devices used to capture images which can immortalize a dish and provide a graphic record of kitchen and laboratory experiments, and save for later comparison. Modern-day chefs love to display stunning photos of their creations on their Web sites.

A simple digital camera (or even that of a cellular phone) is the perfect tool. Pointillist painters discovered that reality can be described as a series of neighboring points in different colors that fuse into a picture when observed from far away. A digital image is just the same. It's an array of columns and rows (also called a "matrix") in which each element is called a *pixel*, and can take different but fixed values characterizing a single color. A color image consists of three matrices, each representing one axis of a color space. Thus, the images on a TV are formed by combining red (R), green (G), and blue (B) coordinates within each pixel, which thus takes on a specific color, exactly like what the pointillist painters did. In black and white images, things are simpler because each pixel can take values on a grayscale ranging from 0 (black) to 255 (white) and the total image is formed by $i \times j$ pixels

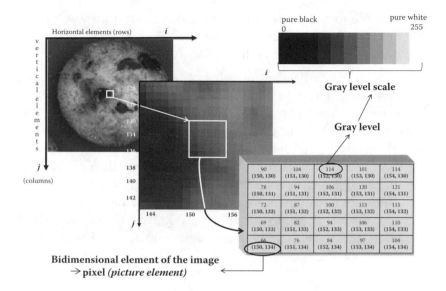

FIGURE 5.7   DIGITAL IMAGE OF A CHOCOLATE CHIP COOKIE. TOP LEFT: ORIGINAL PICTURE AND SELECTED SQUARE; CENTER: PIXELS OF THE SELECTED SQUARE CORRESPONDING TO ROWS 143 TO 162 AND COLUMNS 126 TO 145 (20 × 20 PIXELS). BOTTOM RIGHT: MATRIX SHOWING THE VALUE OF EACH PIXEL IN GRAYSCALE VALUES AND THE PIXEL COORDINATE (*i, j*) IN THE ORIGINAL DIGITAL IMAGE. TOP RIGHT: GRAYSCALE. (FIGURE ADAPTED BY G. LEIVA.)

(Figure 5.7). Each pixel has a coordinate (*i,j*: *i* represents the row number and *j* represents the column number) and a gray value.

When images are generated using digital cameras or scanners, they can be processed and analyzed on computers with special software, some of which are available for free on the Internet. This is because operating with matrices is a well-established technique in mathematics and fast computers make the task quite easy. The information in the integrated system may then be evaluated in a similar manner that the human eye and brain would interpret the image, so you have a form of *digital vision*. It becomes a simple matter to quantify the number, length, width, area, color, and so forth of any element of a food, after recognizing and isolating it from the rest, and counting pixels. Just as it is possible to calibrate an image by the size of each pixel, it is easy to determine several geometric features.[22] If you examine a chocolate chip cookie with digital photography (as shown in Figure 5.7), you can count the number of chips (which are darker so their pixel values are closer to zero), calculate their individual sizes, determine the color of each one as well as the rest of the cookie, and so forth.

Digital photography has had broad applications in the food industry in the area of quality assurance because of its noninvasive nature and the possibility of automation in the production line. Among the specific examples include the determination of color and location of blood spots (hematomas) in salmon fillets, the detection of bones in chicken and fish fillets (in combination with x-ray images), the evaluation of color in baked goods and of fat in pork chops, and even analyzing the distribution and quantity of pizza toppings. In the future, every bit of food that reaches your mouth will probably have been inspected ex ante for its quality by an array of noninvasive imaging techniques and computer software.

NOTES

1. Some of the very basic math needed by chefs is found in the book by Arroyo, S.L. 2010. *How Chefs Use Math*. Chelsea, New York.
2. This, H. 2007. Formal descriptions for formulation. *International Journal of Pharmacy* 344, 4–8.
3. Though it's a bit more complicated, I have retained the nomenclature that is more conventionally used in engineering. The forces applied to a solid are generally compression (loading or squeezing) or tensile (pulling), and the deformation (change in dimension) is designated as ε. Liquids are deformed by shearing or cutting forces, and the deformation is called γ (gamma). The rate of deformation or $\dot{\gamma}$ (gamma dot) is the variation of γ over time.
4. The unit of viscosity is the pascal-second (Pa·s), named after the French physicist Blaise Pascal (1623–1662). It is equivalent to 1 kg/(m·s). Water has a viscosity of 1 mPa·s, while the viscosity of cooking oil is around 70 times greater.
5. Very large σ values indicate that the distribution is very "wide" and that there are many individual values that fall far from the average.
6. The 9-point verbal hedonic scale is the most used by industry. The range of the scale includes the following nine values: like extremely, like very much, like moderately, like slightly, neither like nor dislike, dislike slightly, dislike moderately, dislike very much, dislike extremely.

7. In this case the variation of the glucose concentration (C) over time (t) is given by a slightly more complicated expression: $C = C_\infty(1 + e^{-kt})$, where C_∞ equals the baseline value, which is the equilibrium concentration of glucose in the blood (the glucose level before eating a meal). The constant k gives the shape to the curve.

8. The equation that is normally used to predict the effect of temperature on reaction kinetics was developed by the Swedish scientist Svante August Arrhenius (1859–1927), who received the Nobel Prize in Chemistry in 1903. The activation energy of the reaction is obtained from the value of the slope of a line in a plot of the natural logarithm of the kinetic constant k for each temperature T (°K), *versus* $1/T$.

9. The complete experiment can be found in Petersen, M.A., Tønder, D., and Poll, L. 1998. Comparison of normal and accelerated storage of commercial orange juice: Changes in flavour and content of volatile compounds. *Food Quality and Preference* 9, 43–51.

10. This figure was adapted from the article by Jin, T., Zhang, H., Boyd, G., and Tang, J. 2008. Thermal resistance of *Salmonella enteritidis* and *Escherichia coli* K12 in liquid egg determined by thermal-death-time disks. *Journal of Food Engineering* 84, 608–614.

11. The data in this figure are generated by introducing the contaminated food into thin tubes and instantly heating them (in this case to 52, 54, 56, and 58°C), maintaining the tubes at those temperatures for various periods, then quickly cooling them. The contents of the tubes are prepared in various dilutions and inoculated onto microbiological plates supplied with special nutrients for the bacteria in question. The plates are incubated at a temperature favorable for the bacterial growth. The surviving microorganisms, which grow on the plate as dots known as colonies, are later counted. Using the calculation for the dilution, the results are expressed as colony forming units per milliliter (CFU/mL).

12. The logarithmic axis (vertical axis) of Figure 5.3 can never reach zero CFU/mL but can only reach very small numbers such as 0.001 (10^{-3}) or 0.0001 (10^{-4}), which means that the probability that one bacteria will survive the treatment is very low.

13. *Thermal diffusivity* (α) is a concept analogous to mass transfer diffusivity (Section 7.2). It is defined as the ratio between the thermal conductivity, k (Section 6.6) and the product of the specific heat (Cp) and the density (p) of the material. In other terms $\alpha = k / \rho c_p$.

14. If you were Einstein, you could predict outcomes based on theoretical arguments and skip the experiments. Einstein suggested that gravity could bend a ray of light, which was corroborated years later (in 1919) through an experiment performed during a solar eclipse.

15. A more detailed explanation of a partial experimental design to optimize the properties of a textured vegetable protein produced using extrusion cooking is presented in Aguilera, J.M., and Kosikowski, F.V. 1976. Soybean extruded product: A response surface analysis. *Journal of Food Science* 41, 647–651.

16. When particles (of sugar, for example) are in a container, movement of the container produces a phenomenon called *segregation*, in which the smaller particles fall to the bottom. After a period of time, sugar from the top of the container will be of different size than sugar removed from the bottom. Segregation can be frustrating for those who end up with the last serving of breakfast cereal from the box.

17. You can see a picture of the dish at http://farm1.static.flickr.com/124/353643929_23e82a1e98_b.jpg (accessed December 21, 2009).

18. Fractal Recipe. Welcome! http://fractalrecipe.wikidot.com/ (accessed August 12, 2009).

19. Mandelbrot, B.B. 1982. *The Fractal Geometry of Nature*. W.H. Freeman, New York.

20. Mandelbrot, B.B. A multifractal walk down Wall Street. *Scientific American* 280(2), 50–53.

21. One example of our joint collaboration is the article Briones, V., Brown, C., and Aguilera, J.M. 2006. Effect of surface topography on color and gloss of chocolate samples. *Journal of Food Engineering* 77, 776–783.

22. Image Tool 3.0 is a free online image processing program that can be downloaded at UTHSCSA Image Tool. http://ddsdx.uthscsa.edu/dig/itdesc.html

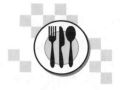

CHAPTER 6

Nutritional and Culinary Thermodynamics

Molecules move and constantly collide, and are a source of energy that we can capture as heat. The laws of thermodynamics that describe this phenomenon can be applied in food and cooking as well as explain why we gain weight. Heat is crucial in the food industry and is sometimes referred to as the main "ingredient" in the kitchen. But thermodynamics also deals with two intriguing concepts in our lives: equilibrium and entropy.

6.1 THERMODYNAMICS AND SOME OF ITS CHARACTERS

Thermodynamics is present in our food, though in an imperceptible way. It explains why coffee and milk never separate, why hot soups always cool down, and why people who eat too much tend to get fat. It also makes clear why the simple thermos box always behaves correctly: it keeps refrigerated foods cool and heated products warm.

Thermodynamics (from the Greek *thermos*, meaning "heat") is one of the most important branches of engineering. It deals collectively with the macroscopic properties of the world (rather than at the level of individual molecules) and the relationships between various forms of energy (electrical, chemical, mechanical, etc.). This book can only scratch the surface of this topic, but without some concepts of thermodynamics it would be difficult to understand how food is fundamentally a process of energy conversion: from the sun's energy into that of edible raw materials, and finally into the energy that we use to power our bodies. Thermodynamic principles regulate the cooking of our food as well as any variations in our body weight.

Until the seventeenth century, natural philosophers believed that heat came from the movement of small corpuscles, whose activity increased with temperature. While digging hollows for cannons in Munich, Benjamin Thompson Rumford (1753–1814), who later became Count Rumford, realized that hollowing a metal piece immersed in water with a steel drill produced enough heat to generate steam. This suggested the possibility that heat could be converted back into mechanical energy, which gave rise to the development of the steam engine and eventually the industrial revolution.[1] Count Rumford presented his seminal article to the Royal Society in London, describing his theory that heat was produced by molecular movement.[2] But that's not Rumford's only contribution: food science scholars also recognize his invention of the home oven and the pressure cooker, among other culinary innovations, as well as the development of a soup for feeding the poor. He has even been credited with the invention of the famous dessert called baked Alaska, for which ice cream is covered with a layer of sponge cake and meringue, then flambéed without melting the ice cream. In his old age he married the widow of the famous French chemist Antoine Lavoisier, who was also interested in food and cooking. Rumford bequeathed part of his fortune to Harvard University to establish a professorship in "the application of science in the useful arts."

It is now well understood that heating something introduces energy to its molecules. When a soup is placed on a stove, the molecules begin to move faster, and the temperature is a measure of how fast the molecules move. Once the hot soup is served, the rapidly vibrating molecules escaping from its surface start to interact with the slower molecules in the surrounding air, transferring energy and retarding their own movement. The heat is "transferred" from the hot soup to the colder air.[3]

There are many events in our daily lives that involve thermodynamics and seem obvious today, but they have only been explained in the last two centuries. In 1824 the French military engineer Sadi Carnot (1796–1832) concluded that the heat in a steam engine flowed from the place of higher temperature to a lower temperature, generating the movement of the piston. The Englishman James Prescott Joule (1818–1889), a brewer from Manchester, postulated that the different forms of energy could be converted into one another. Later the German scientist Julius Liebig (1803–1873), famous for his meat extract factory, proposed that the movement of animals and their body heat derived from combustion of the food they ate. But it was the German Rudolph Clausius (1822–1888) who brought us down to earth by stating that some heat dissipates into the environment as we perform work, and we cannot recover it; he called this loss of energy *entropy*. The American physicist Josiah Willard Gibbs (1839–1903), a strange figure in the history of thermodynamics, used this concept to define *free energy*, which is the maximum amount of useful work that can be obtained from a system that exchanges heat or mass with its surroundings, the rest being lost and unavailable for future work. Free energy is a property of the system and is not dependent on the environment, and in equilibrium, free energy is always at its minimal value.

Although the concept of thermodynamic equilibrium has allowed us to study the properties of macroscopic systems independent of time, like soup that has completely cooled or ice cream that has spent weeks in the freezer, the real world has little to do with equilibrium (more on equilibrium and food balance in Section 6.3). Life on this planet requires a state of nonequilibrium. The formation of ordered, functional structures involves continually exchanging matter and energy with the environment, therefore generating entropy or disorder in their surroundings. For living beings, thermodynamic equilibrium is only achieved after death.

6.2 COMPLYING WITH LAWS

Traffic law includes speed limits for highway driving. Many people exceed these limits without any consequence (unless they have a collision or an encounter with the police). But no matter how hard we try, we cannot violate the laws of nature. If we take an object that is denser than air and throw it up toward the sky a thousand times in a row, it will fall back down a thousand times, pulled back by the mass of Earth.

The *First Law of Thermodynamics* states that energy is conserved, but it can be transformed from one form to another. This is expressed as "what goes in equals what goes out, plus whatever is accumulated." When applying the first law of thermodynamics to food energy, it means that the energy we obtain from our food is either used, removed (e.g., urine and feces), or accumulated in our bodies. People gain weight when they consume more calories than they expend or remove as waste.

The First Law of Thermodynamics can be expressed by a balance between energy (E) and its conversion into work (W):

$$E_{in} = E_{out} + E_{stored} - W_{performed}$$

This equation can be roughly explained in the following way. When humans eat food, the energy input (E_{in}) is released from the food molecules and used for metabolism, which is a set of chemical reactions that occurs in our cells. The "average" daily caloric intake for Americans (their E_{in}) is around 2200 kcal for women and 2800 kcal for men. Energy output (E_{out}) is the energy expended on basal metabolism (e.g., the energy needed just to keep us alive), plus the energy used for physical activity and that discarded in the urine and feces. The stored energy (E_{stored}) is the glycogen and fat stored in our adult bodies plus that needed for growth at an early age. Incredibly, from the point of view of thermodynamics, the work ($W_{performed}$) balances out to zero in this case.

E_{stored} accumulates in our bodies over time. There are nutritionists who say that an average imbalance of only 20 kcal per day (equivalent to around a teaspoon of sugar) can cause someone to become overweight over the years. Energy output (E_{out}) includes physical activity, which has declined significantly in recent decades. Based on body weight, hunter-gatherers had an energy expenditure associated to physical activity of about 20 kcal/kg/day, but most modern-day, sedentary office workers only spend around 5 kcal/kg/day, or four times less, and so do people who spend most of their time chatting at the computer (see Figure 12.1). In fact, it is quite strange that most of the blame associated with obesity is placed on the high caloric content of some foods and not on reducing caloric expenditure in physical activity. Some high-performance athletes may require as many as 5000 kcal per day or more just to maintain their weight.

If the First Law of Thermodynamics was the only factor in play, an energy source could be used again and again without end, and perpetual motion would be part of our lives. But the *Second Law of Thermodynamics* imposes a penalty every time a source of energy is transformed into another: the amount available to do work is always less. We call the difference that is lost *entropy* (sort of "energy that is dissipated into the surroundings"). This second law, that places a restriction on the first law, is also known as "the arrow of time." A drop of milk can fall into a cup of tea and mix, but the likelihood that the reverse process would occur—that the drop of milk would re-form and rise from the tea back into the milk carton (as if you were running a video of the process backwards)—is so infinitely small that we assume it has never been observed and will never happen. Now you understand the meaning of the expression "don't cry over spilled milk": there is no possible way that the milk will spontaneously go back into its carton. Both laws of thermodynamics, which are empirical, can be summarized in the simple phrase, "The total energy of the universe is constant, and total entropy is constantly increasing."[4] Human beings need food to obtain the energy required to remain vital and active.

When a piece of bread is digested, the starch transforms into sugars and enters the cells, where it is "oxidized" with molecular oxygen, generating energy and releasing carbon dioxide. But we must be aware that this process increases disorder in the rest of the universe.

6.3 ESCAPING FROM EQUILIBRIUM

This section is mostly conceptual, but the ideas are fundamental for understanding the transformations that give rise to food structures, and therefore the title of the section is quite explicit. Several times in this book I have emphasized some characteristics that make food unique in our daily life: (a) food is not designed (you won't find "plans" for an ice cream); (b) food is made up of complex biological structures that are susceptible to rapid chemical and biochemical changes from internal or external factors, and; (c) most foods are in a condition of "metastable" equilibrium, thanks to circumstantial barriers that prevent them from falling into inevitable equilibrium (Section 2.3). The intuitive notion of equilibrium is a situation in which different variables that are capable of producing a change are canceled or balanced out. It has also been said that living things only achieve equilibrium in death, so therefore life means keeping oneself out of equilibrium.

There are two important variables that affect the equilibrium of a food: its temperature and the possibility that its components will react or change. A loaf of bread in "equilibrium" is cold and hard. The warm temperature when fresh has become equal to that of its cool surroundings; its starch molecules are now firmly ordered and much of the moisture has been lost and it has a hard texture. It will not change appreciably for a long time. In order to keep bread fresh, it must be kept out of equilibrium by exploiting the conditions that existed before equilibrium was reached, such as retaining its original moisture. A raw steak or a fresh egg can be cooked to different degrees of "doneness."[5] In both cases, once the temperature is fixed the only other variable that can be controlled is the cooking time. If the cooking is stopped after reaching equilibrium, the result is a "well done" steak and a hard-boiled egg, respectively.

Once while having breakfast in a little hotel in the Swiss Alps a man at the table next to mine ordered "poached eggs, three and a half minutes." I had always liked my soft eggs cooked for 4.5 min (in boiling water... at the atmospheric pressure found at the altitude of 600 m). To me the eggs looked quite uncooked but they were ferociously devoured so I concluded that he lived in the highlands and not in the Netherlands.[6]

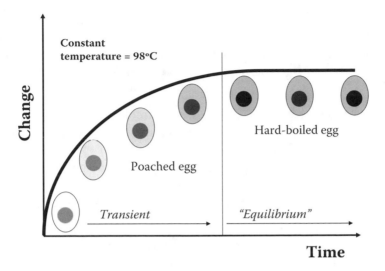

FIGURE 6.1   THERE ARE DIFFERENT STAGES OF "DONENESS" FOR COOKED EGGS, DEPENDING ON WHEN THE EGG IS TAKEN OUT OF THE BOILING WATER (BUT WATER BOILS AT DIFFERENT TEMPERATURES DEPENDING ON ALTITUDE). ONCE THE "HARD-BOILED" STAGE IS REACHED, ALL OF THE CHANGES HAVE OCCURRED AND IT CAN BE SAID THAT EQUILIBRIUM HAS BEEN ACHIEVED.

Definitely the man liked his eggs very soft. He knew that at the altitude we were, water boils at around 92°C instead of 100°C as in Amsterdam, where 3.5 minutes would give firmer eggs. Figure 6.1 shows the example of what happens to an egg placed in a pot of boiling water. During the first few minutes there is a transient period in which the consistencies of the egg white and the yolk are changing. The egg white changes from a gelatinous consistency to a soft gel before hardening, while the yolk goes from a viscous liquid to the consistency of shampoo, until it finally transforms into a solid that crumbles easily. From the cook's point of view, a hard-boiled egg is one that has reached equilibrium, but there were many opportunities during the cooking time that the egg could have been removed from the hot water, resulting in different textures. In fact, when you order a soft-boiled egg, the waiter (or waitress) should ask how many minutes you would like it to be cooked, but that question becomes irrelevant when you order a hard-boiled egg.

This transient period before equilibrium is reached gives the cook endless creative possibilities in the kitchen. If along with cooking time the cooking temperature also becomes a variable, the combinations and possible results increase, like when meat is cooked at a low temperature for a long time (Section 6.8). It is important to control the kinetics, or the path that leads to equilibrium, so as to be able to stop at the desired intermediate state (more on kinetics in Section 5.4).

Most processed foods like baked goods, emulsions, and ice cream are not in thermodynamic equilibrium when we eat them. Instead, as explained above, they are said to be in a metastable state, or momentarily stable (see Section 2.3). They are in the situation of a skydiver who did not open his parachute and is hanging from a tree branch that is slowly bending and soon will break. According to the laws of physics, the skydiver will reach equilibrium when he hits the ground.

An oil/water (O/W) emulsion in a jar will remain dispersed as droplets, as long as the molecules located at the oil/water interfaces are doing their job of keeping the droplets separated (Section 2.6). In equilibrium, the oil and water will separate in two phases. In confectionery things are also kept from reaching equilibrium. Toffees are supersaturated sugar syrups in which the high viscosity of the mixture prevents the sugar from crystallizing (which would result in a grainy texture). But toffees are considered metastable because they have more sugar than they would have at equilibrium, and because sucrose likes to crystallize, it will do so spontaneously given any excuse. Often this metastable equilibrium is achieved using "barriers" that slow the inexorable advance toward the final equilibrium, such as molecules at the interface oil droplets, a high viscosity in a liquid that inhibits mobility of the molecules, or by achieving the glassy state in a solid (Section 2.3).

6.4 AN ACCOUNTING EXERCISE

For those who find the concepts of thermodynamics difficult to understand when they are applied to the realm of food and food consumption, an analogy based on money might be useful. Just like the dollars in our wallet are our units of currency, the joule (J) is the official unit of energy, heat, and work for thermodynamics. We will use the *kilocalorie* (kcal) as our unit of measure from now on, however, because people are in the habit of expressing everything in terms of "calories" (they really mean kcal) when discussing weight management. Just as currencies become devalued and basic goods end up costing thousands and millions of units, we need to use kilocalories because one calorie is a very small quantity. A kilocalorie, which is equal to 4.2 joules, is the amount of heat required to raise the temperature of 1 liter of water from 14.5 to 15.5°C, but it is also roughly equivalent to the energy burned each minute during sleep by a person weighing 70 kg.

The body functions in a way that is similar to our personal finances, except that what the body accumulates in its "bank" is much less desirable. If you have money leftover at the end of the month, after your necessary expenses have been paid, you can invest it in bonds or use it to buy real estate. Similarly, each time you eat, every gram of food is converted into calories according to the following exchange rate (in kcal/g): protein and carbohydrate, 4; alcohol, 7; and fats, 9. The sugar that enters your blood is like cash and can be used immediately by the cells. Part of what is left over is converted into a large molecule called *glycogen* and stored in the liver and muscles. The glycogen is like having shares of stock—it can be converted back into cash, but it takes some time. All of the remaining excess calories, regardless of where they came from, are eventually converted into fat. The fat storage is like an investment in real estate—not easily undone. Fat accumulates around the waistline and chest, or the hips and thighs, resulting in body types called "apple" or "pear," respectively.[7] It is therefore important to have an idea of how many calories are in the foods we regularly consume. Just like we need to do a bit of mental bookkeeping when we shop at a supermarket, it is important to recognize when we are reaching the "overdraft" point in our daily calorie limit. Table 6.1 provides some benchmark values to keep our calorie budgets more or less up to date, because like a credit card, sooner or later you have to pay it off.

There are many ways to determine and measure energy expenditure. Fortunately, the mere act of staying alive expends between 1500 to 1800 kcal daily, or the equivalent of two double cheeseburgers, just to be at rest.[8] Resting metabolic rate (RMR) is the energy expenditure per unit of time (kcal/day) of a person at rest, and it varies somewhat depending on the person's age and weight. When expressed as a function of weight, there are large variations between individuals,

TABLE 6.1
Approximate Calories Spent during an Hour of Activity (*credit*), and the
Amount of Calories in Different Portions of Food (*debit*)

Credit	kcal	Debit	kcal
Sleeping	63	Teaspoon of sugar	48
Working on the computer	110–140	White wine (150 cc)	87
Watching television	145	Fried egg	108
Driving a car	192	Icemilk ice cream	211
Housekeeping	190–280	Soda (16 ounces)	204
Walking	317	Fried empanada	315
Gardening	357	Pork chop	336
Playing golf	437	Whisky sour (150 cc)	350
Easy aerobics	460	Pasta (1 cup)	456
Jogging	635	Hot dog with mayonnaise	560
Cycling	635	Potato chips (120 g)	644
Stationary bike	830	Double hamburger with cheese	740
Stationary bike (intense)	1,000	Combo meal[a]	1,550

[a] McDonald's double quarter pounder with cheese (740 kcal), Coca-Cola Classic (310 kcal), and large fries (154 g, 500 kcal). Data obtained from www.mcdonalds.com (accessed June 3, 2010).

particularly between fat and thin people. This is because adipose tissue has a higher metabolic rate than lean tissue or muscles. Therefore, 1 kilocalorie can be redefined as the energy that an adult who is completely at rest spends approximately each minute (there are 1440 minutes in 24 hours, which corresponds to 1440 kcal per day). About 70% of the RMR is used to maintain the basic functions (one fourth of these are spent on the metabolism of the brain, which weighs a little more than 1 kilo) and about 20% go to thermogenesis, which is the energy associated with digestion, absorption, and utilization of food.

If you got up in the morning and went straight from the bed to the sofa and watched TV or sat in front of the computer the entire day, the RMR would be a guesstimate of your daily calorie expenditure. Because Americans consume on average around 2700 kcal per day, you are responsible for the extra 900 to 1200 kcal.[9] Now take a look to the left side of Table 6.1.

In 2004, filmmaker Morgan Spurlock decided to eat all his meals at McDonald's for an entire month, an experience he documented in the movie *Super Size Me*.[10] During the 30 days of this "junk food" regime, Spurlock gained almost 11 kilos (24 pounds). A freshman engineering student could have predicted this outcome based on a simple balance of calories, and saved Spurlock his fatty liver, headache, and obesity troubles, but that would have also deprived him the proceeds from the film.[11] The calculation goes something like this: an accumulation of 11 kilos of fat in 30 days is equivalent to an excess intake of 3300 kcal per day (11 kg fat × 9000 kcal/kg fat = 99,000 kcal, divided into 30 days). Let's go to Table 6.1. The caloric expenditure (eating whatever you like) is based on 14 hours of low activity at 140 kcal/hr (like watching TV, working on the computer, and riding in a car), which equals around 2000 kcal, and 10 hours of sleep, equivalent to 640 kcal, resulting in a total of 2640 kcal/day. For the surplus calorie intake to reach 3300 kcal/day, he would have had to consume about 6000 kcal/day at the fast food chain. You can go to McDonald's Web site (www.mcdonalds.com) and easily put together three or four daily menus that achieve this caloric intake—just two combo meals are more than 3000 kcal. All fast food aside, simple overeating—like having an appetizer of six fried shrimp with mayonnaise and a piña colada—can quickly add up

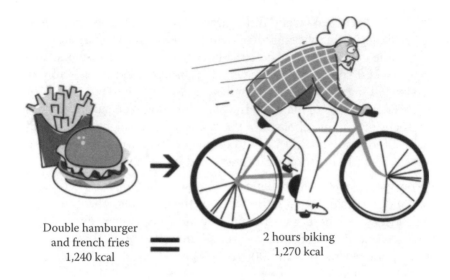

Double hamburger
and french fries
1,240 kcal

=

2 hours biking
1,270 kcal

FIGURE 6.2   CALORIC ACCOUNTING: THE RATIONAL SOLUTION TO WEIGHT GAIN IS TO EAT
FEWER CALORIES AND EXERCISE MORE. A HIGH-CALORIC TREAT HAS TO BE COMPENSATED FOR
WITH A CORRESPONDING EXTRA PHYSICAL ACTIVITY.

(to 1000 kilocalories in this case), to which you have to add breakfast,
coffee and biscuits, lunch, and dinner.

While we wait for a miracle pill that can make these daily accounting
adjustments in our caloric intake accurately and without side effects,
there is only one rational solution for avoiding weight gain: eating fewer
calories and exercising more (Figure 6.2). It's just like keeping a positive balance in the checkbook or credit card, by earning more money
or spending less, or ideally by doing both. For those who struggle with
balancing weight and calories, the best solution involves a change in
food consumption habits.

6.5 APPETITE AND SATIETY

Our body's calorie regulation must be fairly complicated, considering
that an adult consumes about a million kilocalories annually and yet
we do not expect our weight to vary more than a few hundred grams.

Even more surprising is that when we eat, the difference between the first signal to terminate eating and that of feeling "full" may involve no less than 2000 kcal, a hefty amount. *Satiation*, that prompts the termination of eating, determines the amount of food consumed at each sitting but it tells nothing about the time until hunger appears again. To our misfortune, foods that are gladly overeaten have relatively little impact on satiation and are usually highly palatable and energy dense. A single extra slice of pizza "costs" us about 600 kcal, or the equivalent of 2 hours of jogging.[12]

Many people believe that obesity is caused by a failure in the system that regulates the energy balance in our bodies. This regulation is known as energy homeostasis, and the nervous system plays a fundamental role in it, particularly the brain. There is a short-term regulation system that signals the body when it needs to eat, by triggering the physiological response called *appetite*. This system also signals the feeling of fullness that persists after eating called *satiety*. On an equal calorie basis protein seems to have a higher satiation effect than carbohydrate, while fat exerts the weakest effects on both satiation and satiety. Appetite and satiety are triggered by the brain (and transmitted through nerve impulses) in response to endocrine and metabolic signals, such as those produced by hormones secreted into the digestive tract, the levels of glucose and certain lipids in the blood, and the concentrations of the insulin and the hormone glucagon, which helps to raise glucose levels.

It makes sense that the signal telling us when to eat comes from the level of glucose in the blood because this molecule is a good indicator of whether or not the cells need energy (see Section 7.7). Following a meal, the blood glucose level rises and the pancreas releases *insulin* to help cells take in and utilize the glucose. After some time has passed, glucose levels in the blood begin to decrease as do insulin levels (see Figure 5.3). In response, glucagon instructs the liver to break down some glycogen in order to release more glucose to offset the decline (see Section 1.2). This is the system that regulates glucose levels and appetite in the short term, after each meal that we eat. The cells in people that are insulin resistant do not respond correctly to insulin, and their bodies need more insulin to help glucose enter cells. Eventually, the pancreas fails to keep up with the body's need for insulin, and excess glucose builds up in the bloodstream. The cells remain "hungry" while glucose is excreted in the urine. Insulin resistance increases the chance of developing type 2 diabetes.

There is another form of regulation, more long term, which informs the brain about the fat reserves in the body. The hypothesis that glucose levels were the only regulators of food intake succumbed in the 1990s with the identification of the hormone leptin (from the Greek *leptos*, meaning "slender"). Leptin is secreted by fat cells or adipocytes in various tissues to signal that appetite should be suppressed. There is a direct correlation between the leptin levels in the blood and the amount of adipose tissue in the body. The brain can perceive only fluctuations in leptin levels, however, not the total amount of leptin in the blood, which is why obese people still experience hunger, despite having excess adipose tissue.

There are other hormones involved in the regulation of food intake. They are synthesized in the digestive system in response to the presence of nutrients. Cholecystokinin, a satiating hormone that responds to the presence of protein and fat, and ghrelin, is known as the "hunger hormone," as it increases in conditions of fasting and stimulates food intake. All of these regulatory hormones are peptides, as their actions are related to gene expression and they also interact with hormone receptors. Because so many articles in the popular press about appetite and diets mention these molecules, some of them are described in Box 6.1.

For those who do wish to become experts in this area, Box 6.1 shows that we have only recently begun to understand the mechanisms involved in the regulation of our energy balance, both in the short and long term, and that these mechanisms are very complex. It is unlikely that a single substance is responsible for the control of such a complicated system that has been working night and day for hundreds of thousands of years. Therefore it is best to ignore ads about miraculous weight loss from pills or hormones, which can actually have harmful side effects.

Prolonging the sensation of fullness has been one of the most sought-after solutions to overeating. The rate that the stomach empties itself depends on the volume, composition, and state of the gastric contents. Liquids are discharged into the intestine more rapidly than solids, so

---

BOX 6.1   SOME HORMONES AND PEPTIDES INVOLVED IN REGULATING FOOD INTAKE

Insulin. This hormone is synthesized in the pancreas and exerts a dual effect on food intake and body weight, reducing appetite. Insulin allows glucose to enter cells, providing the energy needed to carry out their normal functions. The presence of insulin results in decreased blood glucose levels, which generates a signal that induces appetite.

Leptin. This hormone is mainly secreted in adipose tissue and circulates in blood in direct relation to levels of body fat. Its main effect is the regulation of body weight over time. In the short term, leptin levels rise with consumption of foods rich in carbohydrates and suppress the appetite.

Ghrelin. Also known as the "hunger hormone." Ghrelin is secreted in the stomach and associated with the growth hormone. The circulating ghrelin levels increase during periods of fasting and decrease after eating.

Cholecystokinin. CKK is secreted in the duodenum and jejunum in response to the presence of partially digested fats and carbohydrates from the stomach. It inhibits gastric emptying, contributing to the sensation of satiety.

Peptide YY This hormone inhibits gastric and pancreatic secretion and helps suppress hunger.

---

drinking lots of water does not prolong satiety (another myth). If the volume of food expands once it reaches the stomach, the sensation of satiety tends to last longer. In her book *The Volumetric Diet*, Barbara Rolls discusses how satiety is affected by the consumption of foods with low caloric density and high water content, such as fruits, vegetables, low-fat milk, lean meat, chicken, and fish. The idea behind this diet is that the water retained in the matrices of these foods not only helps to dilute the ingested calories, but also fills the stomach.[13] A diet of bland jellies without sugar is not likely to be popular, however effective it may be. Some current research has used magnetic resonance imaging (MRI) scanners to monitor real-time gastric emptying in individuals who have consumed different formulations that increase the viscosity and fluid retention of the food bolus (Section 3.4). Dieters may someday be able to buy foods that have been reformulated with components that have high water binding capacity, such as fiber and hydrocolloids or gums, which could help prolong the period of satiety between meals and thereby avoid snacking.

As noted, some are hopeful that the solution to weight regulation will come in the form of medication. This route is not presently feasible, given the complexity of the regulation of energy homeostasis. Some drugs do have an effect on appetite, but they also affect other processes and cause side effects. Such is the case with sibutramine, which contributes to moderate weight reduction but also causes hypertension. Currently the most effective treatment for morbid obesity is bariatric surgery, but the mortality (risk) and cost associated with this procedure limits its use to the most extreme cases. Understanding the mechanisms that control satiety is a very important problem in the treatment of obesity, one that may lead to development of new low-calorie foods designed to make your stomach feel fuller.

6.6 CALORIES IN THE KITCHEN AND COOKING

No one knows exactly when humans started using fire to cook food. Historians think this occurred sometime between 1,500,000 BC and 500,000 BC, depending on the location in question.[14] According to anthropologists and biologists, *Homo erectus* was most likely the first hominid to apply fire to food, improving digestion of proteins and starch and providing the caloric intake needed to develop a larger brain. Our brains use about 16 times more energy per unit of weight than our muscles.[15] With the ability to cook, primitive man was able to incorporate new ingredients into his diet, such as certain vegetables whose anti-nutritional compounds are inactivated by heat. Grains and tubers also became more digestible (Section 7.6). Humans moved from being merely omnivores to become *coctivors* (from the Latin *coquere*, meaning "to cook"), and turned into the only species on earth to cook their food.[16] Heat continues to be used today to preserve food; make it safe; and induce changes in texture (tenderized meats, for example), appearance, and taste, thus becoming the "main ingredient" of many dishes. Some of the most significant changes to the major food groups that occur during cooking are shown in Figure 2.3.

In engineering terms there are three basic ways of transferring heat to food: conduction, convection, and radiation, which are simply explained below. Heat by *conduction* involves direct contact of food with a hot surface, like when a steak rests on the grill. The key factors are the temperature difference between the heat source and any point in the food; the thermal conductivity, or the speed with which a material can be heated or cooled; and the size or thickness of the food. *Convection* cooking is mediated by the movement of a high-temperature fluid (usually water, oil, or air) that surrounds the food and heats it. In addition to the temperature of the fluid, the convection coefficient, a parameter related to the agitation of the heating medium, is also very important. This is the way in which kitchen ovens use hot air to bake pizza and cakes. Heat transmission by radiation involves the emission of radiant energy from a surface at high temperature, which is converted into heat when absorbed by an object. Heat by *radiation* uses electromagnetic energy and does not require a medium between the transmitter and the food (e.g., microwave heating). In the case a radiant element is used, as in broiling, heat transfer depends strongly on the temperature of the heat source. In the real world, several heat transfer mechanisms can coexist, but usually one of them dominates. Figure 8.4 illustrates the heat transfer mechanisms in action during deep frying of fish.

Traditional cooking techniques involve applying heat to the outside of the food, either through baking (hot air), cooking in hot water, or grilling. The outside of a solid food always heats up first and reaches higher temperatures than the interior, allowing for desirable characteristics of a roast beef that is well done outside and nearly raw inside, or crusty bread that is soft and moist inside. Once the outside temperature of a solid food rises, the inside cooks mainly by conduction. With liquids such as soups, the heating occurs more uniformly because currents allow mixing between areas at different temperatures.

The cooking techniques that impart flavor, color, and texture to foods have a somewhat confusing nomenclature, depending on the type of food, the utensils required (ovens, frying pans, pots, or pressure cookers), the environment, and the expected results. A full exploration of all of the cooking processes involving heat, along with the terminology (in Spanish and German), can be found in a book by the author Schwedt (2004).[17] To give scientists a general idea, without going into too much culinary detail, various cooking methods and their common names are grouped as follows:

1. When cooking with a hot aqueous medium, there is a distinction between boiling, which usually involves immersion in boiling water, and poaching, which is a slow cooking process. Parboiling involves partially cooking a food before further treatment, while scalding is used to inactivate enzymes and soften leafy vegetables like cabbage and kale. The cooking medium can be water, broth, milk, syrups, and so forth. For double boiling (*bain marie*), a container of food is introduced into another container of hot water, for better temperature regulation.

2. When cooking with a nonliquid medium or with dry heat, without adding water or fat (other than that of the food itself), heat is directly applied to the product. Roasting is an enclosed heat treatment in which the heat is transferred by convection from the hot air and also partly by radiation (from the walls of the oven). If the food is wrapped in a paper or foil, the cooking method is called *en papillote*. With grilling, heat transfer occurs mainly by radiation, and the food is supported on a rack or a griddle. Broiling is done with a high-temperature source, typically located above the food, and is the preferred method for cooking *au gratin*, or any dish whose surface is to be toasted. In the case of toasted bread, metal toasters are placed directly over a flame or slices are introduced within an appliance with which you can control the amount of toasting and then eject the toast.[18]

3. The use of grease or hot oil determines the difference between the surface cooking (*sautéing*) that takes place in a pan with little oil, and deep frying, where the food is completely submerged into the frying medium (Section 8.7). Fried products may be coated with flour (floured); a mixture of egg, milk, and flour (battered); or bread crumbs (breaded).

4. Steam cooking is a process in which food is placed in a basket that is located over a boiling liquid (water or broth). The steam generated by the boiling liquid cooks the food. Although the process is relatively slow, it results in unique food textures and aromas.

Those who love grilled or roasted red meat will be interested to know how the temperature measured at the center of the meat corresponds with its color. Four stages of doneness have been defined for a steak: extra rare, or *bleu* (red, 46 to 49°C); medium rare (pinkish red, 54 to 60°C); medium (pink, 60 to 66°C); and well done (gray, 70 to 80°C). More on meat cooking can be found in Section 6.8.

There are some more unconventional methods of cooking in which the food is brought into direct contact with the primary heat source. Mexican stone soup, for example, is prepared by placing a hot stone into the soup in order to heat it. Not surprising really, and hardly any different than when you add ice to cool a drink (except that the ice melts). There is also the Peruvian *huatia*, in which potatoes and other ingredients are surrounded with hot clumps of dirt, and the Chilean *curanto*, where a hole in the earth is filled with hot rocks in order to cook layers of fish, shellfish, meats, sausages, and potatoes, all covered with Chilean rhubarb.[19] In the latter two cases the indigenous tradition is to bring the cooking of food back to the land that produced it.

6.7 HEATING WITH WAVES

In 1945 a fortuitous event occurred in a research lab that was followed by an astute observation. A distracted physicist (typical) accidently left his sandwich inside of a wave-transmitting device, and when he returned he noticed that his sandwich was hot. The waves had penetrated the food (just like they penetrate elevator walls to reach cell phones) and had transferred their energy to the water molecules in the sandwich, which transformed the energy into heat. Microwaves are electromagnetic waves. This spectrum also includes visible light whose wavelength ranges between about 400 nm (violet) and 700 nm (red) and can be detected by our eyes. Microwaves have much larger wavelengths (e.g., the distance between two successive wave crests) ranging from 1 millimeter to 1 meter. Microwave ovens operate at frequencies of about 2450 million cycles per second, or 2.45 gigahertz (GHz), to avoid interference with other signals used for communications.[20]

Microwave heating is a unique cooking method. Instead of heating food from outside, the microwaves penetrate the food and cause liquid water molecules to oscillate rapidly, generating heat by friction. The heating action is performed by energy that dissipates as microwaves travel through the food. Some materials are transparent to this radiation and do not get hot, while others like metals and some ceramics reflect the waves and stay cool. Foods that contain water let the microwaves pass through them for a few centimeters and heat is generated along their path. From there on, heating in solid foods is mostly by conduction, and that is the reason on/off cycles are recommended when programming a microwave oven. During the period that the oven is off, heat at any hot spot flows by conduction to a colder portion inside the food (Section 6.6).

The microwave oven operates through a device that raises the household current (110 or 220 volts) to around 3000 volts or more. The key component is the magnetron, a vacuum tube that generates microwaves powerful enough to be used for radar and in cell phones. Microwave cooking opens up countless possibilities for food preparation, used alone or in combination with other conventional heating methods (Section 6.6). It is the first heating device in history that is able to heat the interior of a food while keeping the outside cold (if the outside does not absorb the microwaves). This makes it possible to create foods with different layers of "transparency" to the microwaves in order to produce differential heating. This effect would be temporary, because after removing the food from the oven (or turning it off) the heat would flow from high-temperature areas to colder areas by conduction, until the food reached an intermediate temperature throughout. As stated before, this is why short cycles are recommended for cooking food in the microwave, allowing the food to come to equilibration during the periods in between, and preventing water from boiling in certain areas (bursting). This allows time for the heat to transfer by conduction to the parts of the food that absorbed fewer microwaves (such as those containing fat or oil and dry portions). Microwaves are especially useful for rapidly thawing food, by penetrating through the ice and heating the water as the ice melts. Microwave energy passes through ice four times faster than through liquid water.

Some heating methods use waves from other regions of the electro-magnetic spectrum. Infrared heat is produced by the energy emitted in a range of wavelengths greater than the upper limit of the visible light spectrum (which corresponds to the color red), or between 780 nm and 1 mm. Our eyes cannot see infrared waves, but our bodies can feel them as heat. Infrared energy is transferred by radiation to a food's surface (but without penetrating much into the interior of the food), where it causes the surface molecules to vibrate and induces heating. Most home ovens come with an electric grill that heats or browns food with infrared radiation, the same way heat lamps keep food hot.

Using ohmic heat to cook food would be like connecting the food to a socket and electrocuting it.[21] This heat is produced by the action of an electric current, which is transferred into the product through a pair of electrodes. The food acts as an electrical resistance that does not let the current pass and accumulates the resultant energy as heat throughout its volume. Though this method has some commercial applications, modern cooks rarely include it in their repertoire, despite its capability for volumetric heating.

A discussion of the electromagnetic spectrum would not be complete without touching on irradiation, a process in which food is exposed to the radiation energy from extremely small wavelengths: x-rays (0.10 to 10 nm) and gamma rays (<0.1 nm). Food irradiation does not generate heat, but it has a penetrating power that is used to pasteurize and steril-ize cold foods and sterilize foods while keeping them cold (Section 1.12).

6.8 BARBECUE AT THE LAB

Cooking meat can be a "tough" challenge for a cook. There are many different types of meat as well as different cuts from the same animal, all with different qualities. But once the cooked meat is removed from the grill, oven, or pot, the expected result is always the same: it should be tender and juicy. How can we help the cook achieve this?

Going back to Section 2.1, it all starts with the structure of muscle tissue (Figure 2.1, right) and the proteins that compose 80% of its dry weight. Muscle is made up of fibers, as well as the connective tissue that glues the fibers together. Like many other natural foods, cooking meat fits the brick wall analogy: it involves dissolving the cement and softening the bricks (see also cooking of dry beans, Section 3.8).

We will assist the cook doing a small experiment in the lab. Let's take a tiny piece of meat (i.e., few milligrams), place it in a sample holder, and introduce it into a differential scanning calorimeter (DSC) (Section 2.14). With this instrument the temperature change can be set at any constant value (in °C per minute), and the equipment will increase the temperature of the meat at exactly that rate, by continuously and automatically adjusting the heating power. We can't do this in our home kitchen, because our appliances supply a constant amount of heat (set by the knob regulating the gas or electricity in the stove or range), and the temperature is the response. A DSC operates in just the opposite way—it supplies the necessary heat to raise the temperature at a fixed rate.

The output of the experiment, called a *thermogram*, is a tracing like the one in Figure 6.3, consisting of several peaks at different temperatures. Each downward pointing peak indicates where extra heat was introduced to the sample during a certain temperature interval because some "unusual" thermal event took place. The area under the peak is proportional to the amount of heat required (calories per gram of sample) to keep the experiment going at the preset rate. If pure water had been placed in the sample holder, the readout would be a straight, negatively sloping line without any peaks (unless we reached 100°C). In fact, the dotted line in Figure 6.3 is related to the specific heat of the meat, or the amount of heat necessary to raise the temperature of 1 gram of meat when no other thermal phenomena occur (as between 35 and 45°C). This value is around 0.6 and 0.75 cal/g °C.

So far we haven't provided much help for the cook, because raw data mean nothing if not interpreted correctly. The first change that we can observe in the thermogram is a peak at around 30°C, which indicates the heat necessary for fat to melt. From then on a series of peaks begin to superimpose one another because more calories are needed for the globular sarcoplasmic proteins to denature, aggregate, and coagulate,

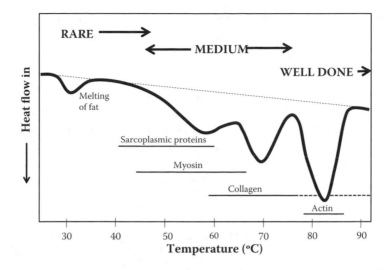

FIGURE 6.3   DIFFERENTIAL SCANNING CALORIMETER (DSC) THERMOGRAM OF MEAT, SHOW-
ING THE RANGE OF TRANSITIONS OF THE DIFFERENT COMPONENTS IN RELATION TO HOW MUCH
THE MEAT IS COOKED.

and so a second peak appears around 45°C. The myofibrillar proteins
in the meat fibers have a wide range of denaturation temperature, starting at around 50°C and ending past 60°C, while collagen (the cement)
denatures between 55 and 65°C as it softens and shrinks. If the animal
is not too old, collagen will form a gel after it denatures (gelatin); if not,
it continues to hold the fibers together which makes the meat tough.
Actin, the other protein in muscle fiber, has a well-defined denaturation
peak that appears between 80 and 86°C. The important conclusion is
that each of these phenomena requires heat, and the DSC thermogram
shows how much heat and when. As noted in Figure 6.3, the culinary
conditions for cooking meat to "rare," "medium," and "well done" are
related to the denaturation of myosin, the denaturation of myosin plus
some connective tissue, and the denaturation of all skeletal proteins,
respectively. This is another important difference between "DSC cooking" and real cooking. "Real" meat pieces are much larger than our
sample, so that during cooking the outside of the meat heats faster than
the interior and the temperature is not uniform. This allows us to cook
our steaks "medium-rare" (seared on the outside but juicy and tender
inside). Incidentally, boiling meat for several hours (like a "pot roast")

is the only way to solubilize the cross-linked connective tissue of old animals.[22] Now is probably a good time to jump to Section 11.14 and read about why chefs cook meat at low temperatures for long periods of time (hours).

The thermogram doesn't show us how the water-holding capacity of the meat proteins decreases as they denature (meat is roughly 75% water), so that valuable meat juices are lost as the temperature increases. This means that you can end up with a tender but dry steak. One chef suggests cooking tough cuts of meats under vacuum for 48 hours at 57°C, instead of the traditional several hours at 80 to 90°C.[23] To determine if that method works, we would need an instrument that could quantify the loss of juiciness by determining changes in the weight of the meat sample in relation to temperature changes. Unfortunately no such instrument exists.[24] The thermogram also doesn't tell us much about color and toughness. The red pigment myoglobin starts turning pink at about 60°C and gray at 75°C, while toughening decreases at around 60°C and then gets worse as temperature increases (largely because of shrinkage of the myofibrils). Because heating is so important in cooking, it's time for cooks to visit the lab and learn what to expect from the other foods they purchased at the market.

NOTES

1. The life of Count Rumford is described in Brown, G.I. 1999. *The Extraordinary Life of a Scientific Genius.* Sutton, Gloucestershire.
2. The original paper is signed as Benjamin Count of Rumford. 1798. An inquiry concerning the source of the heat which is excited by friction. *Philosophical Transactions of the Royal Society of London* 88, 80–102. The text can be accessed through www.jstor.org.
3. The thermos bottle is a fascinating apparatus. If we put hot food inside, the thermos keeps it hot, but if we fill it with a cold drink instead, the drink stays cold. How does it know what to do?
4. Rifkin. J. 1981. *Entropy: A new world view.* Bantam Books, New York.
5. Optimal cooking temperatures (in °F) for meat, poultry, seafood, as well as for the different cooking stages can be found at http://whatscookingamerica.net/Information/MeatTemperatureChart.htm (accessed January 10, 2011).

6. At 600 m altitude water boils at 98°C while at 2500 m the temperature is 92°C, a large difference for cooking an egg for a fixed time.
7. Abdominal fat is visceral if it surrounds the abdominal organs, or subcutaneous if it is located between the skin and abdominal wall. Several studies suggest that visceral fat is more closely associated with risk factors for certain diseases. Magnetic resonance imaging (MRI) can locate and quantify the amount of fat in any part of the body within minutes.
8. There are many Web sites that allow you to determine resting metabolic rate (RMR) based on sex, height, weight, and age.
9. Forty years ago the average daily calories per capita from food adjusted for losses were less than 2400.
10. Spurlock won the Documentary Directing Award at the Sundance Film Festival for *Super Size Me*. The student who made the calculation only earned an "A" on the assignment.
11. This was actually an exam question for one of my courses. Students were required to see the film, plan a daily diet from the McDonald's menu, consult the McDonald's Web site to determine calorie intake, estimate daily physical activity, and calculate the energy balance. On average, their responses predicted a weight gain of 10 to 11 kilos.
12. Protein-rich foods (fish, meat, and eggs) and carbohydrate-rich foods (pasta, rice, beans, wholegrain breads and cereals) are among the most satiating foods. On the contrary, fat-containing foods (french fries, cream cheese, croissants, cakes, and biscuits) exert the weakest effects on both satiation and satiety.
13. Rolls, B.J., and Barnett, R.A. 2005. *The Volumetrics Weight-Control Plan*. HarperTorch, New York.
14. Tannahill, R. 1988. *Food in History*. Crown, New York.
15. Leonard, W.R. 2002. Food for thought: Dietary change was a driving force for evolution. *Scientific American* 287(6),106–115.
16. The term *coctivor* was coined by J. Muth and U. Pullmer in 2010 to describe human beings, based on the theory that people were designed to cook their food. An interesting talk on this topic by H. Watzke can be found at www.ted.com/talks/heribert_watzke_the_brain_in_your_gut. html (accessed January 22, 2012).
17. Schwedt, G. 2004. *Experimentos en la Cocina. La cocción, el asado, el horneado*. Editorial Acribia, Zaragoza. The original book is in German and there is no English version.
18. The word *toast* can be used to mean both toasted bread as well as a verbal tribute. In England, in olden times, if someone wanted to speak at a banquet, he would let everyone know by dipping a piece of toast in his cup

(nowadays we just stand up, rather than contaminating our drink). This custom has also been attributed to the ancient Romans.

19. There are at least two meanings of the Mapuche word *kurantu*: a collection of stones and stones heated by the sun. Both are good descriptions of how food is cooked in a traditional *curanto*.

20. The *electromagnetic spectrum* is the set of waves traveling through the air all around us, which are characterized by their wavelength (λ), frequency, and energy. The electromagnetic waves that are of interest with regard to food include microwaves (λ of the order of centimeters), x-rays (λ of the order of 1 nm), and radiation γ (gamma), which is used for food irradiation. The visible spectrum of light is the range of wavelengths between 350 nm (violet) and 780 nm (red). An outline of the electromagnetic spectrum can be found at http://imagine.gsfc.nasa.gov/docs/science/know_l1/emspectrum.html (accessed January 12, 2012).

21. Do not confuse the word *ohmic* with the suffix *-omics* (as in proteomics or metabolomics). George Ohm (1787–1854), a professor from Munich, related the flow of electric current with voltage and electrical resistance. As the current circulates, the resistance dissipates energy in the form of heat.

22. See more on meat cooking and structured meats (e.g., comminuted meat products) in Dobraszczyk, D.J. 2008. Structured meat products. In *Food Materials Science: Principles and Applications* (J.M. Aguilera and P. Lillford, eds.), Springer, New York, pp. 501–523.

23. See Keller, T. 2008. *Under Presure: Cooking sous vide.* Artisan, Singapore, p. 3.

24. There is a technique called *thermogravimetric analysis* (TGA) that quantifies weight loss as a function of temperature but due to vaporization of compounds. This may help to see losses of water as vapor but not of juices from a piece of meat.

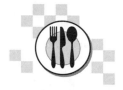

CHAPTER 7

Between Brain and Cell

Food structures must eventually break back down into molecules because these are the units that are needed by our body. Their collapse begins in the mouth, where molecules are released and interact with receptors in the brain, thus unleashing a cascade of sensations. The destruction continues in the digestive system, an essential but relatively complex and unknown reactor that prepares the molecules to enter our body. This closes the food cycle: all starts as molecules created by nature and will be converted back into molecules again (inside our bodies). After completing this chapter you will have one secret: Eat less and enjoy the food more.

7.1 STRUCTURES THAT MUST BE BROKEN

Food is just about the only thing, besides medication, that we put into our mouths and consciously swallow, but unlike pills and other pharmaceutical products, we expect food to taste good. No matter how attractive a meal appears, and even if it is prepared from the highest quality and healthiest ingredients, it still must face a very sensitive and biased judge—the mouth.

Food engineering is somewhat different from the more conventional engineering fields, such as mechanical and structural engineering, that aim for strong, resistant products. Food engineering involves working with soft materials that will end up being broken. A primary goal of mastication is to break up the food so that it can be swallowed. This process also exposes the internal parts of the food and increases the available surface area, releasing flavorful and aromatic molecules.

The chewing process varies greatly among individuals. For example, a serving of peanuts can undergo between 15 and 70 chewing cycles before being swallowed, depending on whether someone wolfs their food or patiently chews it before swallowing. The next process that occurs in the mouth is the lubrication of the particles with saliva, which is also quite variable among individuals. Saliva is essential in food tasting in order to dissolve certain flavors, exposing them to the taste buds (Figure 7.2). Saliva secretion varies from less than 0.2 milliliters to almost 4 milliliters per minute (a milliliter is approximately 15 to 20 drops), depending on the individual. Another important variable is the movement of the bolus of disintegrated food and saliva within the mouth. As the food is exposed to different parts of the oral cavity, the food molecules come in contact with the taste receptors. It is said that people of Asian descent appreciate flavors in a "circular" way, in the sense that food moves all around the mouth to access the appropriate receptors, whereas food tracks in a more linear way (straight to the pharynx) through the mouths of Westerners. All this suggests that the period of time an individual food spends in our mouths—its "residence time"—is very important for the complete perception of its sensory attributes.

While taste has to do with chemistry and molecules, texture is directly associated with food structure and physical characteristics that can be appreciated by the sense of touch. When a panel of blindfolded judges sampled familiar foods that had been ground into the consistency of baby food, a number of the testers failed to recognize the foods by taste alone.[1] When apples are made into juice, most textural properties of the fruit are destroyed so that you can no longer appreciate the crunch of the apple as you chew, or the crisp noise caused by the rupture of the apple's turgid cells as you bite into them. But with texture, everything is relative. *Al dente* noodles (the interior of the pasta is still firm) may mean perfect to an Italian, while others might find that same pasta to be hard and under-cooked (see Section 3.7). The firmness of meat is absolute, yet people differ in how they perceive it. The Inuit are used to eating dried meat and chewing animal skins before stitching them. Any of our meats seem tender to them, as their jaws can exert twice the force as most other people.

The forces generated in our mouths don't need to be as strong as those of the Inuit, because most solid foods contain water or bubbles that make them softer. In addition, the adhesive between the cells of vegetables and meat fibers softens with cooking. Solid food can also fracture easily through the propagation of faults or cracks produced during processing (as happens with some cookies). This latter process is similar to cutting glass: first the glass is scratched with a hard object, creating a fault, so that the glass can be broken with minimal force. Food engineers are very interested in how food breaks down in the mouth (sometimes in odd ways such as licking a lollipop and eroding it with saliva, for example), as this phenomenon is important in the perception of texture. Variations in particle size at several intervals during mastication can give information on certain desirable physical characteristics of a food. A minor complication in these studies is that the tasters must spit out the contents of their mouths at certain time intervals or after a designated number of chewing cycles, in order for the particle size to be determined by sieve analysis or by examination of photographic images.

Heat transfer (cooling or heating) between food and the tongue and palate occurs simultaneously with the mechanical breakdown of the food. In this case, the heating of this results in the melting of certain food components, cocoa butter being one of the most flavorful examples. The rapid change that chocolate undergoes in our mouths (from a solid to a viscous liquid) provides unique sensations, as chocolate fat finishes melting at a temperature just slightly lower than body temperature (36.5°C). Ice also melts in our mouth, and an interesting example of this thermal effect is the sequential release of flavor from a scoop of vanilla, chocolate, and pistachio ice cream. Initially we taste vanilla as the ice melts and releases the vanillin first, which is soluble in water. The milk fat, which contains the liposoluble pistachio and chocolate flavors, takes longer to melt and so these flavors are appreciated a bit later.[2]

The mouth is the entry point into the digestive system—the place where chewing occurs, where odors and flavors are released, where we appreciate the texture of food, and where the changes in structure occur before impending digestion. Because of all of this, understanding what happens in our mouths when we eat is high on the agenda of food researchers.

7.2 MOLECULES ON THE MOVE

Few things are more pleasant than the aroma of freshly brewed coffee in the morning. In order for us to enjoy this phenomenon, about 800 types of aromatic molecules must be released from inside the particles of roasted coffee beans, extracted in hot water and get transported through the air to our noses. The perception of aroma in our nose depends on two factors: the concentration of the aromatic compound in the air and the odor threshold of each type of molecule. Concentration has to do with the number of odoriferous molecules per unit volume, while threshold is the stimulus level at which an odor can be perceived. This combination means that when molecules with a very low detection threshold are present in a low concentration, we may still be able to "smell" them more easily than a higher concentration of molecules with a high stimulus level. Even gas chromatography analysis, which can separate, identify, and measure the amount of many of the aromatic chemical compounds in coffee, is not sufficient to describe their perception in the nose because of these stimulus-level properties.

Engineers define as *mass transfer* the phenomenon by which individual molecules move from one place to another, which will be discussed with reference to frying in Section 8.7. Dehydration, the escape of water molecules from wet solids, reduction, or the evaporation of some water from soups, and extraction of sugar from beets, are all operations involving mass transfer. Molecules in any medium will move spontaneously from where they are most highly concentrated into areas where they are less concentrated, until they reach equilibrium and the concentration in space becomes uniform. This phenomenon is called *diffusion*. Adolph Fick (1829–1901) proposed that the flow of molecules is proportional to the concentration gradient (difference in concentration between two points divided by distance).[3] This relationship, known as Fick's *First Law of Diffusion*, is very important in engineering, biological sciences, and food processing. This is the reason why water vapor migrates from wet food (where it is more concentrated) to dry air (low concentration) during dehydration. In contrast, the water molecules in humid air congregate on unprotected dry cookies and potato chips, making them soft and less crisp. Diffusion is also the relevant phenomenon involved in the salting of cheeses and hams, the distillation of spirits, the wetting of tea bags, and even the mating of insects attracted to pheromones.[4]

There is another event, independent of concentration, which also causes the molecules to move from one place to another, but should not be confused with diffusion. Convection is the displacement of large masses of fluid due to differences in pressure or temperature. When a soup is heated on a burner, currents are created in the liquid from the temperature differences inside the pan. The exhaust vent removes molecules from the kitchen because the blower creates a lower pressure (suction) in the outlet pipe. Air pollution is transported over long distances mainly by winds, while diffusion plays a very minor role. As discussed in Section 7.6, the process of nutrient absorption in the intestine makes use of several diffusion mechanisms for the transport of the molecules into the body.

The *diffusion coefficient*, or diffusivity (D), is the characteristic parameter for the diffusion process, and it represents how easy it is for a molecule to move in a given medium. In traffic terms, a motorcycle has a greater diffusivity in a jammed highway than an automobile as it can slide through the slow-moving cars. When things get back to normal both face a similar condition. In foods, the diffusion coefficient is a unique characteristic of each type of molecule and the type of matrix in which it moves (Figure 7.1). *Ceteris paribus*, a high diffusivity is synonymous with a greater flow of molecules. For example, the makers of perfume have the advantage that fragrance molecules are small and volatile and can move swiftly throughout a thin medium (like air), so people perceive them quickly. These aromatic perfume molecules, as well as those in the aroma of coffee, have a high D value in air (Figure 7.1).

But the manufacturers of food flavorings do not want their aromatic molecules to escape until they are right under our noses. As ingredients,

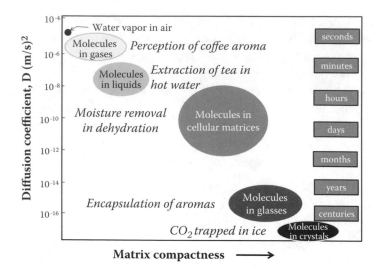

FIGURE 7.1   THE RATE AT WHICH MOLECULES DIFFUSE DEPENDS ON THE MATRIX WHERE THE MOVEMENT OCCURS. APPROXIMATE VALUES OF DIFFUSION COEFFICIENTS OF MOLECULES IN DIFFERENT MEDIA AND THEIR RELEVANCE IN CERTAIN FOOD PROCESSES. NOTE THAT THE SCALE IS LOGARITHMIC AND THAT THE EXPONENTS OF 10 ARE NEGATIVE (E.G., 10^{-4} IS 1 DIVIDED BY 10^4 OR 0.0001). THE HIGHER THE VALUE OF D, THE "FASTER" THE MOLECULE WILL MOVE IN THAT MEDIUM (RIGHT).

aromas are "encapsulated" inside the dense matrix of a sugar glass (and look like a powder), delaying their release until the precise moment when the matrix dissolves in water or saliva. Encapsulated aromas are trapped and show a very low diffusivity through the matrix, as shown in the bottom of Figure 7.1. This figure also depicts the wide range of mobility that molecules can have depending on the type of food matrix (structure) in which they are dispersed, be it gas, liquid, rubber, glass, or crystal (see Section 2.3 and below). Molecules of different sizes trapped inside the same compound may be released at different speeds (or not be released at all) depending on their D value. Regarding the matrix, it is possible to find a particular food ingredient, such as sucrose, in a molecular solution (syrup), as a rubber (toffee), in a glassy form (cotton candy), or as a crystal (table sugar). Explosive candy is pressurized CO_2 captured inside a glassy sugar matrix and it will remain as such because of its low diffusivity in such a compact structure; however, the same gas will readily escape from a sugar solution such as a soda. A cappuccino coffee powder develops a wonderful foam when hot water is added, because the water rapidly dissolves the glassy matrix of particles that contain a gas trapped at a high pressure. The sudden release of gas generates abundant bubbles that produce the foam.

Air gets trapped as minute bubbles in ice during the freezing of ice popsicles (or ice pops) with no apparent consequences. But the relevance of gas bubbles being trapped in ice crystals (bottom of Figure 7.1) is that by drilling ice cores in Antarctica scientists have been able to determine the composition of air as far as 500,000 years ago. They can then study the correspondence between climate change and the CO_2 concentration in the atmosphere through time.

In the end, the molecules must escape from their food matrices, either to be perceived in the mouth and nose, or to become available so they are absorbed in the intestine. The latter is of great importance because a chemical compound does not become a nutrient until it is released from the food and can be processed and absorbed in the digestive tract (Section 7.6). A pertinent example is that of polyphenol antioxidants in grapes. The crushing of grapes releases polyphenols from the cells, and maceration in the presence of the skins facilitates diffusion of polyphenols into the juice, as occurs during the making of red wine. These processes explain why the polyphenol content of red wine is 10 times higher than that of white wine (which is not macerated), and is also higher than that of grape juice.[5] Sometimes food processing does things better than our mouth and gut.

The First Law of Diffusion, like the First Law of Thermodynamics, does not address the effect of time. So, there is a Fick's *Second Law of Diffusion*, which allows for the calculation of the concentration profile of molecules in the interior of a product that is incorporating or losing a certain component over time (e.g., a piece of cod that is immersed in brine or a portion of salt cod being desalted in pure water). Intuition tells us that the outside edges of a product will first notice the entry (or exit) of the molecules and that the center will be the last to experience the phenomenon. Refer back to Figure 3.5 and corroborate visually how the diffusion of hot water into pasta during cooking proceeds slowly from the outside to the center.

In fact, this second law is identical to the law that governs heat transfer by conduction, or Fourier's law. In this case, Fourier's law shows the profile of temperatures within a body being heated (Section 6.6), which varies from hot in the external areas to cold in the center (cooling has the reverse profile). This is why a steak can be at the same time cooked on the outside and raw in the center. An important equation is derived from Fick's second law, which is used to estimate a representative time for the advance of the molecules in a medium when they move by diffusion:

$$t_{c=1/2} = \frac{x^2}{2D}$$

where $t_{c=1/2}$ is the elapsed time (in seconds) from the beginning of the process until the concentration at x is equal to half the concentration at the point where molecules started and x (in meters) is the distance traveled by the molecules. D, of course, is the diffusivity of the molecules in the medium in which they move. When applied to aromas and food, this formula makes it possible to estimate how much time will elapse from when you open the oven door in the kitchen until the smell of the roast arrives in the dining room (as long as you omit the convection of air in the home). It also states that diffusion is a slow process (given the low values of D), so be sure to stir your coffee with a spoon if you want the sugar to dissolve before the coffee cools. Don't forget that in order for the molecules to diffuse, they must escape from the matrices that trap them in the food and begin a journey into unoccupied space. We will see more about how molecules move after digestion when they are ready to leave the intestine and enter our cells (Section 7.6). Thereafter and since diffusion is such a slow process (but quite selective), our body uses convection and a potent pump—the heart—to rapidly propel the nourishment of cells (also known as bulk flow). Molecular diffusion, a more selective transport mechanism, will be utilized again to let the right metabolites enter the cells of the different organs.

7.3 FOOD IN THE MOUTH
AND IN THE NOSE

Most food connoisseurs appreciate the work of a great chef who can create a progression of sensory effects that complement one another and develop over the course of the meal. But when we consider that hundreds or even thousands of different kinds of small molecules are responsible for the tastes and aromas of food, we wonder how we can possibly discriminate between them.

The concept of *flavor* combines the experiences of taste and smell, and in this sense the word flavor is used often in this book, although flavor is often confused with taste. *Taste* has to do with the properties of certain molecules to elicit taste sensations on the tongue and palate, or to trigger smell in the nose. It comes from the sensations produced in the mouth by certain nonvolatile components, which are solubilized in saliva. The perception of a food's taste occurs when the protein receptors in the cells of the taste buds (which already exist in the fifth month of gestation) are activated by reversible interactions with sapid molecules, much in the same way a key fits tightly and uniquely into the lock of a door. This coupling between a molecule and the receiver generates an electrical signal that is transmitted to the brain via the gustatory nerves. The brain "reads" these signals and determines if the food is bitter, sweet, salty, acidic, or savory. It is possibly false that taste cells have evolved to ensure that we eat things that keep us healthy and reject foods that could poison us, but most toxic substances do not taste good.

Contrary to popular belief, the tongue does not have specified zones that recognize certain tastes, but there are greater numbers of specific types of receptors in certain sections of the tongue and oral cavity. There are five basic taste sensations: sweet (sugar), salty (salt), sour (lemon), bitter (quinine), and *umami* (savory). The latter was characterized by Japanese scientists and is related to the enhancement and increased "fullness" of certain flavors. Monosodium glutamate (MSG) and some nucleotides provide umami taste.[6] Meats and their juices, soy sauce, Parmesan and other pungent cheeses, some seaweed, anchovies, tomatoes, and mushrooms all have umami flavor. Chefs take advantage of these characteristics and enjoy combining ingredients to develop their unique "tasty melodies."

The molecules that we are able to smell are volatile—under environmental conditions they disperse in a gaseous phase like air. In physicochemical terms, the molecules have a high vapor pressure and seek to escape from the liquid state into the air, where they can have more mobility (Figure 7.1). We first perceive the scent of our food directly through the nose by sniffing, even before it enters our mouth (Section 7.2). This pathway of perception is known as *orthonasal* detection. Once the molecules are released from the food during mastication, they can move more freely and dissolve in air. This allows them to reach the nose quickly through small currents that convey odoriferous molecules dispersed in air from the back of our mouths into the nasal passages. This second pathway of perception involving the travel of odor molecules from the mouth to the nostrils is known as *retronasal* smell and appears to be the main mechanism by which we perceive odor during eating. Don't forget that while we are chewing we are also breathing.

Odoriferous substances carried by air currents from the mouth to the nose interact with the olfactory receptors in a slightly different way than sapid substances combine with taste receptors. It appears that molecules are trapped in a binding pocket rather than in a tight cavity, resulting in a broader spectrum of associations. Nevertheless, a minimum number of molecules is necessary to produce a perceptible stimulus (the *detection threshold*, Section 7.2), but only some molecules have a chemical structure that elicits an odoriferous response. Water molecules, for instance, produce no recognizable stimuli (or smell), despite the fact that they are volatile and abundant in the air, and many reach the nose. The olfactory region of the nose is called the olfactory mucosa and has 10 to 20 million olfactory receptor cells equipped with receptor proteins for odor molecules. As should be clear by now, the olfactory receptor proteins are encoded by olfactory receptor genes, a discovery that won the 2004 Nobel Prize in Physiology for Richard Axel and Linda Buck. Throughout our evolution we have lost a large number of the genes that encode the formation of olfactory receptor proteins, and today we have less than 1,000 in our genome. Signals from the olfactory cells are transported by the olfactory nerve to an area below the front of the base of the brain called the *olfactory bulb*. There the corresponding synapses occur, sending impulses to the cerebral cortex, which then generates the response that we identify as smell.

While the messages of the five basic taste sensations (which are hardwired from birth) flow directly to our brains, flavor is constructed into patterns by associating the flavors with signals received from the sense of smell. These interactions set up patterns of activity in the brain that translate into "flavor images," which are the basis for perception of flavor and are analogous to the images of the visual world (Figure 7.2). Interestingly, scientists are discovering that flavors in food and addictive drugs activate similar brain mechanisms.

It must be emphasized that the perception of tastes and odors starts at the molecular level, and in order for that to happen, the molecules must be released from inside the food (or drink) and presented to the respective receptors. Figure 7.2 attempts to summarize the temporal events related to the perception of taste and smell. The velocity of the

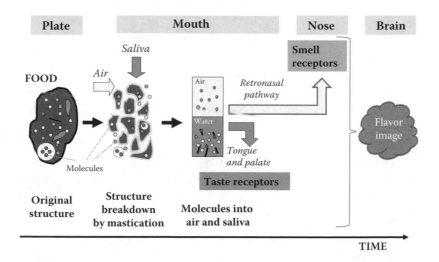

FIGURE 7.2 A TIME-SPACE DIAGRAM FOR FLAVOR PERCEPTION IN THE MOUTH AND NOSE. THE MOLECULES THAT CONTRIBUTE TO THE FLAVOR (TASTE AND ODOR) OF A FOOD MUST BE RELEASED FROM THE FOOD MATRIX SO THAT AIR AND SALIVA WILL CARRY THEM, ACCORDING TO THEIR PARTICULAR AFFINITY (PARTITION) AND DIFFUSIVITY, TO THE RECEPTORS IN THE NOSE AND TONGUE.

molecules (related to the diffusivity D, Section 7.2) provides chefs with a unique opportunity to create symphonies of tastes and smells by taking advantage of the fact that the molecules trapped within food matrices can be released at different times. Figure 7.2 may appear complicated, but it demonstrates how the tastes and scents from a morsel of food finally combine in a unique and personal arpeggio after the period of time it remains in the mouth.

But not all food perception takes place in the mouth and nose. The senses of sight and hearing are also involved. Chefs know this well and place great emphasis on the visual presentation of their dishes and may even consider the sounds emitted during mastication of different foods (Section 11.7). The trigeminal nerve has three branches that innervate both sides of the face, adding tactile, thermal, chemical, and pain sensitivity to the perceptions of smell and taste.

7.4 EXPERT AND ELECTRONIC NOSES

There can be a surprising number of versions of the same food product, and some people are able distinguish very subtle differences among them. Thanks to refined tastes, tradition, and even legend, certain fundamental elaborations have evolved into different kinds of the same product. There are over two thousand varieties of cheese recognized worldwide, all derived from about 20 basic types, which are prepared according to similar processes. One current example of this phenomenon of differentiation is the appellation of origin, which identifies a product as originating in a particular country, region, or locality, where certain natural, historical, or human factors have become characteristic of the product.

The book *Salumi d'Italia*, for example, contains photos and descriptions of more than 250 Italian hams and salamis, whose differentiations arise from the great culinary culture of the Italians.[8] The *Culatello* is the quintessential cured ham from Parma and is prepared by artisans from the thinnest and most tender back section of the pork leg. A *Culatello di Zibello* does not exceed 4 or 5 kilos but costs more than 100 euros per kilo. In addition to its tender texture, the *Culatello* is famous for its delicious fragrance that is said to come from the pigs' natural diet, careful handling during the salt curing process, and the favorable climate conditions of the region around Parma, ideal for the long curing that lasts more than a year. The Spanish Iberian ham is notable as well, prized around the world for its aroma and flavor. The best of the Iberian hams is the "acorn ham," which comes from pigs that have been fed a diet of antioxidant-rich acorns, which protect the fat from oxidation.[9] During the maturation of a *Culatello* ham, the process and development of aromas is carefully managed by a master "ham *sommellier*," who occasionally introduces a needle-sharp horse bone into the fatty areas (in the fat are the largest contributors to the flavor) and takes a sniff. His expert nose is able to recognize the desirable aromatic characteristics that are produced by the biochemical processes of maturation and only he knows why a bone from a horse is necessary. But the magic behind this ancient practice is threatened by the use of modern electronic instruments that attempt to measure these same sensory characteristics that our mouths and noses appreciate so easily (Section 2.14).[10]

An electronic nose may sound like an implant from the Six Million Dollar Man, but it is an actual instrument, capable of detecting and characterizing odors in a manner that approximates what our noses can do. These devices are equipped with sensors whose surfaces react with volatile molecules, generating an electrical signal that is transmitted to a processor that identifies the type and quantity of molecules present. Although an odor may encompass hundreds or thousands of substances, these devices make use of only a dozen sensors at a time, such as semiconductors of oxidized metals, quartz microbalances, and superficial acoustic waves.[11] In the laboratory, gas chromatography coupled with mass spectrometry (GC-MS) equipment is also used to separate odoriferous compounds according to their molecular weight or affinity with specific adsorbents. The readout is a sequence of several peaks of different sizes, each one corresponding to a different substance. The data are then analyzed by computer algorithms to see if there are correlations between the concentration of molecules (area under a peak) with the perceived strengths of different odors. In the future, electronic noses may enter the kitchen and help to evaluate spoiled products much in the same way we do when we sniff a suspicious food but with much lower levels of detection and specificity.

There are also electronic tongues made of an array of chemical sensors that are capable of determining the composition and recognizing the taste of various natural food substances. However, the results from the electronic noses, electronic tongues, and GC-MS instruments do not always match what our senses appreciate. Our senses of taste and smell are still much more sophisticated than any of these modern devices.

7.5 A WELL-FED BRAIN

People who feel good and enjoy positive emotions appear to live longer lives. In 1930, young nuns were asked to write personal essays about their lives for a study on aging. In 2001, these writings were reviewed by psychologists who classified them according to moments of happiness, love, and hope. The now famous *Nun Study*, which inspired the positive psychology movement, revealed that those nuns who expressed more positive emotions in their writings lived 10 years longer than those who expressed more negative emotions. This increase in life expectancy resulting from a positive attitude may be even greater than the increase attributed to smoking cessation.[12]

It is not easy to find a definition of wellness or well-being in the context of nutrition and health. Part of the problem is that health is already defined as "a state of complete physical, mental and social well-being." But it is clear that the concept of overall well-being is broader than health and includes other facets of human life, such as the ability to correctly express and manage one's feelings, interest in knowledge and creativity, work satisfaction, social recognition, and good spousal, family, and societal relationships. For the context of this book, well-being is equivalent to "feeling good in life."

How can foods contribute to well-being? While health is normally associated with the body and is somewhat quantifiable, well-being is more related to what happens in the mind, which is subjective and more difficult to assess. From a neurobiology standpoint, what we eat does influence brain behavior and the neurotransmitters that regulate its operation. Accordingly, we should theoretically be able to follow the effects of the food we eat by following the subsequent neural signals that are transmitted to and from the brain. In reality this is quite impossible, as the active connections or synapses between neurons occur at a rate of 10 quadrillion (10^{16}) of connections per second. It would require something like a million Intel Pentium computer processors (which take up a lot of space) and several hundred megawatts of energy for their operation to achieve something equivalent outside of the body.

In fact, there are very few food molecules that are known to directly affect behavior. One of them is caffeine, an important component in energy drinks, which is related to states of animation like alertness and fatigue. Certain effects in the brain that result from eating can be measured, however, using newly developed techniques. Functional brain imaging allows visualization of the regions of the brain that are involved or activated when an individual prepares to eat, smells and tastes food, and during digestion. There are two preferred techniques for these purposes which are commonly used in medicine and research: positron emission tomography (PET) and functional magnetic resonance imaging (fMRI). Both use images to show blood flow changes in regions of the brain in response to a stimulus, or the increase in brain activity. Thus, it is possible to study responses to the intake of certain foods in the brains of obese subjects, or locate the precise place in the brain that is affected by the consumption of a food associated with positive (or negative) emotions (Figure 7.3).[13]

Food selection plays important cultural, social, and physiological roles. Understanding how the brain works in relation to food choices means unraveling how people assign a reward value to a food product, above and beyond its intrinsic properties. This facet of consumer behavior is a topic of great relevance to the food industry and health authorities because of its relation to eating habits and eating disorders (obesity, for example). Information from neuroscience labs is pouring out daily. In one study using fMRI it was shown that two areas of the brain of individuals who make healthy food choices were activated sequentially: one that assigned a hedonic value to the food (e.g., based on its flavor), and a second one that took into consideration the long-term consequences (healthiness). People that chose unhealthy foods exhibited a dampened brain activity in the second area involving long-term effects (i.e., they

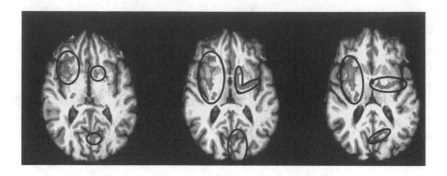

FIGURE 7.3   SET OF SECTIONS OBTAINED BY fMRI AT DIFFERENT HEIGHTS OF THE CERE-
BRAL CORTEX OF THE AUTHOR'S BRAIN, SHOWING THREE AREAS THAT ARE ACTIVATED BY
EATING CHOCOLATE. (COURTESY OF G. ROJAS AND M. GÁLVEZ, CLÍNICA LAS CONDES,
SANTIAGO. WITH PERMISSION.) (A MUCH-QUOTED ARTICLE DESCRIBING THE POSITRON
EMISSION TOMOGRAPHY [PET] DETECTION OF THE BRAIN REGIONS THAT RESPOND TO THE
PLEASANT SENSATION THAT OCCURS IN ANTICIPATION OF THE CONSUMPTION OF CHOCOLATE
IS SMALL, D.M., ZATORRE, R.J., DAGHER, A., EVANS, A.C., AND JONES-GOTMAN, M.
2001. CHANGES IN BRAIN ACTIVITY RELATED TO EATING CHOCOLATE: FROM PLEASURE TO
AVERSION. *BRAIN* 124, 1720–1733.)

had little or no self-control over eating).[14] Another recent investigation
suggested that overweight/obese individuals made poorer food choices
than lean people make, due to impairment in cognitive functions (e.g.,
those related to decision making) that might be the result of a reduced
volume of the orbitofrontal cortex (the frontal area of the brain immediately above the cavities containing the eyes).[15] A rapid conclusion from
these and other data provided by neuroscientists is that overweight/
obesity may have a component that is hardwired in our brains.

The prefix *neuro* is trendy in food research (and in the rest of science
as well). First it is *neurogastronomy* or how the brain creates the sensations from eating a food.[16] Then is food *neuroeconomics*, the elucida-
tion of the decision-making mechanisms in the brain as they relate
to food choices. Last is *food neurogenetics* that contributes to a better
understanding of food-related behaviors due to interactions between
neural substrates, genes, and internal and external environments. As
mentioned before, the regulation of food intake (Section 6.5) and the
networks involved in the hedonic perception (gratification)[17] will be
active areas of investigation with regard to food and the brain.

To close this section, reference must be made to a term representing all those macrofactors that influence our eating behavior. The expression *obesogenic environment* refers to "an environment that promotes gaining weight and one that is not conducive to weight loss, within the home or workplace."[18] One example of the obesogenic environment is the advertisement and "induced purchases" of unhealthy food. In fact, some people think it is ironic that chronic food-related illnesses are referred to as "nontransmissible" when the direct cause of them— an elevated consumption of food having high levels of fat, sugar, and salt—is so effectively "transmitted," particularly to children, through advertisement in the media, promotions, and induced purchases.

7.6 BACK TO MOLECULES: DIGESTION

There is a saying that goes "to make an omelet, you have to break some eggs," meaning that in order to obtain certain desirable results, you must sometimes be willing to destroy something else, without regret. The same goes for food. Although it is true that we eat food structures, our body requires molecules to function. In order to replace tissues and provide energy, the bolus of food structures that passes through the esophagus must be broken down in the stomach and small intestine, and the released small molecules must be absorbed, or they will pass on through. From an engineering standpoint, digestion is a fascinating topic that brings us to the frontier of our knowledge. Allowing for a certain amount of license, the digestive system can be assumed to function as a series of reactors; in fact, as an extremely versatile biochemical reactor. Considering that each meal brings different proportions of ingested food with diverse chemical compositions and structures, it is amazing that after digestion the same basic molecules are always delivered: amino acids, sugars, monoglycerides, and fatty acids.[19]

Food is made up of heterogeneous structures that contain nutrients in complex forms, a system that is much more complicated than a vitamin pill dissolving in a glass of water. During digestion, nutrients must be released from the tissues of plants and animals, or from the structures formed during processing and cooking, which nutrition experts and food technologists now call the *food matrix*.

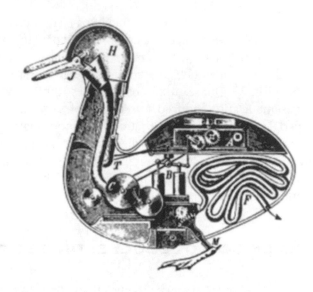

FIGURE 7.4   THE VAUCANSON DUCK (1739), WHICH ATE AND DEFECATED AUTO-
MATICALLY, SYMBOLIZES THE SIMPLISTIC UNDERSTANDING OF THE DIGESTIVE PROCESS HELD
BY MANY SCIENTISTS.

Historically the process of digestion has been undervalued and over-simplified. For Hippocrates, digestion was nothing more than a second cooking session, this time with human body heat. In one extreme example of reductionism, in 1739 Jacques de Vaucanson devised a mechanical duck that supposedly ate and metabolized grain, and even defecated (Figure 7.4). It was obviously a fraud, but it sparked debate among physiologists about whether digestion was a chemical or mechanical process.[20] Today it is well understood that the digestive tract is the second most complex organ of our body (after the brain), an extraordinary defensive barrier against rotten or contaminated food, a harbor for a symbiotic bacterial ecosystem, and a direct connection between our bodies and the external environment.

Digestion has been described in many nutrition books as a relatively simple process, in which large molecules must be cut by enzymes (hydrolyzed) into smaller molecules that can be absorbed and then metabolized by the cells. What has been overlooked until recently is the fact that in order for hydrolysis to occur, the large molecules must have been previously released from the matrices where they are located in food. Even at the molecular level, certain forms of chemical compounds are more accessible by enzymes than others. The beta-lactoglobulin in milk is more digestible when it is denatured than in its original or native state (see Section 2.4). Absorption is not a simple process and compounds like lycopene are better absorbed in the cis configuration (as opposed to the trans configuration), because they fit into the molecular "cages" called *micelles* that are spontaneously produced from the monoglycerides released by digestion (see Section 1.2 and Appendix for more on *cis* and *trans*). Micelles are efficient transporters of nutrients to the lining of the small intestine. The restructuring of the food components and the molecular interactions during digestion are actively being investigated in academia and industry as they may be as important in nutrition as the nutrients themselves.

It is useful to briefly review the process of *digestion*, which begins in the mouth, continues in the stomach, and ends in the small and large intestines. In the first reactor (the mouth), where the pH is close to 6, food structures undergo a partial disintegration as a result of chewing. Despite the short time that food spends in the mouth, much of the starch that is already degraded by the processing can be further solubilized and hydrolyzed by the amylase in saliva (e.g., to shorter molecules called dextrins, Section 1.13). This can be observed outside of the mouth by leaving a starchy snack in contact with saliva. The lingual enzyme lipase also has a small reductive action on triglycerides. The action of chewing is very important for breaking down the cell walls of plant material, because unlike herbivores, the human digestive system cannot rupture the plant cell walls farther along in the process. For example, studies have shown that incompletely chewed almonds have many intact cells that pass right through the digestive system unabsorbed and end up in the stool.

The second reactor is the stomach, which operates at a quite acidic pH, between 1 and 2, causing the denaturation and coagulation of some proteins. The enzyme pepsin hydrolyzes the accessible proteins, breaking them down into peptides and amino acids. The fats end up in an emulsified state, either because they were emulsified in the food (e.g., as in mayonnaise) or because the stomach movements break down the oil phase into small droplets ranging from less than 1 micron to about 100 microns. Gastric lipase hydrolyzes triglycerides, generating fatty acids, monoglycerides, and glycerol (Section 1.2 and Appendix). However, if the oil droplets are coated with proteins or polysaccharides, the access of the gastric lipase to the triglycerides is slowed or partially hindered.

The third reactor is the small intestine, which functions at a pH between 6.8 and 7.5. The final breakdown of food into potentially absorbable units occurs here. In the small intestine, starch is split into glucose molecules by the enzyme alpha-amylase. Some polysaccharides reach the colon (large intestine) intact, such as cellulose, pectins, galactomannans, and glucans (part of dietary fiber), because they are resistant to degradation and therefore slow the transit through the intestine. Later these polysaccharides can be fermented and converted into volatile fatty acids by the kilogram of bacteria that reside in the large intestine. Pancreatic enzyme lipase continues the hydrolysis of the surviving triglycerides (unless it is inhibited by the drug *Xenical*®, thus reducing the digestion and absorption of triglycerides). The enzyme trypsin concludes the breakdown of proteins, liberating more amino acids and some peptides.

The fourth reactor is the large intestine, which harbors the bacterial flora that are responsible for metabolizing not-yet-digested carbohydrates and proteins, as well as the cells that are shed from the intestinal mucosa. The products of bacterial metabolism and much of the water are absorbed here. Finally, the rectum stores everything that was not digested and prepares for the evacuation of the feces.

Once food has been broken back down into molecules, the molecules must reach the wall of the small intestine in order to be absorbed. Some molecules must travel in an aqueous medium, which is not ideal for those that are hydrophobic (don't like water). Vitamin E is not soluble in water and requires the simultaneous presence of fat in order to reach the intestinal wall. If you take a vitamin E capsule at breakfast and then consume two pieces of buttered toast, your absorption of vitamin E is 60% higher than it would be if you ate breakfast cereal with skim milk instead. Similar studies have shown that the same amount of fat in different foods results in different rates of absorption of vitamin E.[21] The likely explanation is that the properties of the foods that are consumed with the vitamin affect retention time in the stomach. It is known that high-fiber foods containing protein are more viscous and retard gastric emptying, allowing more time for an emulsion to form which can safely carry vitamin E to the intestine. In order to be absorbed, this vitamin must travel to the intestinal wall inside lipid vesicles or micelles, true molecular "cages" formed by monoglycerides, with a hydrophilic exterior and a hollow hydrophobic core (Section 2.2). This mechanism is similar to the transport of lycopene discussed earlier in this section. As will be concluded later, proper nutrition requires more than the presence of a single nutrient, and several cooperative mechanisms may be needed to get the nutrients into our cells.The absorption of nutrients in the epithelium lining the small intestine, essential for their incorporation into the cells, is quite complex and includes some of the following mechanisms: (a) movement across differences in concentration or diffusion (see Section 7.2); (b) enzyme-mediated transport against a concentration gradient; (c) facilitated diffusion, which involves using a carrier molecule to operate against a concentration gradient; and, (d) endocytosis, in which the cell directly absorbs nutrients by engulfing them within its membrane and moving them into its interior (e.g., in the case of some lipids). Note that mechanisms (b) and (c) are contrary to the laws of diffusion that act under the impetus of a concentration gradient. The advancement from a lower concentration to a greater concentration requires external help (and therefore energy).

We can conclude several important things from the preceding paragraphs: (a) digestion is a much more complex process than previously thought and food structures play an important role; (b) the accessibility of many nutrients to enzymatic action depends on their timely release from the food matrix; (c) the absorption of certain nutrients requires the simultaneous presence of other compounds (synergy) or dissolution and transport in an appropriate phase; and (d) if the foods are structured in certain way it would be possible to adequately protect some molecules or microorganisms from the stomach's action so that they could later be released more slowly in the intestine. This is why probiotic microorganisms are "encapsulated" in protective matrices, so that they will still be viable when they arrive at the intestine. We are just beginning to understand the effect of food structure on nutrition (see Section 7.9) as well as the additional food "structuring" that occurs within the digestive system.

Meanwhile, engineers and scientists lead the way in an attempt to design a modern version of the Vaucanson duck. Laboratory digestive systems made of peristaltic pumps, transparent plastic tubes, and permeable membranes try to simulate the physical effects and chemical reactions that take place in model foods during digestion. The plastic "stomachs" can even simulate real muscular contractions and their effect on food breakdown, while software controls the doses of gastric juices. The idea is to better understand in the laboratory how different food structures are processed in the digestive system and how the released nutrients become absorbed or interact between them, before doing experiments with humans.[22]

7.7 STARCH GETS TO THE BLOOD

Starch is the main source of energy in most diets. Under normal circumstances, starch is quickly split into glucose, which is absorbed into the blood and distributed to the different tissues. In previous sections we have seen how the starch is synthesized in nature and accumulates in the form of small granules that swell with water and partially dissolve during cooking (Section 2.4). Now we will see how it is digested. Like all chemical reactions, digestion occurs at the rate in which molecules are converted into other molecules. In the case of starch, the kinetics of its digestion and conversion to glucose depends on the type (origin) of starch, the degree of cooking, and the food matrix in which it is found. Our understanding of these relationships has increased greatly in the past 20 years.

Section 5.4 shows how to calculate the glycemic index (GI) that measures the extent to which a certain amount of complex carbohydrates (usually 50 g) are transformed into sugars during digestion. In practice, the GI allows us to rank foods on a scale, assigning an arbitrary GI value of 100 for white bread as a reference. The scale ranges from carbohydrates with low GI (<55) that release glucose slowly to those with a high GI (>75) that are rapidly digested.[23] The concentration of glucose in the blood is regulated by insulin, and the amount of insulin released from the pancreas depends in turn on the amount of glucose in the blood. When starches are digested quickly, a large amount of insulin is released and stays in the blood, producing hunger a short time later and increasing the need to eat food again (Section 6.5). High levels of blood sugar over prolonged periods of time increase the risk of developing type 2 diabetes and cardiovascular disease, as well as weight gain.[24]

Until recent years, complex carbohydrates such as the abundant starch in bread, potatoes, rice, and pasta, were included in the recommendations for a healthy diet, and were even located at the base of the U.S. Department of Agriculture (USDA) Food Pyramid (Section 12.6). But the increase in type 2 diabetes (it is estimated that by 2025 some 300 million adults will be diagnosed with this disease worldwide) has moved starches onto the same blacklist as certain fats, given their effects on the GI. Type 2 diabetes is caused when the body lacks the proper insulin response to move glucose from the blood into the cells. As a result, the blood sugar concentration reaches abnormally high levels (hyperglycemia) that can cause arterial hypertension, damage to blood vessels that irrigate the legs and feet, stroke, high cholesterol, cataracts and glaucoma, among other ailments. Bread is the most common starch-containing food in most Western diets and is quite high in calories. One slice of white bread (25 grams) contains 67 kcal, while a croissant (50 g) provides almost three times as many calories due to the fat content (some of which are saturated fats).

Starch occurs in many forms and not all of them are digested in the same way. From a nutritional standpoint, the starches are classified into three groups: rapidly digestible starch (RDS), slowly digestible starch (SDS), and resistant starch (RS). The rate at which the starch is converted into sugar during digestion depends on the accessibility of the digestive enzymes to the amylose and amylopectin chains in order to transform them into glucose. Figure 5.3 shows typical postprandial kinetics of sugar released into the blood by different types of starch. If a fraction of starch does not undergo digestion in the small intestine (e.g., RS) and is therefore not converted into glucose, it ends up being consumed by intestinal bacteria and converted into short-chain fatty acids (some of which may not be highly desirable). This is good news in a way, because the absorption of short-chain fatty acids produced by bacterial starch degradation provides only 2 kcal/g of energy, half the amount released by RDS and SDS starches. Moreover, RS along with other nondigestible polysaccharides are considered dietary fiber, which means they decrease the insulin and glucose concentration of the blood plasma, and generate a positive effect on satiety.

The structure that a starchy food acquires during processing plays a fundamental role in the release of sugar during digestion and its possible role as RS. Processing and cooking induce swelling and partial rupture of starch granules, a process called gelatinization (Section 3.5), thus preparing them for digestion by enzymes. In general, smaller granules of gelatinized starch are digested faster than larger ones. Food products formed by extrusion, like some "puffed" snacks, in which the starch granules have been almost completely degraded to dextrins, have a high GI because amylases find a ready access to the molecules. Noodles, by comparison, have starch granules that are surrounded by a strong protein matrix (gluten) that restricts their expansion during cooking (Section 3.7 and Figure 2.6) and later physically limit the accessibility of the intestinal enzymes. As a result, there is less hydrolysis of starch during the digestion of pasta (GI between 50 and 70) compared to the digestion of white bread (GI = 100). Amylose and amylopectin molecules released during cooking (see Section 3.4) may recrystallize or retrograde (arrange themselves in an ordered and compact molecular form) over time, hindering penetration of digestive enzymes in these dense areas and lowering the GI. During digestion of a potato that has been cooked, cooled, stored, and reheated, sugar is produced more slowly and to a lesser amount than during the digestion of a recently cooked potato, whose starch has not had the opportunity to retrograde.[25] Retrogradation of starch is a natural phenomenon that has not often been exploited as a way to modulate the glycemic effect of traditional foods. High-amylose starches derived from special corn varieties as well as some chemically modified commercial starches are also available to consumers who want to eat a more resistant starch.

It is good to know that not all the starches in nature behave the same way. Starches in grains and tubers contain different proportions of amylose and amylopectin, packaged inside the granules in different ways. Because starches are important components of many foods, the study of their transformation into food products and of their digestion is a highly active area of research, whose results are expected in the coming years. In addition, the search is on for special varieties as is the case of thousands of native varieties of the potato, each with its own unique taste, nutritional value, and disease-resistant and climate-resistant traits. This may lead to the design of starchy foods with better nutritional properties, while still maintaining the desirable character-istics that have nourished us for centuries.

7.8 WE RECEIVE LESS THAN WHAT WE PAY

We might feel deceived to some extent by the fact that when we pay for a certain amount of vitamins and nutrients that are supposedly present in our food, only a fraction of them actually reach our cells. The content of various nutrients in a serving of food (100 g or 100 mL for example) is listed in the *Food Composition Tables* that many countries publish in order to provide information on the most commonly consumed foods. The data from these tables come from chemical analyses that have been refined and improved over the years in order to extract, separate, and purify specific nutrients contained in a food in an efficient way. The end results go to the Food Composition Tables and onto the nutritional information that appears on packaging and product labels.

Our digestive system is far from being a chemical laboratory in which powerful machines can be used to pulverize the samples and after-ward soak them in different solvents for the amount of time necessary to extract the chemical compounds of interest. The amount of beta-carotene that can be physically and chemically extracted from a raw carrot in a lab is quite different from the amount that is available to be absorbed in the intestine and appears in blood plasma after chew-ing, eating, and digesting the same carrot. Our digestive system only absorbs about 20% of the beta-carotene that the raw carrot originally contained; the rest is unavailable after normal digestion. Studies show that the amount absorbed depends on how the carrots were processed before they were eaten.[26]

This discrepancy is expressed as the *bioavailability* of a nutrient, which is the ratio between the amount of the nutrient that is consumed and the amount that finally appears in the blood plasma after consumption.

This gives us a way to measure how well the human digestive system grinds, extracts, dilutes, mixes, and finally absorbs a nutrient, and is not the result of a laboratory test apparatus. Returning to the example above, the bioavailability of beta-carotene increases as you go from raw carrots to grated carrots, and finally to carrot juice, because our digestive apparatus is unable to break every cell in a carrot and recover all the beta-carotene by itself. Some beta-carotene may end up in the stool, and bacteria in the gut may use some of it. The bioavailability of lycopene is higher in tomato paste than in fresh tomatoes for the same reason (see Section 1.8). With regard to these two nutrients at least, the consumption of fruits and vegetables in processed form may be more "nutritious" than in their raw form.

Nutrients may have low bioavailability values for different reasons. Nature does not synthesize the compounds just to be nutrients, but to perform metabolic functions within the cells of plants. Therefore, these compounds are often linked to or form part of structures that must be destroyed during processing, mastication, and digestion, to make them available for absorption.

It is likely that during these events certain reactions or interactions might occur between molecules of the released nutrients and other food components, reducing their effectiveness. One well-understood example of this phenomenon is the inhibition of the absorption of non-heme iron (i.e., all iron that isn't present in foods as hemoglobin or myoglobin) by phytic acid found in cereals and legumes. Also, it has been reported that palmitic acid (C18:0) in the fat of maternal milk and liberated in the intestine by hydrolysis of triglycerides interacts with calcium, producing a soap that is unavailable for absorption and goes into the stool.[27] But when the palmitic acid stays connected to the glycerol backbone, it cannot bind with calcium. There is more on this subject in Section 7.8. It is also known that some forms of dietary fiber may entrap or bind with minerals and inhibit their absorption in the small intestine.

When triglycerides come into contact with digestive enzymes, the two fatty acids at extreme positions of the glycerol molecule are detached and "freed," while most at the central position stay connected to the glycerol backbone (and become part of a monoglyceride) (see

Appendix). Now the fat energy can be absorbed into the bloodstream. But as this is happening, the free fatty acids can also start binding with other compounds.

But our bodies can also act like spendthrifts and discard things we have purchased. In addition to the inefficiency with which we use certain nutrients once they reach our mouths, there are nutrient losses that happen earlier, during the food processing that occurs industrially and in our homes. We know about the loss of vitamins, minerals, and fiber found in the outer layers of whole grains that are absent in refined flour. Several bioactive compounds are concentrated in the peel and seeds of certain fruits and are usually discarded. If you add to this list the compounds that are sensitive to heat and oxygen, and whose retention depends greatly on processing, packaging, and storage conditions, very often the food that we finally consume contains much lower amounts of certain nutrients than it should (see Section 4.13). The issue of bioavailability is currently a top priority in nutrition and food technology research, as it is directly related with the health benefits derived from the way in which we consume nutrients.

7.9 WHY DO WE AGE?

Human aging can be defined as the lifetime accumulation of biological changes that render people progressively more likely to die. Over the past two centuries, human life expectancy has more than doubled in developed nations due to advances in medicine and public health, meaning that we now age for longer periods. Aging appears to be a pressing question in science given the large amount of journals devoted to this topic, including, among others, *Aging, Journal of Ageing and Health, Age and Ageing*, the *Journal of Ageing Studies*, the *European Journal of Ageing*, and so on.

It is difficult to miss all the talk about antioxidants present in foods or of functional foods that takes place in the press and on TV. Do they play a role in delaying aging? It all starts when the molecules from our food finally reach the cells. As mentioned in Section 1.1, the energy contained in the chemical bonds within certain molecules is released inside each of our cells through a process called *cellular respiration*. Oxygen acts as the oxidizer in this reaction. This combustion that occurs in the mitochondria is not perfect and produces highly reactive, short-lived (in the order of nanoseconds) molecules called *free radicals*, including reactive oxygen species (ROS) molecules. Free radicals are destructive because they lack an electron, which leads them to remove electrons from other molecules to become stable, in a process called *oxidation*. In doing so, free radicals generate more free radicals, so they are self-perpetuating, amplifying their destructive action. Free radicals act like bullets in the way that they cause biological damage to cell membranes, genetic material, and proteins. They are capable of damaging cells of the body, despite its large battery of antioxidants, including proteins, enzymes, vitamins, and several other metabolites. As we age, the body's mechanisms of maintenance and repair become less effective, so that DNA mutations and other cellular damage start to accumulate and interfere with normal activity. This is one of the proposed explanations for why we age. Another hypothesis suggests that certain genes are programmed to work only for a certain time and then stop.

Antioxidants prevent or slow the damage caused by oxidation. Because of their chemical structure, they have the ability to react with free radicals and transform them into products that are relatively stable and harmless. Under normal metabolic conditions, there is a balance between ROS production and our natural defense systems (antioxidants and free radical scavengers). *Oxidative stress* is the name for the condition that occurs when our protective effects diminish or the amount of free radicals increases. Oxidative stress is associated with pathologies such as atherosclerosis, certain cancers, Parkinson's disease, and Alzheimer's disease. The antioxidants in our diet, such as vitamins C and E, carotenoids, and the polyphenols and flavonoids found in fresh fruits and vegetables and in wine should help protect us from oxidative damage. But there are some skeptical scientists who believe such a conclusion is premature and very difficult to prove.[28] Moreover, laboratory tests measuring antioxidant capacity of food compounds are varied and give different results for the same compound, so that the information derived from *in vitro* tests must be considered carefully. It's safer to conclude that antioxidant action may be due to synergistic effects between several antioxidants rather than caused by one single type of molecule.

But, back to the genes—when there is sufficient food and stress levels are low, many genes sustain growth and reproduction. Under unfavorable conditions, genes turn to physiological protection and cell maintenance. This change protects the body from environmental stress and also extends the organism's life span. The best known of these adverse conditions is dietary or caloric restriction, which has been proven to extend life in many species ranging from yeast to primates.[29] That's quite something to keep in mind as we enjoy lunch.

7.10 NUTRITION: *QUO VADIS?*

The science of nutrition began with the study of specific deficiencies and the identification of nutrients to compensate for the deficits. The impact produced by this approach has been remarkable, as evidenced by the history of vitamin C (L-ascorbic acid). A diet deficient in vitamin C causes scurvy, a condition that can be fatal. During Vasco da Gama's voyage around the world, more than half of the crew may have died of scurvy, due to the absence of fresh fruits and vegetables on board. The relationship between vitamin C and scurvy was discovered in the 1930s, and since then the vitamin has been industrially produced by chemical synthesis from glucose (and more recently from fermentation), and sold in tablet form. Nowadays scurvy is only found in situations of general malnutrition or in unusual cases. In retrospect, the almost miraculous effects of vitamins to cure some nutritional diseases gave the nutrition profession a high profile. Unfortunately, the simple relation between one disease and one nutrient evolved into a research methodology among many nutritionists that focused only on single components of foods, ignoring the fact that we eat a complex mixture of chemicals that vary with every meal, even with the way in which we prepare foods (see the case of starch in Section 7.7).

Michael Pollan must be acknowledged for bringing the concept of nutritionism back into the public attention.[30] The term *nutritionism* was coined to represent the reductionist view that the key to understanding foods is to know about their nutrients. Basically it establishes that there are right nutrients and wrong nutrients, but only the right ones make you healthier, which is the sole reason for eating. Pollan concludes intrepidly that "putting the nutritionists in charge of the menu and the kitchen has ruined our meals and done little for our health." (Note 30; pp. 40–41.)

It is true that some links have emerged between certain types of diseases and the consumption of particular food groups or whole diets (see the case of the French Paradox, Section 12.6). But what these relationships strongly suggest is that we have to change the fundamental unit of nutrition from a specific nutrient to the whole food and groups of foods that we regularly consume. It has become obvious that studying the effect of isolated nutrients does not necessarily provide an understanding of how they function when they are consumed as part of a whole meal. Synergies are the positive or negative interactions between different compounds once they are dispersed at the molecular level, like during digestion. For example, antioxidants seem to have synergistic effects, as the action of a mixture of several of them is more effective than one in particular, no matter how abundant.

But even studying mixtures of isolated nutrients may not give sufficient clues about their action in our bodies. For the first time in the history of nutrition, the role of food structure has come to the forefront of research, and it is now accepted that the effectiveness of a nutrient is not independent of its surroundings. Nutrition experts call the microstructure of a food its "matrix," or the spatial arrangement in which nutrients are embedded in the food (Section 7.6). From the point of view of a nutrient, the matrix in which it is immersed undergoes changes during the processing and preparation of food in the kitchen, and then disintegrates during digestion, releasing the nutrients into the gastrointestinal contents. From then on, the nutrient is able to interact positively or negatively with the hundreds of other components released from the food, which can alter its nutritional effectiveness. The *bioaccessibility* of nutrients (how they are released from the matrix), their interactions with other compounds present in the digestive tract at the same time, as well as their *bioavailability* (proportion absorbed by the gut) will be of utmost importance in the field of nutrition and health in the coming years. One recent study illustrates the point; it suggests that the antioxidants in blueberries interact with proteins (e.g., like those in milk) causing the antioxidant levels to appear diminished in the blood plasma.[31]

As the basic nutrient deficiencies have already been identified and the supplements and strategies have been developed to correct them, the current objectives for human nutrition are aimed toward preventing certain diseases (protection) and achieving greater well-being (promoting health and quality of life) through our foods. This interface between nutrition, health, and well-being leads to a two-pronged approach. The first is related to the study of the individual components that may have a favorable biological activity and their behavior within whole foods and diet, where benefits to health and well-being result from synergisms and interactions with other compounds. This top-down perspective on nutrition is complemented by a bottom-up approach that stems from genetics and cell biology. This view recognizes that the effects of food can be better understood if we know how nutrients act at the molecular and subcellular levels. These scientists study these effects using post-genomic technologies such as metabolomics (the study of biochemical pathways and their metabolites), proteomics (the relationship between genes and expressed proteins), and transcriptomics (analysis of gene expression), among other "omics."[32]

As you finish this chapter, you should be left with the understanding that food processing doesn't end when we buy foods at the store or cook them in the kitchen. The processing continues inside of our bodies. Newly available scientific research techniques such as genomics and real-time body imagery should help us to investigate the role of nutrients in the axis that runs from the brain to the cells, producing dramatic breakthroughs. But the act of eating remains voluntary and will always depend on each individual. Figure 7.5 summarizes what happens to the microstructure of a food from the time it enters your mouth until it becomes deconstructed in the gut, and is a good synopsis of the main contents of this chapter.

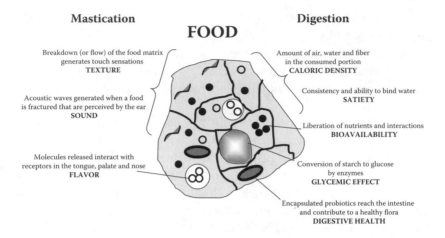

Mastication   **Digestion**

FOOD

Breakdown (or flow) of the food matrix generates touch sensations
TEXTURE

Acoustic waves generated when a food is fractured that are perceived by the ear
SOUND

Molecules released interact with receptors in the tongue, palate and nose
FLAVOR

Amount of air, water and fiber in the consumed portion
CALORIC DENSITY

Consistency and ability to bind water
SATIETY

Liberation of nutrients and interactions
BIOAVAILABILITY

Conversion of starch to glucose by enzymes
GLYCEMIC EFFECT

Encapsulated probiotics reach the intestine and contribute to a healthy flora
DIGESTIVE HEALTH

FIGURE 7.5   EFFECT OF A FOOD MATRIX ON PERCEIVED SENSATIONS DURING MASTICATION AND ON SOME OF THE PHENOMENA RELATED TO THE DIGESTION AND ABSORPTION OF NUTRIENTS. BRACKETS MAKE REFERENCE TO THE WHOLE FOOD, WHILE LINES POINT TO SPECIFIC STRUCTURES AND MOLECULES.

NOTES

1. The text describing the entire experiment can be found at Bourne, M.C. 2002. *Food Texture and Viscosity: Concept and Measurement.* Academic Press, San Diego, pp. 2–3.
2. This example appears in Lister, T., and Blumenthal, H. 2005. *Kitchen Chemistry.* Royal Society of Chemistry, London, pp. 101–102.
3. Acerno, L.J. 2000. Adolph Fick: Mathematician, physicist, physiologist. *Clinical Cardiology* 23, 390–391.
4. An excellent book on diffusion (requiring a certain level of scientific and mathematical understanding) is Cussler, E. 1997. *Diffusion: Mass Transfer in Fluid Systems.* Cambridge University Press, Cambridge.
5. Manach, C., Scalbert, A., Morand, C., Rémésy, C., and Jiménez, L. 2004. Polyphenols: Food sources and bioavailability. *American Journal of Clinical Nutrition* 79, 727–747.
6. Excessive consumption of monosodium glutamate (which normally should not exceed concentrations of 0.2 to 0.8%) can produce the "Chinese restaurant syndrome" in hypersensitive individuals, characterized by dizziness, headache, stomachache, and joint stiffness.
7. Holley, A. 2006. *El Cerebro Goloso.* Rubes, Barcelona. (The Sweet Toothed Brain). This book is an entertaining examination of the tastes, aromas,

and flavors found in food in relation to the chemical and biological mechanisms involved in their perception.

8. The book is part of a compilation by *Slow Food Editore* in 2007.

9. Toldrá, F. 2009. *El jamón curado. Investigación y Ciencia* 399, 39.

10. My friend from Milan, Professor Roberto Giangiacomo, gave me an article entitled *The Nose of Romeo* that describes the preparation of *coppa*, another famous Italian cured ham, which comes from the neck and shoulder of the pig. In the article he describes his experience tasting these hams alongside a master pork *sommelier*, and some of his observations have been transferred into the main text.

11. An interesting review article about the technology and applications of electronic noses is Röck, F., Barsan, N., and Weimar, U. 2008. Electronic nose: Current status and future trends. *Chemical Reviews* 108, 705–725.

12. The story and reported results can be found in Fredrickson, B.L. 2003. The value of positive emotions. *American Scientist* 91, 330–335.

13. There are a growing number of contributions to the scientific literature in this area, such as del Parigi, A., Chen, K., Salbe, A.D., Reiman, E.M., and Tataranni, P.A. 2005. Sensory experience of food and obesity: A positron emission tomography study of the brain regions affected by tasting a liquid meal after a prolonged fast. *NeuroImage* 24, 436–443.

14. Hare, T.A., Camerer, C.F., and Rangel, A. 2009. Self-control in decision-making involves modulation of the vmPFC valuation system. *Science* 324, 646–648.

15. Cohen, J.I., Yates, K.F., Duong, M., and Convit, A. 2011. Obesity, orbitofrontal structure and function are associated with food choice: a cross-sectional study. *BMJ Open* 2011;1;e000175.doi:10.1136/bmjopen-2011-000175.

16. Several concepts of Section 7.2 were adapted from the book by Shepherd, G.M. 2012. *Neurogastronomy*. Columbia University Press, New York.

17. Kringelbach, M.L. 2004. Food for thought: Hedonic experience beyond homeostasis in the human brain. *Neuroscience* 126, 807–819.

18. Swinburn, B., Egger, G., and Raza, F. 1999. Dissecting obesogenic environments: The development and application of a framework for identifying and prioritizing environmental interventions for obesity. *Preventive Medicine* 29, 563–570.

19. Our recent article on the relationship between structure and digestion is Aguilera, J.M., and Troncoso, E. 2009. Food structure and digestion. *Food Science and Technology* 23, 24–27.

20. Riskin, J. 2003. The defecating duck, or, the ambiguous origins of artificial life. *Critical Inquiry* 29, 4.

21. Jeanes, Y.M., Hall, W.L., Ellard, S., Lee, E., and Lodge, J.K. 2004. The absorption of vitamin E is influenced by the amount of fat in a meal and the food matrix. *British Journal of Nutrition* 92, 575–579.
22. Details about one of the many artificial digestive systems in development can be found at http://news.bbc.co.uk/2/hi/health/6136546.stm (accessed June 12, 2010).
23. Because the glycemic index (GI) is based on the glucose generated by the consumption of 50 grams of carbohydrates, it's preferable to use the *glycemic load* (GL) (which is equal to the GI multiplied by the amount of carbohydrates in grams, divided by 100) in the case of small portions or with foods that are low in carbohydrates.
24. Witwer, R. 2005. Understanding glycemic impact. *Food Technology* 59(11), 22–29.
25. Fernandes, G., Velangi, A., and Wolever, T. 2005. Glycemic index of potatoes commonly consumed in North America. *Journal of the American Dietetic Association* 105, 557–562.
26. Van het Hof, K., West, C.E., Weststrate, J.A., and Hautvast, J.G.A.J. 2000. Dietary factors that affect the bioavailability of carotenoids. *Journal of Nutrition* 130, 503–506.
27. Innis, S.M., Quinlan, P.T., and Nelson, C.M. 1998. Structured triacylglycerides in infant nutrition. In Huang, Y.S., and Sinclair, A.J. (eds.) *Lipids in Infant Nutrition*, AOCS Press, Champaign, IL, pp. 268–281.
28. Willett, W.C. 2003. *Eat, Drink and Be Healthy*. Free Press, New York, p. 158.
29. For more on genes and aging, see Kenyon, C.J. 2010. The genetics of aging. *Nature* 464, 504–512.
30. Pollan, M. 2008. *In Defense of Food: An Eater's Manifesto*. Penguin Books, New York, pp. 27–36.
31. See article by Serafini, M., Testa, M.F., Villaño, D., Pecorari, M., van Wieren, K., Azzini, E., Brambilla, A., and Maiani, G. 2009. Antioxidant activity of blueberry fruit is impaired by association with milk. *Free Radical Biology and Medicine* 46, 769–774.
32. For those who would like to delve more deeply into the issue of food as the basic unit of nutrition and the impact of *omics* platforms on nutrition and health, the following articles are recommended: Jacobs, D.R., and Tapsell, L.C. 2007. Food, not nutrients, is the fundamental unit in nutrition. *Nutrition Reviews* 65, 439–450; and Kussmann, M., Raymond, F., and Affolter, M. 2006. OMICS-driven biomarker discovery in nutrition and health. *Journal of Biotechnology* 124, 758–787.

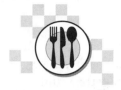

CHAPTER 8

Culinary Technologies and Food Structures

There is a lot of engineering involved in the storage of food in the kitchen, where temperature and humidity are key factors, and in the culinary preparation for cooking. Certain ingredients are better prepared by industry than in the home kitchen, but don't give up. As food structures develop, it's possible to measure the effect of the different variables involved in their formation in order to have better control over them. We use examples in this chapter to explain the science and engineering behind the creation of some of these desirable properties found in various foods.

8.1 THE CONSERVATION MAP

Strawberries go in the refrigerator but bananas don't. Leftover meals can go in the freezer but never sea urchins. Cookies and potato chips belong in tightly closed containers at room temperature, but rice and flour are fine in bags (like the old days). The way we store our food in the kitchen has more to do with concerns about the perishability of food structures than how often we use them, and this section seeks to explain why. The next few pages may seem a little bit complicated, but they nicely demonstrate how the stability of foods has to do with their material nature and justify some of the technologies that are used to keep them for longer times.

There are two variables that are very important to keep in mind when thinking about preserving our foods: the water content and the temperature of the storage area. Engineers can't resist graphing two variables onto x and y axes, and that is precisely what I will do here. Before continuing, it might be helpful to review the concepts about the states of foods discussed in Section 2.3, which are important for understanding the information on the graph.

The x axis will be the moisture content of the food, expressed for simplicity as % moisture content.[1] Thus, 0% represents a totally dry food (right side) while 100% is pure water (left side). You may also find moisture defined as W (g water/g total matter). "Dry" foods like pasta and dried beans, which have a very low W (around 10 to 20 g of water per 100 g of dry matter), have near 10% to 15% moisture. Foods like vegetables and meat are "wet" and have a high W value (about 300 g of water per 100 g dry matter) or a moisture content of approximately 70% to 80%. The y axis will show the temperature T, at which the food is stored. This information will give us the ability to construct a *food conservation* or *food preservation map*, as in Figure 8.1. The temperature of food that is stored in the kitchen can vary from the temperature of the freezer (approximately –18°C, dashed line on the graph) to "room temperature," which ranges between about 15 and 30°C (hatched area on the graph). The temperature of the refrigerator is in between (about 5°C, dotted line).

Foods that contain lots of water such as milk, juices, soft drinks, and sauces also contain dissolved solutes and particles, and are therefore solutions or suspensions. These products are located in the top left corner of the diagram at temperatures above 0°C (the *Solution* zone). Conservation of these types of products depends on factors such as the pH, the amount of dissolved solutes, and the presence of preservatives. Meats, seafood, fruits, and vegetables also fit into this area of the graph, and they are discussed below.

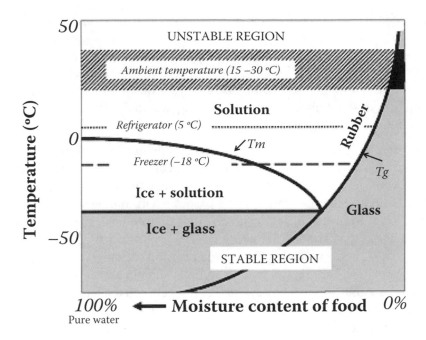

FIGURE 8.1 FOOD STABILITY DEPENDS ON STORAGE TEMPERATURE AND MOISTURE CONTENT. THE GRAY AREA REPRESENTS CONDITIONS UNDER WHICH FOODS ARE STABLE FOR LONG PERIODS. NOTE THAT AT AMBIENT TEMPERATURE ONLY DRY FOODS SATISFY THOSE CONDITIONS (BLACK AREA); MOST OF THE FOODS THAT WE KEEP IN OUR KITCHENS ARE LOCATED IN THE UNSTABLE REGION (WHITE).

The glass transition temperature (T_g) curve (see Section 2.3) is the most important reference of the conservation diagram when it comes to food structures. This curve crosses the graph almost diagonally, separating the glassy state (*Glass* zone) from the rubbery state (*Rubber* zone) when there is no ice present in the food. Very dry foods lie just under the T_g line, if they are stored at room temperature and are therefore in the glassy state under those conditions (black area, top right). A food structure in a glassy state is very stable, but if it passes into the rubbery state (if the storage temperature rises or the humidity increases, for example) it becomes unstable. Low-moisture foods such as cookies and instant coffee are found to the right of the diagram. When you purchase these foods, they are usually in a glassy state within their container (i.e., in the black area). But if these products are directly exposed to the atmosphere, like when you open their packaging for the first time, they absorb humidity from the air and W moves to the left, which means danger. How much water is exchanged between dry foods and the moist air from the kitchen? It continues until equilibrium is reached in which the exposed food stops acquiring water molecules and the weight of the food stops increasing, which depends on the relative humidity of the air.[2]

An extreme case of this kind of moisture exchange between dry foods and moist air is when powders like instant coffee start to "cake." Every time you open a jar in an environment in which the air has a high relative humidity, the space around the particles within the jar is renewed and water from the air is introduced into the product. This moisture gain causes the particles that were in a glassy state to change into a rubbery state. In this state, the particles deform and stick together, forming a compact solid inside the jar (Section 3.8). Low-moisture foods need packaging that acts as a waterproof barrier between the food to be kept dry and the moist air. Canned foods, oil and vinegar, and foods with high sugar content like jams and honeys are more shelf-stable and can be stored at room temperature, because they are well protected and water exchange does not affect them significantly.

Let's move to the left side of the diagram which is more complicated. At high moisture contents and temperatures below 0°C (as in the freezer), the ice melting temperature curve, T_m, appears. Foods with high W values as they cool start forming ice at a temperature below T_m, and the part that is not frozen remains a concentrated solution (*Ice + solution* zone). As the temperature continues to fall below the T_m curve, more ice forms and the solution becomes more concentrated (and viscous).

Foods with high moisture content (left side in Figure 8.1) are perishable and must be stored in the refrigerator or freezer. This lowers the temperature of the food, which reduces the rate of growth of microorganisms as well as the rate of deterioration reactions, but the food is not stable indefinitely. Bread should not be stored in the refrigerator, because it turns stale more quickly at about 4°C, and some fruits can be damaged by the cold of the refrigerator. Despite these exceptions, the rule of thumb is that deterioration rates are reduced by about half for each 10°C drop in temperature. Meat and fish, processed meats (ham, pâté, etc.), eggs, pasteurized milk, and fruits and vegetables can be preserved almost four times longer under refrigeration than at room temperature.

Certain high-moisture foods are stored in the freezer, but not only for the effect of the lower temperature on deterioration rates. Some of the water turns to ice at 0°C and is therefore immobilized and unable to participate in reactions that damage the quality. At –18°C, which is the normal operating temperature for most domestic freezers; only some of the water in "frozen" fish (for example) will be in the form of ice. As the temperature drops, more ice crystals form and the remaining aqueous solution increases in concentration, which lowers the freezing point (moving right along the T_m curve). Until when? The minimum temperature at which the last portion of water turns to ice in fruit and meat is about –40 to –45°C. At lower temperatures the concentrated solution is so viscous that it becomes glassy and the food becomes part ice and part glass (*Ice + glass* zone). When high-moisture biological material is in these conditions, it has the highest possible stability, a sort of cryo-preservation. But food in our homes never reaches this state. It is not necessary to cryo-preserve food—it would be expensive as well as impractical to maintain food at these temperatures. Remains of early humans have become exposed when the ice on high mountain peaks starts to melt as a result of global warming. These remains are in a great state of preservation because they have stayed in the *Ice + glass* zone for thousands of years.[3] Placing the foods you bought on your most recent trip to the supermarket on the diagram would be an excellent exercise to check that you have understood Figure 8.1 correctly.

The frozen foods that we buy go straight to the home freezer. Commercial foods are frozen as quickly as possible in industrial freezers and reach temperatures around –30°C. A slower freezing process produces large ice crystals that can disrupt the cell walls and membranes of fruits and vegetables. The crystals also grow outside of the cells and fibers of the meat, removing the water, and destroy emulsions, which causes the exudation of fluid when the product is later thawed. The answer to the question: "can you freeze this or that food at home?" is invariably yes—anything can go in the freezer. But the home freezer is designed to store already frozen foods and does not freeze food as rapidly and cold as commercial freezers. In some ways, industry can quickly freeze foods much better than nature can. Nature never had to resort to these methods in order to maintain structures.

This section on the conservation of dry food would not be complete without the mention of a notable example of the preservation of "life" in a state of desiccation. In some deserts (like the one in northern Chile) seeds can survive in the extremely dry environment, even though they are intermittently exposed to extremes of cold and heat which irreversibly damage most living things. Just a touch of rain on these seeds is enough to put their whole cellular machinery quickly back into operation and they will produce a "desert flower." Part of this amazing resurrection on the part of the seeds has to do with the preservation of certain vital molecules inside of a matrix of sugars. The sugars remain in the glass state under prevailing dry and hot conditions but pass into the rubbery state when water is available, thus the mobility in the matrix increases and the machinery of life is restarted.[4]

8.2 WAITING FOR DINNER TO BE READY

In a commercial kitchen as well as home kitchens, raw materials and ingredients must undergo some preparation in the process of making a final product or dish. Culinary engineers use a series of operations in order to condition ingredients for further processing, such as thawing, washing, soaking, peeling or shelling, cutting, grinding, agitating liquids, mixing powders, kneading, and so on. Most of these steps have an equivalent in chemical engineering, so there are plenty of empirical knowledge and developed concepts already available.[5] It's very helpful to consult these sources before beginning any serious study of the processes of culinary preparation. One common characteristic is that these steps are typically carried out at room temperature.

Removing the skins or peel from products like potatoes, tomatoes, carrots, and certain fruits is performed in the kitchen by physical means (e.g., peeling them with a knife). But peeling can also be done chemically, with a caustic solution that diffuses into cells that attach the peel to the fleshy part. The solution partially dissolves these cells, and pieces of the peel are then easily removed with brushes or water jets. This is how the potatoes are peeled for commercially prepared french fries. Although the removal of shells and peels results in little physical loss, the nutrient losses can be significant. Many vitamins and bioactive compounds are located in the parts that are removed. Engineers have developed machines that separate the inedible parts very quickly and accurately on the processing lines, where tons of product passes through quickly. To produce white wheat flour and peeled rice the outer part of the grain (the bran) is physically removed from its attachment to the inner endosperm. Peeling almonds and asparagus, separating pebbles from lentils, picking meat from the bones, and squeezing oranges to make juice are all very tedious work but can be done with amazing speed by automated equipment in a factory. Sometimes, however, peeling shrimp or shelling crabs at the table is part of the enjoyment of a dish.

Size reduction (slicing, dicing, etc.) is a frequent intermediate stage in the kitchen, as it increases the surface/volume ratio and makes the transfer of heat (cooking or frying) and mass (extraction or impregnation) much faster. For example, when beets are processed into refined sugar, they are sliced into triangular "noodles" to facilitate the rapid diffusion of sucrose from the interior cells (whose cell membranes remain intact and act as filters so that the larger molecules don't migrate). The industrial preparation of frozen french fries involves propelling the peeled whole potatoes by a fast stream of water so they hit head on with a set of sharp knives that are arranged horizontally and vertically. Thus, the knives cut the potatoes into long strips with a square section. Water jets can now be used to precisely cut solid foods such as potatoes and frozen products as well as softer foods like cakes that would otherwise deform under the pressure of the most sharpened knife. This reduction in size allows foods to be mixed until they reach a more or less homogenous state. But breaking the cell walls of plants releases enzymes that can lead to reactions that alter the color and taste; therefore, applying a mild heat treatment beforehand (blanching) or protecting the vegetables from the air once they are cut is recommended.

Grinding reduces ingredients to a finer size, resulting in a powder or a collection of particles that can be as small as a few microns. Engineers know that not all grinding machines produce the same type of particles. Wheat flour and cacao nibs are ground between smooth cylindrical rolls separated by a narrow gap, while roasted coffee grains are pulverized at home with high-speed blades, but commercially they are ground between two rotating hard plates that rub together. Colombians claim that the best "arepas" (a kind of thick tortilla) are only prepared with mortar-ground corn (never in a blender). Particle size is often controlled by periodic sieving and removal of the already disintegrated small fraction while the coarse particles continue the process. Not all disintegration processes are equal: Parmesan cheese should be shredded, and garlic cloves are crushed with a press.

Some people prefer home-cooked meals and enjoy the tranquility of eating in a calm setting, far from the bustling food courts with their plastic utensils and disposable materials. But many people, especially young ones, only like to cook sporadically or as a hobby. It's clear that people are less willing to dedicate much of their free time to meal preparation. A reasonable alternative is to buy safe, preprocessed products that can be quickly "assembled" into tasty meals at home, or to make in the kitchen those pleasing fast food alternatives more "gourmet" and lower in calories. In the first case, there will be more distance between the farm and our dinner table, and in the second case, a higher cost involved. If these options are not being adopted as time-saving alternatives, in the first place, and a healthy adaptation of an acquired habit, in the second, we will definitely be facing a paradigm shift in how we think about cooking our food at home.

Preprocessed foods are currently available: pre-chopped, precooked, partially baked, and so on. You can even purchase precooked meats that need only to be warmed before eating. Fresh produce that has been cleaned, chopped, disinfected, and packaged for consumption is labeled "cuarta gama" (fourth generation) in Spain, and "ready-to-eat" in the United States. These products retain their natural properties and freshness for about 7 to 10 days. Ready-to-eat foods are normally consumed in the same condition as they are sold, while the concept of cook-and-chill corresponds to foods or preparations that have been cooked and then rapidly cooled to 4 to 6°C. These foods are often placed into modified atmosphere packaging (containing gases such as CO_2 and nitrogen) or are vacuum sealed to maintain the natural aromas and flavors, and ensure a safe shelf-life. The cooling process is critical because cook-and-chill products (and also *sous-vide* foods) are not sterile and must be protected to ensure microbiological safety.

Certain kitchen operations require the application of brute force. In artisan bakeries and pizzerias you can observe bakers vigorously mixing the flour and water to develop the dough. Ice cream used to be churned by hand with a wire whisk and potatoes mashed with a potato ricer, but nowadays these utensils hang as ornaments in many kitchens. Modern kitchen equipment makes use of electrical energy rather than human energy to mix and disperse ingredients, but cooks are losing some of the innate "feeling" that comes from working with their hands.

Cleaning of utensils and plates is another task that should undergo considerable progress in terms of the effort involved and the use of potable water and detergents. Compared to other water uses in the home (clothes washing machines, showers, toilets, etc.), dishwashing requires much less water, probably less than 5% of total water use, but the organic matter in the drain water requires further treatment. In the future, nanotechnology may enable the development of special coatings that would make the surfaces of utensils and dishware more "self-cleaning" or able to repel solids, reducing water use.

The introduction of new technologies for the home kitchen will help boost convenience and save time during meal preparation. The popularization of information technology will lead to remote activation devices for kitchen appliances, further speeding up the work. Smart packaging that interacts directly with ovens and other kitchen devices is another area of development in the convenience arena.

8.3 MATERIALS AND UTENSILS IN THE KITCHEN

Until the Middle Ages, kitchens were very rudimentary spaces, equipped only with a fireplace for cooking over a flame or with embers. There were no ovens or cooking ranges. There was no refrigeration— items like butter, lard, bacon, and milk were kept fresh by storing them in cool places. Meats were ripened at room temperature and had to be boiled before roasting to kill microorganisms growing on the surface and to wash away the slime. There was plenty of manpower for cooking tasks, however. A typical kitchen brigade in a palace could easily exceed a hundred people. In the eighteenth century, people began facilitating the logistics of cuisine and service, using dumbwaiters to move food from the basement to the upper floors and acoustic tubes to transmit orders.[6] Eating utensils were pretty basic. It wasn't until the sixteenth century that the fork made its way to France from Italy. Starting in the seventeenth century, wood carvers and European lathe operators produced delicate dining utensils for everyday use, such as nutcrackers, cups and glasses, lemon squeezers, butter molds, and stamps for bread, among others, which are now eagerly sought after by collectors or housed in museums (Figure 8.2).[7]

Today, cooks and chefs have a huge battery of materials and equipment in their kitchens, ranging from stainless steel counters and knives

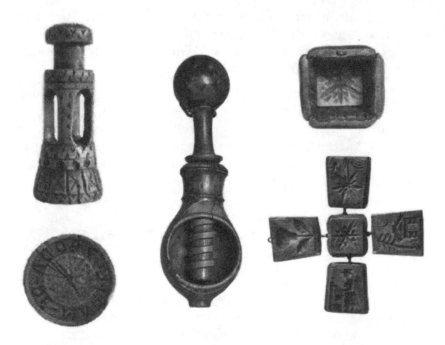

FIGURE 8.2   CARVED WOODEN ANTIQUES (NINETEENTH CENTURY) USED FOR THE PREPARATION OF FOOD: BREAD STAMP, NUTCRACKER, AND BUTTER MOLD. PROPERTY OF THE AUTHOR. (PHOTOGRAPH BY A. BARRIGA A.)

to sophisticated electrical equipment and electronics for cutting, mixing, and heating.[8] More specific devices like siphons for making foams, syringes for injecting liquid, torches for making the hard caramel shell on top of a *crème brûlée*, and surgical tweezers for decoratively placing flower petals and herbs on a finished plate are showing up in modern kitchens. Even vacuum chambers for expanding the bubbles in a foam are becoming popular.

Now we come to some materials. Copper transfers heat most efficiently compared to all the metals used in the kitchen. The copper ions that are shed from copper utensils make cooked vegetables more intensely green.[9] Copper bowls are great for beating egg whites, because the metal ions help one of the egg proteins (conalbumin) to denature (see also Section 2.7).[10] Teflon® is a material that has changed the lives of the people whose fried eggs always stuck to the pan, as well as those who now have Teflon artificial aortas or kneecaps. A trademark of DuPont, the giant of the U.S. chemical industry, Teflon was discovered accidentally in 1940 by a chemist who observed that a depleted gas cylinder that had once contained tetrafluoroethylene, had a white and waxy substance inside. The tetrafluoroethylene molecules had polymerized, creating this solid. But it was not until 1960 that the first cookware appeared on the market, and not until 1986 until a Teflon coating was developed that could withstand the same cleaning procedures as metal pots and pans.[11] Resistant and transparent glass cookware was developed by Corning in the 1920s and was followed by the introduction of glass ceramics (a glass with partly crystallized regions) utensils in the 1960s. Polycarbonate, the tough and transparent plastic used in almost every form of rigid packaging from baby bottles to 5-gallon water containers (as well as in shields that protect presidents and the Pope), was also discovered by chance, this time at a General Electric research lab.

8.4 BRINGING INDUSTRY
INTO THE KITCHEN

The food industry produces many high-quality intermediate ingredients and final products that would be somewhat complicated, expensive, or simply unnecessary to create in a home kitchen (at least for now). Drying out a liquid to produce a powder, for example, is a relatively simple industrial process but would be almost impossible to do at home. Imagine the possibility of being able to make dehydrated juices from your favorite fruits or encapsulating delicate aromas in your home kitchen. For most industrial equipment there is a laboratory version with which one can prepare a small amount of a product, and these bench-top devices could be accommodated perfectly in the chef's laboratory. Although many industrial technologies aren't applicable in the kitchen, Box 8.1 describes some of the most important technologies that could make up part of a culinary engineering laboratory.

Because it's unlikely that many of the chef's laboratories have these devices in their bench-top version, the most practical alternative is to approach the food technology departments at universities and research centers. It won't be long until cheaper and less-sophisticated types of some of this equipment are available for the more technological kitchens.

There are many emerging technologies in the food industry intended for producing higher-quality products.[12] Two already have varying degrees of commercial applications. High-pressure processing (HPP) is used to pasteurize and gel foods. Supercritical fluid extraction (SCFE) exploits the high diffusivity and solvent power of pressurized CO_2 in order to remove solutes, as CO_2 is a natural solvent. Pressure is a thermodynamic variable just like temperature, but special technology is required to design equipment that is resistant to pressures that might be hundreds of times greater than atmospheric pressure. Proteins and microorganisms experience a similar response to increased pressure as they do to higher heat. The advantage of HPP is that its effect is mainly produced by pressure, and it does not require high temperatures. If a gas is compressed at high pressure, it transforms into "fluid" and acquires certain desirable properties of liquids, such as the ability to retain solutes, while maintaining a high diffusivity (ability to penetrate the food matrix) and low viscosity. This phenomenon occurs with CO_2 when the pressure exceeds 73 atm and the temperature is above 32°C. These conditions are typical of SCFE and are ideal for extracting solutes like caffeine and hops (for beer) using a "friendly" solvent, and other potential applications continue to emerge.[13]

BOX 8.1   SOME INDUSTRIAL TECHNOLOGIES THAT CULINARY LABORATORIES COULD ADOPT

Spray drying. Method for drying liquid foods or extracts in which a nozzle distributes the liquid as droplets (like a garden hose spray nozzle), which fall into a chamber of flowing hot air (between 120 and 180°C). The droplets lose water to the warmer air and become dry particles (e.g., powdered milk and instant coffee) that must be quickly removed from the dryer (e.g., powdered milk and instant coffee).[15] Chefs could use laboratory-size spray dryers to convert juices, extracts, and sauces into a few hundred grams of delicious powders.

Lyophilization (freeze-drying). Involves removing water in the form of vapor from a frozen product.[16] As water passes directly from ice to vapor (sublimation) the boundary separating the nearly dry layer from the frozen area moves. Because there's never any liquid water present, the product's matrix doesn't collapse. The food never reaches very high temperatures. Freeze-dried foods maintain the shape, texture, color, and flavor of the natural product much better than other methods of drying. Used in astronauts' foods, to make freeze-dried instant coffee and dry berries to a fresh-like appearance.

Extrusion. A technology adapted from the plastics industry where it is used to make pipes and plastic wrap. In foods, the process consists of continuously dosing a barrel or tube with wet corn or soy flour. Inside the barrel a tightly fitted screw turns and pushes the mass toward an exit. The rotation generates friction heat which raises the temperature of the dough above 100°C (hence the name *extrusion cooking*). Extruded products can be expanded by violent vaporization of water from the dough as it exits the extruder, producing starchy puffed snacks. Fibers formed from denatured proteins orientated in parallel layers by shearing the last section of the screw, making texturized vegetable protein or soy meat.

Centrifugation. Is the application of a centrifugal field induced by rotation at high speed which induces separation of materials with different densities (Section 5.2). The centrifuge can "skim" (i.e., separate cream and skim milk), clarify suspensions (e.g., removing particles from juices and broths), "drain" wet pulps (as in the household clothes washers), and even filter.

Homogenization. Homogenizers and colloid mills can finely disperse particulate matter and make emulsions containing very small droplets. Homogenizers break up the fat globules in milk, forming smaller ones that do not separate as quickly in the carton or bottle, giving the milk a more "homogeneous" appearance. Homogenizers have one or two valves in the form of narrow channels where the droplets are driven under pressure so that they collide and break. They are also used to make mayonnaise and sauces.

Membrane processing. Polymer or ceramic membranes with different pore sizes (less than 100 microns) make it possible to filter and separate particles ranging in size from microscopic molecules to those suspended in liquid. Microfiltration can remove fine particles in suspension to produce clear and transparent liquids. Ultrafiltration separates the macromolecules from small solutes, such as whey proteins from lactose in milk. Reverse osmosis removes salt ions from water and has been used to desalinate seawater.

The industry is increasingly using quality sensors, or devices that can rapidly detect certain conditions in the products and issue an alarm signal. A number of commercial sensors give information about freshness, ripeness, gas content, and even the presence of certain microorganisms in packaged food. Time-temperature indicators (TTIs) are the most widely used of these sensors. They attach to packaged food and change color to indicate the "thermal history" or abuse that products might have suffered during storage or distribution. There are also radio frequency indicators (RFIDs) that can be used to monitor products remotely. Other technologies come from the development of micro- and nanotechnologies, such as "smart" food containers with sensors that report on the condition of the packaged product or even activate and program kitchen equipment for its preparation. The future methods for assessing the quality and safety of food will undoubtedly involve biosensors or compact analytical devices with high biological specificity. When these sensors come in contact with food, they convert a biochemical signal into an electronic response. It won't be long until we may have our own quality control laboratory in the kitchen, with a battery of inexpensive and easy-to-read microsensors to ensure the safety and quality of our food.

And then there are all of the gadgets.[14] Internet sites offer products for "the kitchen of the future." One of the more useless devices is a display for outside the refrigerator that lets you see what's inside. You save energy by not having to open the door, but sticking your head in the refrigerator in search of a snack is one of those sacred pleasures that many will be reluctant to give up.

8.5 MEASURE OR MAKE MEASURABLE

An important difference between scientists and chefs is that scientists like to measure things with precision and accuracy (two terms that should be clarified). *Precision* refers to the dispersion of the set of values obtained from the measurements. The lower the dispersion, the greater is the precision. *Accuracy* means how close the measured values are to the actual value. Therefore, something can be precise but not accurate. Precision and accuracy are critical when working with the temperature of a sugar syrup and color changes, in the pH of the curd and quality of a cheese, and in the consistency of gelatin and the costs for a dessert manufacturer.

A company dedicated to providing culinary ingredients or any chef interested in science needs a basic laboratory with instruments for measuring parameters and controlling important variables in the development of food structures. Some of these are listed in Box 8.2. If they need to perform more elaborate studies, they can seek help from the food laboratories at universities and research institutes.

BOX 8.2   ESSENTIAL MEASUREMENT TOOLS FOR A CULINARY LABORATORY

Thermocouples. These are insulated flexible cables (as thin as 0.1 mm in diameter) shrouding two thin wires made of different materials attached at one end, and are used to measure temperature (see, e.g., www.omega.com). When inserted into a food a small voltage is generated, which increases with temperature. The temperature is read on a digital display or stored in a computer. Alternatively, infrared thermometers measure the temperature of hot surfaces from a distance without contact.

pH meters. The pH or hydrogen potential is a measure of the acidity or alkalinity of an aqueous solution. The pH can be measured accurately with a pH meter, an instrument that consists of glass electrodes and an analog or digital display. pH also can be estimated in the kitchen with special solutions or litmus paper.

Viscosimeters. These measure the viscosity or flow characteristics of liquids or quasi-liquids such as creams, dressings, sauces, jams, and so on, as a function of the speed of deformation (Section 5.2). There are simple devices that measure "consistency" or the time required for a material to flow a certain distance (the Bostwick consistometer, for example).

Colorimeters. Portable colorimeters measure a color by assigning it a point in a "color" space and mapping it with three coordinates, like the red (R), green (G), and blue (B) colors of digital cameras and TV. The color space that is more frequently used for food has three axes: L (luminosity), a (going from green to red), and b (covering blue to yellow). With digital photography and image analysis software (some of which is available online for free), color measurement of foods is no longer a problem (Section 5.8).

Water activity meters. These are instruments that measure the "availability" of water or a_w (Section 2.2) and range from devices as simple as hair hygrometers to automated and

thermostated (controlled temperature) equipment (see, e.g.,
www.decagon.com/water_activity/).

Magnifying glasses and microscopes. These instruments allow
investigators to observe and record with images (digital or
video camera) things that the naked eye can't see (Section
3.3). Possible applications include the observation of surfaces, the detection of certain impurities in ingredients,
measuring droplet size in emulsions and fine particles in
powders, and so on.[17] Quantification of morphological characteristics, counting objects, and so on can be performed
through the analysis of digital images (Section 5.8).

Refractometers. They measure the concentration in degrees Brix
(°Bx) of a soluble compound, usually sugar, in a solution
using the index of refraction (Section 11.10).[18]

Precision balances. Essential for any laboratory experiment,
precision balances are capable of precise measurements of
weight to within one hundredth of a gram.

Many of the physical properties of food ingredients and products can
be measured, providing information that can be used to characterize
processing and quality. Examples of these properties include viscosity (already mentioned) and the viscoelastic behavior of gels (Section
2.5) which is measured with a rheometer; thermal properties such as
specific heat, thermal conductivity, phase transitions, and the glass
transition temperature T_g (Section 8.1) which are determined using
different types of calorimeters, including the DSC (Section 2.14);
mechanical or textural characteristics obtained with mechanical
testing equipment (such as a texture analyzer, Section 2.14); the size
and shape of particles and droplets (determined by various methods,
among them image analysis, Section 5.8); and fine porosity which can
be measured in a mercury (or other type) porosimeter. Certain tests
may require the construction of a specific *ad hoc* device (for measuring the hydration of a powder or the stability of a foam, for example).
Many databases list representative values of physical properties for
different products. Research on the physical properties of food has
been of great interest to many food technologists, as they work to
characterize traditional foods and new ingredients.

8.6 WHY DOES POPCORN POP?

For most Americans, a trip to the movies is not complete without popcorn, a practice that has spread to other countries as well.[19] Cinema owners are happy with this business deal, as over 90% of what they sell is air. Popcorn qualifies as "junk food": a large bag of movie popcorn has more than 1000 kilocalories, as much as 1.5 grams of sodium, and often lots of saturated fat.

Although the scientific literature has given much consideration to certain factors that influence the expansion of a kernel of corn, such as the variety of corn, the method of heating, the physical properties of the grain, and so on, the variable that seems to have the most importance for popping is moisture. To understand what is happening when the corn kernels "inflate," we must consider the structure of the grain. Starch-filled cells are located within the tough skin or shell called the pericarp. When the kernel is heated and its internal temperature rises, two important phenomena occur: the water in the cells converts into steam, which increases the pressure inside the kernel, and the starch passes from the glassy state to a rubbery state and then to a molten state, in which it can flow (Section 2.3). At a certain point, the internal pressure produced by the vapor exceeds the resistance of the shell and the shell violently breaks, allowing the mass of hot starch to flow and expand by the escaping water vapor. As the steam exits to the atmosphere, the moisture drops and the product cools, allowing the starch to return to the glassy state, which makes the expanded product crispy. For all of this to happen properly, the initial moisture content of grain should be between 10% and 18%, and the maximum expansion occurs at about 14%. In short, every grain of corn acts like a tiny pressure cooker that operates safely within pots and microwave ovens.

There are other ways to expand whole grains that don't have a shell, but working with "shelled" grains requires heavy-duty equipment, as it must support the high pressure generated by the steam and the subsequent violent explosion that spews both grain and steam. Rice, wheat, and amaranth, for example, can be placed into a steel cylinder that is directly heated by an external fire as it turns. When the cylinder reaches a certain pressure from the evaporation of water, remotely operated doors open, allowing the product to expand or "inflate" as it is being shot out. Frying can also cause volume expansion. The principle is the same: steam generates inflation of the product. Inflated french fries (*pommes de terre soufflés*) undergo two rounds of frying. Cooling them after a first short frying period forms a plastic and waterproof crust of gelatinized starch that covers the still raw center of the fry. The second time the fries enter the hot oil, the remaining internal moisture changes to steam and inflates the fries like balloons.

If there were an exam on food expansion or inflation, the preparation of a soufflé would be it. This impressive foam is formed by multiple thin-walled gas cells stabilized by egg protein and inflated by steam. The soufflé starts forming when a base of flour is added to the egg white foam. It should be baked at a temperature that is high enough to coagulate the proteins before the foam reaches its maximum volume. A softer or drier interior can be obtained at temperatures between 160 and 205°C. The expansion of air inside the foam does not cause the soufflé to inflate (pardon the redundancy), but the evaporation of the water contained in the egg white becomes the steam that escapes from the freshly baked soufflé. Everything works perfectly when the egg whites have just coagulated at around 70°C.[20] When the soufflé comes out of the oven, the air and the water vapor inside start to cool and the volume begins to contract (as the temperature decreases, so does the volume). The process of preparing a soufflé is surprisingly similar to that used to make expanding foam for pillows, and the structures of both appear similar under a magnifying glass. Guidelines for experimenting with soufflés in the kitchen were presented in Section 5.6.

8.7 DECIPHERING FRYING

The first known references to frying in the Western world come from the Aegean basin, where frying was used as a conservation method for fish. The shallow ceramic pans exhibited in museums suggest a "stir-frying" type of cooking method, in which a small amount of hot oil was used to decontaminate the surface of the fish pieces and create a protective crust (Figure 8.3).[21] Stir-frying was probably originally developed in China. A round-bottomed wok is very efficient for mixing

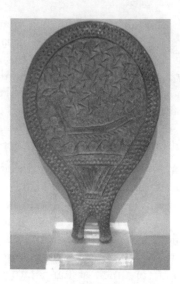

FIGURE 8.3   CERAMIC FRYING PAN WITH DECORATION (AROUND 200 BC). (PHOTO BY
AUTHOR, NATIONAL ARCHAEOLOGICAL MUSEUM, ATHENS, GREECE.)

chopped food in hot oil so that vegetables stay crisp and retain their
original colors while meat browns and its natural juices are preserved.

Frying is an excellent example of a contribution by culinary engineers
to the unit operations of process engineering.[22] Frying is a thermal
treatment that uses a liquid (oil) at high temperatures (170 to 190°C) to
produce important chemical and physical changes in a product. Frying
not only removes the surface water and permeates part of the solid with
hot oil, but from the mechanical point of view it changes a piece of raw
potato into a semirigid beam in just a few minutes.

A basic analysis of the engineering involved in the process of hot oil
immersion frying (deep frying) begins with a physical model that represents heat transfer and mass (or matter) transfer. Figure 8.4 is a diagram showing a piece of fish that is frying, surrounded by hot oil. The
mass transfer occurs when water boils off the outside of the fish, leaving behind a dry, porous crust through which oil can enter. Because
water does not dissolve in oil, it exits from the hot oil in the form of
water vapor bubbles. Mass transfer also occurs when oil sticks to the
surface of the final product.

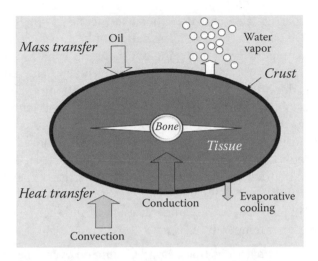

FIGURE 8.4   THE DEEP-FRYING PROCESS OR IMMERSION OF A PIECE OF CONGER EEL IN HOT
OIL. TOP, OIL IMPREGNATES THE SURFACE, AND BOTTOM, HEAT IS TRANSFERRED BY CONVECTION
FROM THE OIL AND THEN BY CONDUCTION INSIDE THE PIECE. MINOR COOLING IS PROVIDED BY
HEAT TO EVAPORATE WATER.

Heat transfer involves the mechanisms that bring heat to the interior
of the piece of fish so that it cooks. Heat flows by convection from the
high-temperature oil (180 to 190°C) to the surface of the piece, and
then penetrates by conduction from the hot surface to the cold interior
of the food (Section 6.6). The food experiences a small heat loss, in the
form of the energy needed for the water to evaporate from the crust
(evaporative cooling). The dry crust gradually reaches the temperature
of the oil as the process advances (the crust begins to brown and may
eventually burn), while inside, the area from which the water evaporates maintains a temperature of 100°C, and the central portions are
heated and steadily cook. An interesting scientific finding is that the oil
does not enter into the crust by diffusion (Section 7.2). Instead, the oil
that remains on the surface after the food is removed from the fryer is
sucked inside the food as the crust starts to cool.[23]

The crust of the fried eel should be crunchy and golden brown in color
(but not too dark), while the meat inside should be white, moist, and so
tender that it flakes easily with a fork (but never chewy). There should
not be any traces of blood on the central bone if the meat is fully cooked.

In fact, preparing fried eel is another good test of a chef's skill, as it takes a delicate balance of providing sufficient heat to cook the interior without burning the crust or drying out the meat. What variables does the chef have to work with? There are relatively few. The temperature of the oil is important because it affects the formation of the crust and the transfer of heat to the inside of the food. If the oil temperature is too low, a good crust doesn't form, and if the temperature is too high, the crust starts to burn and the product must be removed before the center is cooked through. The frying time is another variable, as not all pieces to be fried are the same size. The expertise, experience, and attention of the cook become essential. In some cases it's advantageous to fry certain foods at a lower temperature first, and then a second time at a much higher temperature.

There are several reactions that degrade frying oil over time, due to the heat and the interaction with the food. The most important of these are oxidation reactions, which produce disagreeable odors and flavors in food, and polymerization, which leads to the formation of compounds that can be toxic. The oil in a commercial fryer must be inspected and completely replaced with new oil (not just topped off) from time to time (Section 5.6).

The information from the previous paragraphs helps us to understand the rise and fall of french fries. The crisp crust forms from the heat that quickly transfers from the oil (at a temperature near 180°C) to the outside of the fry, causing the dehydration of the area and the progressive formation of the crust (measuring no more than 1 mm thick). The heat transfer from the crust to the interior produces the gelatinization of the starch in the potato cells, giving the inside of the french fry a soft, moist texture that is similar to mashed potatoes but very different from baked potatoes. Removing french fries from the hot oil is like writing them a death sentence, as the unstable system seeks to reach an equilibrium with humidity and temperature of the environment. The french fry cools off when exposed to air and becomes progressively softer and less stiff, due to the migration of water from the moist interior out to the dry crust, making it softer and less crisp, a condition known as "limpness."[24] The fast food chains do not serve fries that have been out of the fryer for more than 10 minutes, even though they can be kept warm under an infrared lamp. Once water migrates to the crust, it can't be returned to the center (see Section 6.3).

Just as the boiling temperature of a liquid drops under conditions of lower pressure, foods can be fried under vacuum at temperatures around 110°C. With vacuum frying it's possible to obtain products with less oil, higher retention of temperature-sensitive nutrients, and a more natural color and appearance due to the lower temperature (which also helps in reducing the acrylamide content, see Section 1.11).

Are oils the only liquids that are edible and can be heated at temperatures above 150°C at atmospheric pressure? Sugar crystals melt at temperatures around 160 to 170°C, so it's theoretically possible to "fry" food in hot sugar syrup. One problem is that sugar syrup changes color as it heats, becoming increasingly brown from caramelization (Section 2.4). But it's still worth a try.

8.8 IN SEARCH OF THE PERFECT COFFEE

Many people can't start their day without a good cup of coffee. For those who just want a dose of caffeine and aren't worried about appreciating fine coffee aromas, instant coffee fits the bill. Instant coffee is made by dehydrating an aqueous coffee bean extract in a spray drier or by freeze-drying it (see below and Box 8.1). The powders from both methods are distinguishable to the eye: the spray-dried particles are small and rounded (and sometimes agglomerated into granules), while the lyophilized product is made up of small irregular pieces with smooth edges, which are often light brown. In any case, coffee contains appreciable amounts of polyphenols and if consumed regularly can be an important source of antioxidants.

All good coffee begins with careful bean selection and proper roasting. Coffee is roasted at about 185 to 240°C. At these temperatures, a series of chemical reactions (such as the Maillard reaction) combine sugar compounds with amino acids and produce melanoidins that give the coffee its flavor (Section 1.3). Simultaneously other reactions produce series of small volatile molecules that give coffee its distinctive aroma. The aroma of green coffee is made up of about 250 odorant molecules, while the aroma of roasted coffee comes from more than 800. Grinding the coffee beans produces smaller particles and increases the contact area with the water, so that the soluble compounds are quickly and completely extracted. The surfaces of the coffee grinds are composed of broken cells that release their odorous components quickly, while the cells in the interior of the particles remain intact, and the odor molecules must be recovered from inside of them.

There are two phenomena that occur when ground coffee beans brew. The first is the extraction of soluble polysaccharides, caramelized products, lipids, volatile aromas (which are a minute fraction of the weight), soluble acids, and caffeine from the coffee grinds, which is done with hot water. The second process is the filtration, in which the extract must flow through the bed of particles without getting trapped while the spent grinds remain behind. Drip coffee makers use medium ground coffee and receptacles lined with filter paper. Experts recommend rinsing the filter paper with boiling water first to remove the paper smell. The water used for the extraction should be almost boiling, and the process should take no more than 4 to 6 minutes. The filtration time depends on the size of the particles, the thickness of the particle layer, and the pressure. Turkish coffee is made by mixing equal proportions of coffee and water (and sugar if desired) in a special pot (*ibrik*) that is placed directly over the fire so that the mixture boils slightly. The coffee is shaken and stirred when it begins to boil, and this process is then repeated at least twice.

Espresso coffee deserves special mention. The secret of this coffee lies in a combination of several factors. The coffee is ground very fine (with particles averaging 350 to 450 microns in diameter) and there is a greater proportion of coffee grinds to water. Moreover, the water temperature should be between 92 and 94°C, and applied under pressure (nine times atmospheric pressure) so it passes quickly through the grinds (for 30 milliliters of coffee, the optimal extraction time is 30 seconds). The shorter filtration time means that less-soluble acid and caffeine are extracted, and the pressure removes oil droplets and pieces of cell walls that give the espresso a velvety body and intense flavor. The pressure also breaks the oil droplets and releases the carbon dioxide that was produced during the roasting process and is trapped inside the cells that survive the grinding process. The freed carbon dioxide produces a stable creamy foam. If the foam is light in color, the extraction is not complete; a dark foam indicates that the grind was too fine or that too much coffee was used.[25] Good baristas and coffee quality specialists are becoming almost as famous as some chefs.

The subject of instant coffee production was briefly addressed earlier in this section. Water is used to extract the soluble compounds from coffee grains (much like a home coffee machine), and the solids in the resulting extract are then concentrated by evaporating the water. As mentioned, there are two methods for producing a coffee powder. The first method is to spray dry the concentrate, exposing small droplets to hot air which evaporate the liquid water and result in rounded dried particles. A more sophisticated technology is to freeze the concentrate and then remove the water by sublimation at low pressure (the ice passes directly to vapor), which is known as freeze-drying. Freeze-dried coffee particles have irregular edges because they are produced by breaking up the dried mass. Freeze-dried coffee retains more aromas because during freezing the odorous molecules become part of a viscous concentrated solution occluded between the ice crystals (Figure 8.1). After drying, these molecules are trapped in amorphous micro regions and cannot diffuse out until particles are dissolved by hot water (see Section 7.2). Some instant coffees (e.g., *capuccino* coffee) produce abundant foam with the addition of hot water. The secret here is that scientists have been able to encapsulate gas under pressure within a glassy matrix (see Section 2.3). When the granules dissolve in the hot water they quickly release a large amount of gas, creating multiple bubbles that form the foam.

NOTES

1. A binary system is a mixture containing only two components, for example, water and a solute (e.g., sugar). The percentage of moisture (or water content) of the system can also be defined as [water (in grams)/solid (in grams)] multiplied by 100.
2. The *relative humidity* in the air (RH) is a term that needs clarification. For practical reasons we don't use the actual water or moisture content in a

volume of air (e.g., the kilos of water per m³ of dry air), but instead we measure how close the air is to being saturated with water vapor, which corresponds to a RH of 100%. The RH of air is a property of the environment and varies in different parts of the world, and from day to night.

3. One of these cases is Östi, a prehistoric man who was buried in the snow of the Austrian Alps at −30°C for more than 4000 years. It is one of the oldest and best-preserved mummified humans ever discovered, beating King Tutankhamen by 1000 years. See the whole story of Östi in *National Geographic* 183, No. 6, June 1993.

4. Remember "sea monkeys" sold in supermarkets? They are desiccated eggs from a brine shrimp (*Artemia salina*) that hatch rapidly when placed in water, causing children to think that an organism has been brought back to life.

5. A classic reference book on unit operations for the chemical industry is McCabe, W.L., Smith, J.C., and Harriott, P. 2004. *Unit Operations of Chemical Engineering,* 7th edition, McGraw-Hill, Boston.

6. Neirinck, E., and Poulain, J.P. 2001. *Histoire de la Cuisine et des Cuisiniers.* LT Éditions, Paris.

7. There is a museum of wooden nutcrackers in Leavenworth, Washington, which houses over 6,000 pieces, both ancient and modern. Details can be found at www.nutcrackermuseum.com.

8. A good chapter on the tools and technologies used in the kitchen can be found in Wolke, R.L. 2002. *What Einstein Told His Cook: Kitchen Science Explained.* W.W. Norton, New York, pp. 269–320.

9. This, H. 2006. El color verde de las judías. *Investigación y Ciencia* 354, 92. Also published as Le vert des haricots, in his book *De la Science aux Forneaux,* Belin, Paris, pp. 88–89.

10. McGee, H. 2004. *On Food and Cooking: The Science and Lore of the Kitchen.* Scribner, New York.

11. Roberts, R.M. 1989. *Serendipity: Accidental Discoveries in Science,* Wiley, New York, pp. 187–191.

12. There is a book on novel food technologies edited by Sun, D.W. 2005. *Emerging Technologies for Food Processing*, Elsevier, London.

13. Details of the SCFE process can be found in the book by Rizvi, S.S.H. 1998. *Supercritical Fluid Processing of Food and Biomaterials*, Aspen, Springer, New York.

14. One of these Web sites is Forbes.com. Greenberg, A. Gadgets for your future kitchen. www.forbes.com/2008/02/08/kitchen-gadgets-luxury-tech-personal-cx_ag_0211kitchen.html.

15. The reason why the particles do not burn in hot air at 180°C is based on the concept of *wet-bulb temperature*. When a wet object is exposed

to large amounts of the hot dry air, the object remains at a temperature below 100°C, as long as liquid water is continuously supplied to its surface and evaporates. The evaporation requires heat that comes from the product resulting in a cooling effect, such that the product temperature is much lower than 100°C.

16. At sea level (at an atmospheric pressure of 1 atm) water changes from ice to liquid water at 0°C and then to steam at about 100°C (depending on the altitude—in La Paz this would happen at about 89°C), but when the atmospheric pressure is less than 0.6 MPa (0.006 atm) the liquid phase disappears. The transition occurs directly from ice to vapor, a phenomenon that is called *sublimation*.

17. McGee, H. 2004. *On Food and Cooking: The Science and Lore of the Kitchen*. Scribner, New York, shows several photomicrographs, including some images of the preparation of mayonnaise.

18. The Brix measurement (in degrees, symbol °Bx) expresses the concentration of soluble solids in a solution. A solution of 20°Bx is one containing 20 grams of sugar per 100 grams of total solution (20 g sucrose and 80 g of water).

19. The statistics show an annual per capita consumption of about 60 liters of popcorn in the United States.

20. For more on soufflés see This, H. 2006. *Molecular Gastronomy: Exploring the Science of Flavor*. Columbia University Press, New York, pp. 38–40.

21. An interesting article about the origins of fried food in the Mediterranean basin and the types of utensils used is Pucci, G. 1986. Il fritto nel mondo grecco. *International Journal for Social & Economic History of Antiquity*, issue V, 159–165.

22. In chemical engineering, unit operations are the basic transformations that occur in industrial processes, such as milling, distillation, drying, and heat exchange. Any process in the food industry involves several unit operations that generally occur sequentially. This concept was developed at the Massachusetts Institute of Technology (MIT) in the early twentieth century to more specifically analyze the fundamentals of each unit operation.

23. The mechanism by which the oil enters the porous crust of a fried product and its relationship with the structure can be reviewed at Bouchon, P., Aguilera, J.M., and Pyle, D.L. 2003. Structure-oil absorption relationships during deep-fat frying. *Journal of Food Science* 68, 2711–2716. Basically, as the product cools, the vapor in the inner pores of the crust condenses, producing a vacuum that sucks the oil wetting the surface into the crust.

24. In the artice by Miranda, M., Aguilera, J.M., and Beristain, C. 2005. Limpness of fried potato slabs during the post-frying period. *Journal of*

Food Process Engineering 28, 265–281, we report the use of a video camera and image analysis to follow the bending of french fries placed horizontally and held on one extreme. The increase in the angle of deflection with time was used to interpret the kinetics of limpness in the post-frying period.

25. Illy, E. 2002. The complexity of coffee. *Scientific American* 286(6), 86–91.

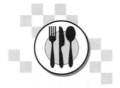

CHAPTER 9

The Pleasure of Eating

Food is presented to us as attractive and tasty structures that we like to eat, normally in a social context. In the past, fine dining was restricted to a few, but in the last two centuries restaurants have democratized access to excellent food (and not so good food). To understand our current situation and the increasing influence of chefs, it is necessary to briefly review the history of traditional cuisine. This chapter introduces some basic culinary nomenclature and provides some references for digging deeper into the topic.

9.1 ENJOYING EATING

No doubt the physiological response of our bodies to food is a result of our evolutionary biology, and the pleasure we derive from eating is based on certain hardwired preferences. For instance, we prefer sweet things and dislike bitter ones, most probably because the first meant calories for survival and the second was a signal for toxicity. Many psychologists agree that when early man began to cook his food, eating became the first actual human pleasure, rather than just an animalistic instinct.[1] In fact, we are not the only species that derive pleasure from eating, but our pleasure goes beyond what our senses perceive: it has to do also with the "essence," something hidden that we want to make contact with.[2]

The sharing of cooking practices between primitive communities is one of the earliest examples that anthropologists have found of the dissemination of empirical knowledge. Anthropologists also believe that cooking made us human, in the sense that more nutritious cooked food enabled early man to progress beyond animal-like activity and helped to distinguish humans as unique creatures.[3] Biologists and nutritionists suggest that cooking was a key feature in the evolution of human beings, as it improved the quality and availability of some nutrients.[4] Food has also influenced our history. In Roman times, the quest for spices inspired the search for better trade routes to the East, eventually leading to the discovery of the Americas, changing the history of mankind.[5] It has been said that Talleyrand, while feasting after he secured great advantages for France, told Louis XVIII "Sir, I need cooking pots more than I need instructions." For Pablo Neruda, the Chilean poet and Nobel laureate, sex and food go well together: "I want to eat your skin like a whole almond" (Sonnet XI).

Socialization and sharing meals with other people at regular times, often referred to by the terms *commensality* or *commensalism*, have been an important dietary ritual since ancient times. Eating was more than just a way of refueling—it was a way to reaffirm family and friendships and to establish social and religious ties.[6] Certain passages from the Bible make clear that eating was about more than just satisfying hunger. During the exodus from Egypt, Yahweh sent *manna* to the hungry Jews, which is described in the Bible as "coriander seed, white and flavored like honeycake" (Exodus 16). After 40 years of eating manna, the Israelites said to Moses: "Who will give us meat to eat? How we remember the fish we ate in Egypt, and the cucumbers, melons, leeks, onions and garlic! But now we have dry souls; our eyes see only the manna" (Numbers 11). The memory of a varied and delicious diet made the Jews forget that they were slaves in Egypt (possibly a consequence of having "dry souls" at the moment). This biblical passage should make twenty-first century nutritionists reconsider the value of certain traditional foods. These foods may be nutritionally "unhealthy" according to present guidelines, but they can also "refresh the soul" if eaten with a sense of remembrance and in moderation.

In *Aphorisms of a Professor*, the gourmet and French intellectual Jean-Anthelme Brillat-Savarin (1755–1826) wrote about food in the middle of the eighteenth century: "The pleasure of the table belongs to all ages, to all conditions, to all countries, and to all areas; it mingles with all other pleasures, and remains at last to console us for their departure" (see following section).[7] In early civilizations the pleasure of food was reserved for the nobility and clergy, while the masses ate to survive. Visitors to the Topkapi Palace in Istanbul can see the ten buildings with tall chimneys that made up the imperial kitchen, which was divided into specialized sections for beverages, confectionery, dairy, and so forth, and where around 800 people prepared daily meals for the 4,000 inhabitants of the palace.

Food has become more accessible thanks to abundance, variety, and relatively low prices. But it's not necessary to consume expensive foods (and drink exclusive beverages) or eat in large amounts in order to take pleasure from eating. The tastes, smells, textures, and other qualities of good food can be found in even the simplest of meals, like a piece of bread with good cheese and a glass of wine, or a fresh salad. Enjoying a meal can be as simple as tasting every bit of what you are eating and drinking, appreciating it with all five senses, sharing the moment with others, and knowing when to stop.

We have a wide range of food options of varying quality available to us, but younger generations in particular seem willing to compromise easily, even on health benefits. Apparently, for them it makes little difference if a food has little nutritional value as long as it tastes good. People often eat alone, distractedly, frequently, and without restriction, which is damaging to their bodies (and possibly to their minds). They are ignoring Aristotle's advice: enjoying the pleasure of eating in moderation, or finding a happy medium, is good and synonymous with virtue.

9.2 GASTRONOMY, GOURMET, GOURMAND, GLUTTON, AND SO ON

It is difficult to establish the beginning of gastronomy, or "the art of eating well." The etymology comes from Ancient Greek (*gastro*, meaning "stomach"; *nomos*, meaning "law"). According to *Larousse Gastronomique*, the bible of gastronomists, the term *gastronomy* became popular in France with the publication in 1801 of *La Gastronomie ou l'Homme des Champs to Table* by J. Berchoux, and the *Academie Francaise* made it an official term in 1835. While eating well is not exclusive to the French people, gastronomy is so ingrained in the culture of that country that it is rare that a French film does not have at least one scene in a restaurant or in the kitchen.

The nomenclature used to classify people who appreciate good food leaves room for some interpretation. The highest level on the scale is occupied by the gastronomers, who are the arbiters of good taste in food. A *gastronomer* appreciates and values the finest dishes of the culinary art, is aware of how to prepare them and recognizes the ingredients, but needs not be a chef. The *gourmet*, however, is a person who knows how to choose a good meal and a corresponding beverage and derive pleasure from their consumption, especially in a social environment. Marco Gavio Apicius was a famous gourmet. In the first century AD he wrote the cookbook *De re Coquinaria libri decem* (cooking in 10 books), but he later poisoned himself upon realizing that he did not have enough money to continue eating well. One level below gourmet is the *gourmand*, who simply enjoys good food. Today the term *foodist* is in vogue to describe someone who is a connoisseur and takes food seriously. The term *foodie* is also popular to refer to someone interested in foods but who does not quite play in the big leagues.

Sybarite is another word that is often used in this context, which derives from the inhabitants of Sybaris, an ancient Greek city on the Italian peninsula famous for its cuisine. Excess wealth led the Sybarites to surrender to sensual pleasures, including food, so the accepted meaning of the word is to describe someone who eats indulgently. At the bottom of the hierarchy is the *glutton*, who represents the total abandonment of reason and unlimited eating. Gluttony is not exclusive to humans. The ancient Egyptians were the first to discover that the wild geese who are about to migrate and travel thousands of miles without possibility of nourishment gobble up large quantities of food and store the energy reserves in their livers. Thus *foie gras* was born. The history of foie gras as a culinary delicacy is on display in bas-reliefs currently located in the Louvre.[8]

Brillat-Savarin (Figure 9.1) is very important for modern gastronomy, as his ambition was to transform the culinary arts into a science, drawing from chemistry, physics, medicine, and anatomy (Section 9.1). He is the author of the book *Physiologie du Gout, ou Méditations de Gastronomie transcendante* (Paris, Sautelet et Cie, 1826), whose cover is shown in Figure 9.1.[9] For its time, this book was an advanced treatise on the pleasures obtained from good food. It ventured in various areas of the human spirit, such as the relationship between gastronomy and conjugal happiness. Brillat-Savarin was the author of the famous phrase "Tell me what you eat and I shall tell you who you are." He is recognized by fans, chefs, and scientists as a scholar and a gourmet who was able to relate in anecdotal and entertaining ways certain scientific aspects of the art of cooking, while reaffirming the compatibility between good food, health, personal well-being, and pleasure.

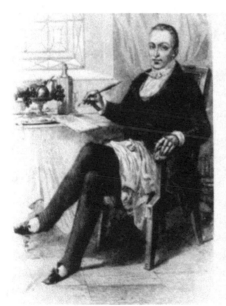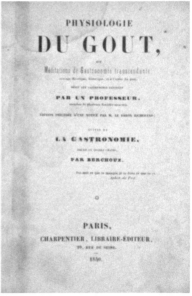

FIGURE 9.1   JEAN ANTHELME BRILLAT-SAVARIN AND THE BACK COVER OF THE BOOK *PHYSIOLOGIE DU GOUT, OU MÉDITATIONS DE GASTRONOMIE TRANSCENDANTE*, 1840 EDITION. (PROPERTY OF THE AUTHOR. PHOTOGRAPH ON THE RIGHT BY A. BARRIGA A.)

9.3 ENGINEERING AT THE TABLE

The relationship of the human body with the various methods for bringing food to the mouth, together with the utensils used for this purpose, form a kind of "gastronomic ergonomics." Through time and across different cultures, people have eaten while standing, sitting, lying down, or squatting. The oval or rectangular table highlights inequalities in access to food, while the round table, used by the Chinese, denotes equality among the people who are eating. The spoon has been the most commonly used utensil, while the fork and knife were introduced by Western cultures. Chopsticks are used in Asia to access food from a common pot (and therefore, should never touch the lips). But the use of the fingers has been (and still is in some cultures) the most common method of bringing food to the mouth, as long as consistency and temperature permit.[10] There is also certain symbolism associated with not using utensils, in that nothing comes in between food and body.

The logistics of the interaction between diners and their food, and the order in which meals are served have changed over time. Greek nobles made a division between the actual meal (*deipnon*) and what happened afterwards, or the *symposium*, which was devoted to drinking wine and talking (Figure 9.2). Today the word symposium is used to describe meetings where scholars come together to make presentations and discuss specific topics (and possibly enjoy some liquor afterwards). As shown in Figure 9.2, the Greek meals and the symposium occurred while the nobles were reclining, a practice adopted from the Assyrian and Persian royalty.

Starting in the sixteenth century, French-style service came into practice. A multitude of dishes were presented simultaneously at three different times during the meal. While diners could choose and serve themselves according to their personal tastes, the foods were not always easy to reach because they were placed on the table in a particular way in order to maintain a symmetry, in which the main course was at the center of the table and the other dishes were distributed around the edges. Therefore, not all of the seats at the table offered the same opportunities to access different dishes. With an oval table, this geometry gave prominence to the central positions at the table, which

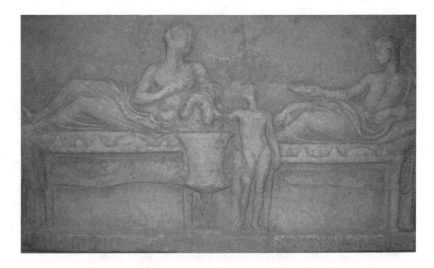

FIGURE 9.2   BAS-RELIEF OF A SCENE FROM A SYMPOSIUM, IN WHICH LIGHT FOOD AND DRINKS WERE CONSUMED IN A RECLINED POSITION AFTER DINNER. (FROM ARCHAEOLOGICAL MUSEUM OF THESSALONIKI. PHOTOGRAPHED BY THE AUTHOR.)

had direct access to vital components of the meal. Those at the end had to rely on neighbors to reach for them or be content with eating just a few dishes.

By the late nineteenth century, French service was replaced by Russian service (still practiced today), in which the various dishes are presented and served one after another in a precise sequence. Everyone ate the same dish at the same time. Reaching the platters of food was no longer a problem, but the diner's position followed in order of importance. Homeowners (the *amphitryons*) sat in the central positions, and the lateral positions were occupied by the guests, whose meal was not to be delayed. The hot serving platters did not come to the table. The food was served in the kitchen, plated, and decorated, then sent to the dining room where each guest was served directly. This system solves a fundamental problem in the French service, which although very pleasing to the eye, was not compatible with the ephemeral conditions of the culinary art, especially the hot dishes. You could say that it was a triumph of taste over the eye, or of time over space, but the diner lost control of selection and size of the portions. Another important difference is that with the French-style service, the food was brought out in order from the most substantial dishes to the lightest. With Russian service, the courses built from lighter appetizers and soups to the main course meat, and then decreased again to desserts and fruits.[11]

9.4 ORIGIN OF RESTAURANTS

There were no fancy restaurants in ancient Athens. Wealthy citizens hired cooks and helpers in the city markets to prepare meals, distinguishing themselves from ordinary people. Poor people were the only ones who ate in public places or bought food on the street.[12] In Europe during the Middle Ages there were taverns and inns where you could eat a simple meal at a common table, but there were no popular restaurants.[13] Instead it was in the kitchens at the court, noble's houses, and monasteries where active culinary innovation was taking place.

It is said that the word *restaurant* originates from around 1756, thanks to a Parisian merchant who provided "restorative broths" or restaurants. The term currently applies to an establishment where meals are served at certain times, either from a set menu or à la carte. The truth is that the emergence of restaurants has much to do with unemployment and entrepreneurship. With the French Revolution (1789) came the abolishment of the privileges of corporations and the prohibition of the manufacture and sale of certain foods. The great chefs who had been serving the nobility found themselves without work and needing to "bring home the bacon," so they had to retrain. Many opened their own restaurants or worked in them.[14] The restaurants quickly filled with the newly rich. These new patrons were wealthy but hardly had a gastronomic culture. In 1803 there were about 400 restaurants in Paris, and by the end of that century, there were around a thousand high-quality restaurants. The first restaurants in London were established around 1830 and served mainly French food.[15]

With the rise of gastronomy, certain dishes began to acquire names, like *Beef Stroganov* (strips of beef with cream sauce, onions, and mushrooms), *Lamb Parmentier* (fillet of lamb with potatoes covered in a wine sauce), and *Chantilly* cream, among many others found in cookbooks. Marie-Antoine Careme (1784–1833) was the first great French chef, and one of the last to work for barons, princes, and tsars. He is credited with double-breasted white jackets (to change sides if staining) and tall hats that chefs wear to distinguish themselves from cooks.

9.5 THE EXPENSIVE RESTAURANT BOOM

Each week several chic restaurants open in big cities, and probably a few close as well. What do you expect from a fine restaurant? You do not expect a good ratio between price and nutrition. The cost of the nutrients that go into a restaurant meal would not exceed 10% of the bill if you bought them at cost.[16] Even if you buy the finest ingredients and assign a cost to their preparation at home, you would still spend less than half of what you would pay for the same thing at a restaurant (unless you are Bill Gates and your time is exceptionally valuable). When we eat in a fine restaurant, we expect great food made with quality ingredients, proper variety and creatively unique dishes, a nice wine selection, personalized service, and most of all, a special atmosphere. Eating well in a pleasant ambiance is something that has been appreciated since antiquity, and therefore it's expensive.

There are no recent published data on the cost of eating in the finest restaurants. According to *Forbes* magazine the basic menu (without wine) at the restaurant *Aragawa* in Tokyo cost about $277 in 2005. *Arpege* in Paris cost $211, and *Eigensinn Farm* in Toronto cost $213.[17] It is said that in 2005 the price for a meal at the top London restaurants rose three times the rate of inflation, and the ones with the biggest price increases were the most expensive. There would have been at least four London restaurants charging over 100 pounds ($190) for a standard meal: two courses, dessert, a bottle of house wine to share, coffee, and tip.[18] The most expensive dish in Germany is a breaded pork (*schnitzel*) coated with 25-carat gold plate and costing about 150 euros.[19]

Magazines and newspaper reviews as well as guides developed by professional food critics and inspectors are good references for choosing where to eat. The role of the professional food critic was born in 1802 with Grimod de la Reynière and his *Almanach des gourmands*, which had 280 pages in its first edition and was an outstanding food guide. Today the French *Michelin guide* is the most respected in terms of gastronomy and haute cuisine. Since 1900 Michelin has awarded its stars on a basis of five criteria (independent of cooking style): product quality, mastery of flavors and cooking, personality and creativity of the dishes, proper value, and consistency. The inspectors, who visit the restaurants in 21 countries anonymously and pay their own bills, can visit the same place several times before granting or removing the famous stars. One star denotes a very good restaurant in its category, two stars reflect an excellent cuisine, and three stars represent an exceptional cuisine, worth a special trip. At the beginning of this century there were no more than 50 three-star Michelin restaurants, and interestingly, half of them were in France. In 2009, 26 restaurants received three-star ratings, 73 got two stars, and 449 got one star.

NOTES

1. Rodrigo Jordan, leader of the first South American expedition to reach the summit of Everest (and a colleague who introduced me to mountain hiking), told me once that the climbers missed their favorite foods more than anything else during the long weeks of an ascent.
2. Bloom, P. 2010. *How Pleasure Works: The New Science of Why We Like What We Like.* W.W. Norton, New York. My dog jumps and wags her tail while I serve her food but she seems not to be very excited while actually eating. Most humans derive pleasure from preparing as well as from consuming food.
3. A more complete account can be found in Chapter 5 (entitled, The kitchen taught how to talk and modeled man) of Cordón, F. 1979. *Cocinar hizo al Hombre.* (Cooking made man). Editorial Tusquets, Barcelona. There is no English version of this book.
4. Wrangham, R., and Conklin-Brittain, N. 2003. Cooking as a biological trait. *Comparative Biochemistry and Physiology,* Part A, 136, 35–46.
5. Corn, beans (*phaseolus*), tomatoes, potatoes, chilis and other peppers, turkey, and of course cacao (chocolate) are among the foods originating from the Americas. Insects were also part of the gastronomic culture of indigenous South American people but were not as well received.
6. This quote comes from the book of Wilkins, J.M., and Hill, S. 2006. *Food in the Ancient World.* Blackwell, Malden, Massachusetts, p. 63.

7. On weekends I have witnessed famous politicians and business leaders standing for over half an hour in line at a bakery in a small village by the sea, waiting for the fresh bread to come out of the oven.

8. In Toussaint-Samat, M. 2005. *History of Foods*. Blackwell, Oxford, pp. 424–434, there is a very complete and entertaining history of *foie gras*.

9. In New York you can get the original version of this classic for the incredible sum of $9,000, but fortunately there are modern versions in English that are much more affordable.

10. Fumey, G., and Etcheverría, O. 2004. *Atlas Mundial de Cocina y Gastronomía*. Ediciones Akal, Madrid.

11. Neirinck, E., and Poulain, J.-P. 2001. *Historia de la Cocina y de los Cocineros*. Zendrera Zariquiey S.A., Barcelona, pp. 43–46, 51–53, and 76–78. Also published in French as *Histoire de la Cuisine et des Cuisiniers*. Éditions LT Jacques Lanore, Paris (2004).

12. Wilkins, J.M., and Hill, S. 2006. *Food in the Ancient World*. Blackwell, Malden, Massachusetts, p. 52.

13. Laurioux, B. 2003. La gastronomía medieval. *Investigación y Ciencia* 320, 58–65.

14. Although there are countless versions of how the restaurant came to be, this section is largely based on what is presented in the book by Gillespie, C. 2001. *European Gastronomy into the 21st Century*. Butterworth/Heinemann, Oxford.

15. Tannahill, R. 1988. *Food in History*. Crown, New York, p. 327.

16. As reference, a perfectly balanced animal feed containing 20% protein, vitamins, minerals, and amino acids in optimal proportions, plus a prebiotic, can cost $1 per kilo.

17. Banay, S. 2005. World's Most Expensive restaurants 2005 (www.forbes.com/2005/10/12/restaurants-mostexpensive-world-cx_sb_1013feat_ls.html (accessed January 20, 2009). The cost of a fixed-price menu at *Eigensinn Farm* is currently about $275.

18. Information obtained from the article, Dinner? That's 100£. *Evening Standard*, August 16, 2005, p. 9.

19. Restaurant in Dusseldorf. *El Mercurio*, Santiago, December 17, 2009.

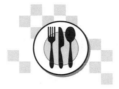

CHAPTER 10

The Empowerment of Chefs

Chefs are the professionals who are the most credible innovators of modern food. Some of them are interested in breaking with tradition, just like the painters of the late nineteenth century, and do not hesitate to use scientific knowledge and even attach "laboratories" to their kitchens. Their creative impact travels to universities and enriches our cuisine.

10.1 GASTRONOMY AND ART

There is a long-standing relationship between art and gastronomy. One could say that the classical arts relate to the ways humans have visually perceived and represented the world around them. Similarly, classical cuisine is related to the perception of smells, tastes, shapes, and textures of natural foods and traditional preparations. *Haute cuisine*, like the fine arts, goes beyond the purely utilitarian function (eating to survive) to include dishes with "aesthetic" value, appreciated by connoisseurs.[1]

In the second half of the nineteenth century, French Impressionist painters managed to capture everyday pleasures. In the famous painting *The Luncheon on the Grass* (1863) by Edouard Manet (1832–1883), food is at the forefront, as it was still art. In the early twentieth century, abstract painting emerged, ending the artists' habit of painting reality just as they saw it. The proposed idea was that what matters in art is not reproduced in nature (nature photography began in 1888), but that inner feelings can be revealed through colors, shapes, and lines. Georges Seurat (1859–1891) studied the scientific theory of color perception and applied paint in tiny dots which could be perceived as known forms when viewed from a distance. The next radical break came with paintings that lacked any recognizable object, appealing to the emotional impact produced with pure colors, simplified shapes, and the use of the line, as proposed by Wassily Kandinsky (1866–1944). No artist took this proposal more seriously than Pablo Picasso (1881–1973), who sought inspiration for his works from other art forms rather than from nature. The Dutch painter Piet Mondrian (1872–1944) wanted to represent the immutable realities of the universe through straight lines and rectangles filled with primary colors. This opened an infinite number of possible representations that were obviously too complex for the lay public, who sees only scratches and stains, to understand. In their childhood and youth, these geniuses painted the classic themes magnificently, as you can appreciate by visiting the Picasso museum in Barcelona or the Hague Municipal Museum (in the case of Mondrian), but their paintings evolved into works that are more difficult to decipher. The same phenomenon takes place with today's modern chefs, who can cook traditional dishes very well but who challenge the traditional with new culinary formats.

It cannot be a coincidence that a first attempt to produce an important break from the traditional cuisine of the twentieth century came from Italian painters and poets, who in 1930 launched the *Manifesto of Futurist Cooking*. Led by Filippo Tommaso Marinetti (1876–1944), the Futurists advocated a change in approach by placing the same importance on form and color as is placed on flavor. They conceived of food as "a special architecture, unusual, possibly unique to each individual." One of their proposals (fortunately unsuccessful) sought to get rid of pasta, as they found pasta dishes to be quite vulgar.[2]

In the last decade of the twentieth century, chefs must have felt just like the painters of the late nineteenth century. How much black sole with butter, steak *au poivre*, and *béarnaise* sauces had they prepared in their lives? Weren't there other ways to explore gustatory, olfactory, visual, tactile, and audible sensitivities through food? Could each person be able to discover and interpret what is in each dish on its own? Similar to trends in photography, new technology was already allowing chefs to explore with some traditional foods, and there was a threat that quick-freezing allowed for the marketing of quality frozen menus prepared under the guidance of renowned cooks. It was the time for chefs to make an offer rather than simply respond to public demands.

The relationship between modern gastronomy and painting can be seen in certain terminology used by some modern chefs. For example, the kitchen deconstructionist dismantles the components of a traditional dish and presents them differently while retaining the essence of the dish, so that the customer "constructs" his or her own flavors in every bite. A "deconstructed" Spanish tortilla consists of eggs, potatoes, onions, and sausage prepared in different ways (like a potato "foam" and mashed chorizo, for example), assembled in layers in a conical glass.[3] As in art, culinary creations are not intended for the everyday public. They become important touchstones for innovation in the kitchen, generating new concepts that enrich everyday meals and enter our lives without us realizing it.

10.2 THE CHEF WHO INVENTED AIR

It's 6:30 P.M. on Tuesday, December 9, 2008, and the Department of Physics at Harvard University is waiting for the speaker to begin. The auditorium is full and TV monitors had to be installed outside to accommodate more people. Who is speaking? A Nobel Prize winner or perhaps Einstein's successor? No, it is a chef who will speak on science and cooking. This is Ferrán Adrià, the Spaniard chosen by *Time* magazine as one of the 100 most influential people in the world in 2004 and the chef at *El Bulli*, voted best restaurant in the world for five consecutive years.[4] El Bulli, which is located near Girona, was rated with the highest possible scores in the Michelin and Gault Millau guides and receives about 500 thousand reservation requests each year from all over the world. "Heck, it's crazy! I can only seat about eight thousand during the season (six months). Some people have been calling for 15 years and still cannot get a table," Adrià said in an interview with local media.[5] The price of the tasting menu at El Bulli is about 275 euros per person. After the conference, the School of Engineering at Harvard decided to introduce the topic of science and cooking into the curriculum, and even created a gastrophysics center in conjunction with the famous chef.[6]

The New York Times proclaimed Adrià the best chef in the world on its front page, and the reporter who wrote the article described the El Bulli menu in the following way:

> Welcoming cocktails of a frozen whisky sour and a foam mojito were accompanied by popcorn that had been powdered and reconstituted as kernels and a tempura of rose petals. An array of seven warm gelatin blocks that resembled watercolor paints, each a vivid hue that proved to be a pure essence of a vegetable. I was handed a fresh vanilla bean to smell while eating vanilla-scented whipped potatoes. And so on, for three and a half hours.[7]

Adrià has been called "the chef who invented air" in reference to his habit of introducing air into food. He says that he applies concepts derived from the paintings of Russian masters in the kitchen. The cover of *The New York Times Magazine* of 2003 shows Adrià posing with an "air," which is nothing more than something that has been liquefied and whipped in the presence of lecithin to make foam. He works in his laboratory in Barcelona for half the year, where he also designs china, cutlery, and cooking utensils. His work is displayed in elegant but very expensive books. Much has been written about this famous chef and more could be written here as well. But unexpectedly, Adrià has announced that he has closed El Bulli to launch a culinary foundation where he will concentrate on creativity.

Not everything is sweetness and light in the world of the star chefs. Adrià's Catalan colleague Santi Santamaría, chef of El Racò de Can Fabes, which also has three Michelin stars, challenged Adrià in 2008 (as well as other "molecular chefs") to "cook things that they themselves would eat," referring to the thickeners, gelling agents, and emulsifiers used in some of the dishes (see Section 11.2). Adrià was even accused of hiding from the public what is served in his restaurant and of supporting a multinational company that sells unhealthy products.[8]

10.3 CHEFS: THE TOP TEN

Each year, the British magazine *Restaurant* presents the S. Pellegrino list of the top 50 best restaurants in the world. Like all rankings based on expert opinions, the results are debatable. In 2011 the list of the top 10 restaurants (including indication of their change in position from the previous year) was as follows: (1) Noma, Denmark (=); (2) El Celler de Can Roca, Spain (+2); (3) Mugaritz, Spain (+2); (4) Osteria Francescana, Italy (+2); (5) Fat Duck, United Kingdom (–2); (6) Alinea, United States (+1); (7) D.O.M., Brazil (+11); (8) Arzak, Spain (+1); (9) Le Chateaubriand, France (+2); and (10) Per Se, United States (=). In the top 20, there are five restaurants from France, four from the United States, three from Spain, two in Japan, and one each in Denmark, Italy, United Kingdom, Brazil, Belgium, and the Netherlands.[9] As mentioned, El Bulli, which won the number 1 spot a record five times, closed at the end of July 2011.

What do these chefs do to become so successful? First, they love what they do and have inquisitive minds, a desire to know more, and a curiosity that distinguishes them from the rest. They are bold and do not feel tied to the classical traditions. Some have found that a teaspoon of science added to their dishes awakens taste sensations and emotions never present in traditional cuisine. For this reason, many of them have their own laboratories for experimentation (like Adrià and Blumenthal of the Fat Duck), maintain connections with scientists (Pierre Gagnaire and Hervé This in Paris, for example), or even contract research in specialized centers (like Andoni Luis Aduriz of *Mugaritz* and Azti-Tecnalia in the Basque Country). They are innate innovators, capable of philosophizing about the food and making propositions that provide meanings and certain symbolism to their cooking.[10] What these chefs have done for the cuisine of the beginning of the twentieth century is proportional to what Kandinsky and Picasso did for twentieth century painting.

Some readers might wonder how much money these elite chefs earn, once their fame approaches the level of rock stars. According to *Forbes* magazine, the Austrian chef Wolfgang Puck, who lives in Beverly Hills, earned about $11 million in 2004, from television programs, food service businesses, his chain of Express restaurants, and sales of books and cooking utensils. In addition, Puck won an Emmy for his television series *Wolfgang Puck* which was broadcast on The Food Network. Emeril Lagasse was second on the list of wealthy chefs, with a yearly income of $9 million. Lagasse appears live seven nights a week on the Fine Living Network.[11] But staying at the pinnacle of world cuisine can be stressful. The French chef Bernard Loiseau committed suicide after the 2003 Gault Millau culinary guide downgraded his restaurant's score to 17 points, or less than perfect. At 52 years old, Chef Loiseau was a prolific and detailed chef, who had said he wanted to be for the culinary arts "what Pele was for soccer."[12]

10.4 THE NEW CUISINES

In the second half of the twentieth century, some of the knowledge accumulated from nutrition and food science research began to influence cuisine. The aesthetic of thinness and preoccupation with health inspired some chefs to gradually shift away from the complex and heavy dishes of classical cuisine, and undertake a search for the natural flavors and textures of each ingredient. *Nouvelle cuisine* began when certain chefs embraced the cause of authenticity and freshness of ingredients, as well as lightness and harmony between the components of a meal and the accompaniments. *Fusion cuisine*, however, was a response to the opportunity to mix foods from diverse backgrounds in a harmonious way, exploring the wealth of culinary cultures from around the world.

Author's cuisine highlights the creativity of chefs looking for new forms of expression in their preparations and giving them a distinctive stamp. This trend includes the rejuvenation of typical or traditional dishes from each country, and the incorporation of indigenous and rarely used ingredients. These kinds of restaurants sometimes have a farm of their own from which to source main ingredients, which then can be offered as natural and reliable.[13] The cuisine associated with agrotourism is one of the most popular expressions of this trend, particularly in Europe, where local chefs offer products made by traditional processes with resources from the area that are often organically produced.

Progressive cooking or *techno-emotional cuisine* are some of the many names for the efforts of modern chefs to include new ingredients, use unconventional cooking methods and instruments, and expand tastes and sensations. As mentioned, some of the most famous chefs who have embraced the modern food movement have added labs to their kitchens. The book *On Food and Cooking: The Science and Lore of the Kitchen* (1984), by Harold McGee, is an important reference for many of these chefs. McGee's book describes the science behind what happens in the kitchen and explains how food structures are born, change, and die.

Success did not come easy to these new cuisines in all parts of the world. Food cultures of different countries are sometimes slow to change, and most people are not prepared to explore foods that are too innovative and they are not willing to accept radical changes. Many young kitchen assistants of famous restaurants, who have become local chefs around the world, have simply adapted to if not copied these new ideas learned at foreign kitchens, without adding much of their own creativity.

The most recent trend among top chefs is to integrate the whole culinary process from the farm to the preparation in the kitchen. This includes aspects such as selection of new varieties of known foods and indigenous crops, control of agricultural practices in small plots, mild methods of harvesting and fast transportation, and so on. It also extends to the provision of seafood, which implies special arrangements with artisanal fishermen. This "culinary" chain is becoming a specialized subset of the conventional food chains.

10.5 IN THE HANDS OF A CHEF

Truly groundbreaking chefs create innovative menus that combine various textures and flavors in stunningly precise designs. A *tasting menu* is the most affordable way to enter the world of one of these chefs. The tasting menu is a series of small dishes or "courses" that are served as an alternative to the traditional menu of appetizer, entrée, and dessert. Some of the courses in a tasting menu might be one single bite, like the oyster and passion fruit jelly with lavender at the Fat Duck. Some people might find the tasting menu disappointing (even a famous chef has agreed) and "just a way of charging a lot for a small amount of food." The tasting menu puts the diner "in the hands" of the chef, in the sense that the diner must accept the chef's choice of creations and the order in which they are served. It is the opposite of the *buffet*, where customers can choose from multiple known alternatives, controlling portion size and deciding in what order they eat various dishes. The tasting menu gives the kitchen staff freedom to create innovative dishes that might be more risky if served in a full portion and the diner did not enjoy it. El Bulli offered more than 20 tasting dishes, but a typical tasting menu has a couple of entrées, four to five main courses, and two to three desserts. Appreciating the creativity of this kind of menu requires a willingness to try new experiences, to listen to the "instructions" before each course, and to arrange the components in each bite, balancing them to suit personal taste.

To some extent the tasting menu is a more formal way to order several dishes for sharing, so that everyone is able to try every one. If Enrico Fermi, the famous Italian physicist was alive, he would say it is "to nibble ... but at a higher level."[14] In a fancy restaurant, a tasting menu normally offers sensational (and instant) preparations, impeccable service, and meticulous presentation, served on special china. There should be a personalized introduction of what is served, and the opportunity for playful surprises (like the diner at a neighboring table expelling nitrogen gas through his nostrils, like an enraged dragon). It is a good way for customers to experience new things and gain a better knowledge of food culture. Beginner gourmets may feel like classical music neophytes at their first opera, as this kind of meal requires an understanding of what the chef is trying to say. The diner must concentrate on tasting the food and be aware that he or she may not find everything delicious or entertaining. Eating at these sophisticated restaurants is a memorable experience, and like the opera, you must wait until the next season for a new menu. Millions of people each year embark on tourism programs that include at least one exceptional dining experience.

Experiencing the creativity of a great chef can be achieved outside of Michelin-class restaurants. I remember a practical degustation of the best of regional Italian cuisine at *Il Granaio*, a countryside *trattoria* near Parma, where dishes were continuously brought to our table over a 3-hour period. As the cook generated the different dishes in the kitchen they were circulated through the tables and you took from them or passed them along. In this way I learned to appreciate pasta *al dente* and fresh pea pods.

10.6 MOLECULAR GASTRONOMY

The relationship between gastronomy and chemistry is not new. Alchemy (from the Arabic *al-kimiya*) took its culinary equivalent in the search of the "vital juice" in foods and the preparation of the osmazome, or the main and absolute flavor in meat. The gastronomic treaty *The Gift of Comus*, published in Paris in 1739, established that "modern cookery is a kind of chemistry. The cook's science consists today of analyzing, digesting, and extracting the quintessence of foods, drawing out the light and nourishing juices, mingling and blending them together."[15] The real "scientification" of cooking may have begun in 1877, when chef Joseph Favre, who conducted research at the University of Geneva, founded the newspaper *La Science Culinaire*, with contributions from chefs. One hundred years passed from then until the emergence of "molecular" cuisine. Put simply, molecular gastronomy is the application of scientific principles to answer questions and uncover the secrets of gastronomy or the culinary arts.[16] Like it or not, the simple fact is that molecules are what we smell and what we eat. Prestigious scientific journals such as *Science* and *Nature* have published articles devoted to molecular gastronomy.

The term *molecular gastronomy* was coined by Nicholas Kurti (1908–1998), a physicist at the University of Oxford and an aficionado of gourmet food. This Royal Society fellow lamented the fact the he knew more about the temperature inside a star than what happens inside of a soufflé. He introduced novel appliances into the kitchen such as syringes to distribute liquor within a food, and proposed a vacuum for making meringues without heat. Kurti also initiated a series of biennial conferences at the Ettore Majorana Center in Erice, Sicily. Chefs from top-rated restaurants (Michelin guide) and a few lucky scientists got together every 2 years to discuss advances and new methods for enriching cooking techniques.[17] The original partner and presumed heir to Kurti is the French scientist Hervé This, who has been associate editor of the French edition of *Scientific American* and an honorary member of the *Academie Nationale de Cuisine*. In his doctoral examination before a jury that included two winners of the Nobel Prize in Chemistry, Pierre Gilles de Gennes and Jean-Marie Lehn, This presented the five key objectives of molecular gastronomy: (a) understand the meaning of culinary tricks and proverbs in empirical gastronomical terms; (b) explain the fundamentals of the recipes and practical methods of classical cooking in order to improve them; (c) introduce new utensils, ingredients, and methods in the kitchen; (d) invent novel dishes as a result of the conducted investigations; and (e) use the kitchen to present science to the public. Today there are a number of chefs who apply concepts of molecular gastronomy in their restaurants.[18] On a visit to the monthly meeting on molecular gastronomy that Hervé This holds with chefs and scientists in a room on the Rue de l'Abbé Grégoire in Paris, the participants discussed the appearance of macarons or macaroons. *Macaroons* are cookies made of almonds, sugar, and egg white, which have a characteristic light-colored, cracked surface once they are baked (French *macarons* are also known as *macarons craquelés*) which is part of the cookie's charm.[19] The theme of this meeting was to investigate how the recipe and baking conditions affected the surface of the cookie, and describe the size, shape, and distribution of the cracks. Our brains find it difficult to quantify these details, but image analysis makes it much simpler (see Section 5.8). The various chefs, clad in spotless white jackets, generously shared their experiences and freshly baked macaroons with one another. The scientist emphasized two important points to the group: that oven temperatures vary and therefore must be determined accurately, and that the instruction "bake cookies with the oven door half open" is not very precise and reproducible.

Although the word "molecular" came into vogue in 1990 and gave a connotation of modernity, some chefs did not feel comfortable with this term because of the association with chemistry as well as with "molecular biology." The term was actually chosen to address the connection between food and increased scientific knowledge, in an effort to understand culinary transformations and expand the range of dining options. In fact, some of the chefs who were initially enthusiastic adherents of this movement, like Adrià and Blumenthal, later declared that molecular gastronomy had died a natural death because it had ventured too far into the use of chemistry and technology. Some experts now prefer to talk about the *scientific* kitchen, while the North Americans invented the word *culinology*, which is a registered trademark of the U.S. Research Chefs Association (RCA) (www.culinology.com), and is defined as an "assembly" of the culinary arts and food science. The American culinologists and the molecular gastronomists across the Atlantic don't seem to get along as well together. For the former, molecular gastronomy is like a "science class," separate from the "art" of cooking.[20]

10.7 FROM THE TEST TUBE
TO THE PALATE

The spontaneous association between gastronomy and science seems to be here to stay. What is at stake is the innovation in new textures, flavors, and sensations for a global market where restaurants sales reach more than $1 billion annually.[21] Modern chefs are aware that access to science and technology will provide new concepts and tools that help them to be more efficient in their experimentation and thus better able to express their creativity. They are convinced that food and science should not be as separate as they have been in the past, but that the synergies between them should be exploited. You could say that the union of science and food is a remarkable case of open innovation, where chefs collaborate with external agents bringing expertise, infrastructure, commitment, and quick development. Food scientists ally themselves with chefs in order to access innovative professionals who are credible with the general public and can offer an effective way to bring science to the people (Figure 10.1).

Adrià and Blumenthal have their own experimental laboratories, and Gagnaire has worked with the French scientist Hervé This (Sections

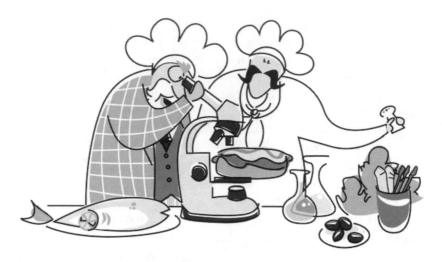

FIGURE 10.1   THE PARTNERSHIP BETWEEN SCIENTISTS AND CHEFS OFFERS SYNERGIES THAT BENEFIT CULINARY INNOVATION.

9.5 and 10.3). The research center Azti-Tecnalia in the Basque Country (www.azti.es) and Andoni Luis Aduriz's restaurant *Mugaritz* have been collaborating since 2006 to develop recipes and create new products. This "laboratory of ideas" combines scientific and technical knowledge with the creativity of the restaurant setting. The *Alícia Foundation*, located in Sant Fruitós del Bages near Barcelona, is a technology research center that is dedicated to the popularization of gastronomy and promotion of good nutrition. Adrià participates actively in this organization (www.alimentacioiciencia.org). Davide Cassi, a professor of physics at the University of Parma and Ettore Bocchia, and the chef of the restaurant *Mistral Bellagio* have worked together for several years and published a book of their experiences working on molecular cuisine together.[22] Our lab and my associates (including graduate students) have interacted with reputed local chefs and made presentations on modern cooking at business meetings as well as in science camps for high school students.

The Experimental Cuisine Collective (http://experimentalcuisine.com) is a collaboration initiated in 2007 by scientists from the departments of chemistry and nutrition at the University of New York with chef Will Goldfarb. It aims to develop a rigorous academic approach for examining the properties of food in the kitchen and to study issues related to health and wellness. Multinational food companies also consult with chefs for help with adding essential flavor to their healthier food options. But not all of these collaborations run smoothly. The European Inicon project involved four chefs (including Adrià and Blumenthal) who worked together with the food industry to develop innovative technologies for modernizing the kitchen and gastronomy. The contributions from this particular project were less substantial than expected, according to some.

As an academic and having worked for nearly five years in close quarters with some local chefs, here are some conclusions I have drawn from the experience. First, the restaurant business is a very important part of the "food industry," which for food technologists usually only includes the companies that manufacture the processed products found in supermarkets. Second, chefs (especially younger ones) are very willing to experiment in the laboratory (while food engineering students prefer to "cook" on a computer). And finally, one of the most important considerations for university scientists: chefs don't need to assess the potential market demand, as their customers are "captive" in their restaurants, nor do chefs seem to have too many cost concerns, as menu prices can be adjusted. Chefs do not have to perform scaling tests on pilot plants that process large volumes because they can serve small portions that are similar to what they prepared in the laboratory, and they can quickly bring their creations to consumers. Working with chefs is the surest way to bring products straight from our research labs into people's mouths.

10.8 THE REASON SCIENTISTS DO NOT WRITE RECIPES

Traditional cuisine is based on recipes that are handed down from one generation to the next. Written recipes begin with an ingredient list and continue with a description of the preparation. While the ingredients are relatively well described, for example, eggs (but, what size?), the procedure is often fairly imprecise. Consider the recipe from the famous French chef Auguste Escoffier (1846–1935), emperor of the world's kitchens:[23]

> *Procedure for preparing a filling of creamed ham:* Finely chop the meat and seasoning, gradually add the egg yolks and pass through fine sieve. Place the stuffing in a deep pan or sauté pan, and keep on ice for 30 to 40 minutes. Then dilute (sic) little by little with the cream, working it with caution, so as to make a mayonnaise.[24]

Instructions like "finely chop," "add little by little," and "keep on ice" abound in recipe texts. These unspecific directions annoy scientists who are accustomed to working with particles of known sizes, using pipettes to dispense droplets in microliter volumes, and measuring temperatures with an accuracy of tenths of a degree. Instructions like "add a pinch" or "a scant teaspoon" are grating to physicists and engineers who are accustomed to precise measurements that go out several decimal places. It is obvious that a young girl's fingers would "pinch" much less ground pepper that a large man's fingers. While this vagueness allows for experimentation and is a source of variability, creativity, and differentiation for professional chefs, it's frustrating for the occasional cook and unacceptable and even offensive to scientists.

Science progresses in small steps based on research contributions that are publically disclosed as scientific articles. In the area of food research there are about 90 major scientific magazines published monthly or bimonthly, as well as books, conference proceedings, professional journals, and patents. This means that, on average, each month more than 1,000 articles are published specifically related to food science and technology.[25] Each manuscript (or paper, as it is known in scientific jargon) is reviewed anonymously by at least two peers (people who research the same topic) before it is accepted for publication. The scientific literature contains a huge amount of information and provides a great opportunity to better understand certain phenomena and gain access to new ideas.

Scientific papers might be equivalent to recipes, because they describe the materials and procedures used to obtain the reported results. They usually include a "Materials and Methods" section, which meticulously details the origin of the reagents used (including batch number), the amounts used, the equipment and conditions of operation, the specific analytical techniques, and the procedures used to carry out the experiments. There is mention of experimental designs and statistical analysis of repeated experiments demonstrating that the results are statistically reliable. The idea is another scientist anywhere in the world should be able to copy the original experiment and determine if the results are reproducible. This feature of the scientific method helps to detect falsified results from unscrupulous scientists as well as poor results from unrigorous research.[26] It would be unthinkable and quite impractical to demand this level of and precision from a recipe that is meant only to satisfy food cravings, not to discover the last particle of matter or cure cancer.

The industrial patents that seek to protect an invention are a bit like the recipes, however, as they describe a process as generally as possible, hiding important secrets in the vagueness of the text. They attempt to disclose only the minimum necessary to prove there is something new while hiding more precise data that could be copied. A patent might read "the concentration of a substance must be between xx and zz grams per liter and the temperature should be between yy and ww °C," with both intervals large enough to prevent someone from reproducing the exact result of the invention. In this sense, engineers are more understanding of the chefs who seek to preserve the secret of their creations by using vague language. Innovative chefs review scientific papers in search of new concepts and even "steal" patent ideas, as an executive publicly acknowledged in a conference at a famous North American cooking institute. The point is that both scientific papers and patents are widely available and are sources of information and inspiration for kitchen scientists. Discounting them would be missing an opportunity, but in order to have a good understanding of their contents, you need to know something about science.

10.9 GASTRONOMY GOES TO COLLEGE

The empowerment of chefs has also arrived in the classroom. Culinology study programs are sprouting like mushrooms all over the

United States, luring students with the attractive combination of food science and gastronomy. One driving force is a wide and tempting job market in a sector that represents about one third of the food industry. The possibility of opening or operating a business is a draw, as are possible incomes, which can exceed $60,000 for an executive chef with five to eight years of experience (equivalent to the salary of a food technologist with more work experience). Some universities have made a place for gastronomy because the food science career market is saturated and schools are desperately looking for programs that will attract motivated students.

There are many varied opportunities related to gastronomy at the university level. Most are for people who want to teach at a culinary school, open a restaurant, or work in product development at a company. Drexel University (Philadelphia, Pennsylvania), for example, offers four-year degrees in hospitality management, culinary arts, and food science. Other programs are less technical, for students who wish to be food and beverage journalists, work in gastronomic tourism, or perhaps be employed in public relations at large hotels or tourist agencies. One very special institution of higher education is the University of Gastronomic Sciences, founded in 2004 by the creators of the Slow Food movement (Section 12.4). This school has two locations in northern Italy. Graduate studies cover food production, and the impact on the environment and sustainability, as well as food culture. The courses include anthropology and food history, photography, culinary techniques, local products, communication and sensory analysis, among others. In keeping with these trends, the university has been accredited by the Italian government. Boston University (Massachusetts) offers a Master of Liberal Arts in Gastronomy, a program developed by Julia Child and Jacques Pépin, which invites students to "explore the role of food and wine in world culture through the arts, humanities, and social and natural sciences." The University of Adelaide in Australia established a postgraduate degree in gastronomy focused on the study of food and beverages in a variety of contexts. One unique "university" is Hamburger University, as it is owned by McDonald's. Founded in 1961, it has over 5,000 graduates. In 1983 the school moved to a campus near the company's corporate offices in Illinois, occupying premises valued at $40 million. The two-year program is recognized in the United States and, as expected, students deal with subjects such as restaurant operation, service, quality, and cleanliness.[27]

But for those who aspire to become renowned chefs, the route has remained the same for 200 years: to become a chef's apprentice. Hundreds of young people intern in famous restaurants where they learn not only culinary skills but also the "philosophy" of the restaurant.

10.10 SOME BOOKS ON GASTRONOMY AND SCIENCE

The food or kitchen section in bookstores keeps expanding to cover more space, suffering a kind of "obesity" that is not necessarily healthy. Faced with such a crazy proliferation of cookbooks, one needs to be a bit selective when creating a personal library. Most cookbooks lack information about how to eat or live better, but are merely collections of recipes, many of dubious taste and quality, with little creativity.

A classic reference and must-have book for foodies, culinary scientists, and chefs alike is the *Larousse Gastronomique*, created 70 years ago (1938). If you can't access the full version, you can content yourself with the concise version.[28] In terms of modern gastronomy, there are also interesting, though rather expensive, illustrated books by celebrity chefs.

The selection of books on science and cooking begins with the obligatory reference for everyone who loves to cook, whether gourmet or chef: *On Food and Cooking: The Science and Lore of the Kitchen* by Harold McGee (Simon and Schuster, 1988, revised edition by Scribner, New York, 2004). In over nearly seven hundred pages McGee has managed to present a rigorous but engaging description of the chemistry of culinary transformations, the properties of different ingredients, and pleasures underlying every dish. His premise is that to understand what happens to food during cooking, it is essential to understand the molecular reactions that take place, and that this in turn is a source of inspiration for experimentation. This book is a must-have addition for any library of modern gastronomy.

It is always good to have a food chemistry text on hand, so that you can consult the basic and fundamental concepts of food science. My favorite text is *Fennema's Food Chemistry* (4th edition, CRC Press, Boca Raton, Florida, 2007). Many of the leading specialists offer their versions of the chemical properties of the constituents and nutrients in food, as well as dispersions, enzymes, vitamins, minerals, animal tissue, toxicants, and pigments. The book *The Chemistry of Cooking* by A. Coenders (Taylor & Francis, Boca Raton, Florida, 1991) is sometimes used as a food chemistry textbook for students of gastronomy. It contains a good description of food ingredients and the chemical transformations that occur during their preparation.

Peter Barham is a physicist at the University of Bristol, United Kingdom, whose hobby (besides kitchen physics) is penguins. In his book *The Science of Cooking* (Springer Verlag, Berlin, 2000) he argues that a kitchen is similar to most scientific laboratories and that many cooking processes are true physical science experiments. This is noted in the chapter on "physical gastronomy" which discusses the effects of different types of heating (grill, microwave, etc.). He even proposes a formula to determine the correct cooking point for a soft-boiled egg. A surprising experiment (which must be done very carefully) is to cook an egg on a piece of paper. It starts by cracking an egg over a piece of paper whose edges are folded to resemble a rectangular pan. The paper must be maintained at a safe distance over a low flame. The paper that is exposed to the flame must always be covered by the egg, otherwise it will burn (obviously). Because the egg whites and yolks contain a lot of water, as it slowly evaporates the temperature of the paper never exceeds 100°C (boiling point of water at atmospheric pressure), and the heat from the flame will cook the egg while evaporating some water. Sauces and cakes are the preferred materials for Barham and their respective chapters are filled with recipes and tips to enhance their appearance and solve problems.

Hervé This, a French physical chemist who works at AgroParisTech in Paris, is an excellent scientist and prolific author who reveals the secrets of the kitchen and demystifies many cooking myths and traditional practices (Section 10.6). Most of his books are in French, although his most popular book, *Molecular Gastronomy: Exploring the Science of Flavor*, has been published by Columbia University Press

(2006). Many of the monthly articles he writes for the French scientific magazine *Pour La Science* have been compiled in a book *De la Science aux Fourneaux* (Belin, Paris, 2007). Here you will find explanations for why we don't perceive the true acidity of foods in our mouths, how to avoid clumps when adding liquid to flour, or why frozen squid become more tender than fresh squid when cooked. This' books are an excellent addition to any library.

Experiments in the Kitchen by the German professor G. Schwedt (in Spanish by Editorial Acribia, Zaragoza, 2006), has an excellent first section that covers the history of cooking and food preparation since Roman times, when different cooking methods were used such as boiling, grilling, hot embers, and "cold cooking" with marinades. He describes famous people in literature who had a connection with cooking, such as Alexander Dumas, who compiled a Dictionary of Cuisine shortly before his death. Schwedt's book describes more than one hundred simple experiments, demonstrating phenomena such as protein coagulation, gel formation, the caramelization of sugars, and the effects of different types of cooking. Moreover, the text is an excellent source of ideas for practical ways to teach physics and chemistry in schools, using food as examples.

Given the relevance of the Spanish experimental cuisine it is not surprising that many books on modern gastronomic science are in that language. The Alícia Foundation and el Bulli Taller have produced *Lexico Cientifico Gastronomica* (Fd. Planeta, Barcelona, 2006), in which the entries are ordered alphabetically and provide definitions, general uses, and methods of use for additives and important food components, as well as reference explanations for scientific concepts, physical and chemical processes, technologies, and so forth. This is a very practical manual and a quick reference resource for both industry and cooks. An English version is available under the title *Modern Gastronomy A to Z* (F. Adria, CRC Press, Boca Raton, Florida, 2010). *Sferificaciones y Macarrones*, a recent book by C. Mans (Ed. Ariel, Barcelona, 2010) addresses the science and technology behind the traditional and the modern kitchen. Another interesting book is *The Sweet Toothed Brain* (*El Cerebro Goloso*, Rubes Eds., Barcelona, 2006) by André Holley, a professor of neuroscience who delves into the current scientific knowledge about the pleasure of eating. Genes, proteins, receptors, ion channels, neurons, and the brain form a hierarchical chain whose links and connections allow odors and flavors to be captured in the nose and tongue in the form of molecules (see Section 7.3). Some suggestive chapter titles include "the signals of satiety," "the brain that tastes and smells," "the delicious synergy between sugar and fat," and so on. He suggests that our problems with obesity and related illnesses may have to do with the fact that our bodies have not changed genetically for hundreds of centuries, while rich food is much more available and accessible than it has ever been.

In *Histoire de la Cuisine et des Cuisiniers* (5th edition, Editions LT Jacques Lanore, Paris, 2004), E. Neirinck and J.P. Poulain review the evolution of French cuisine, starting with its brief relationship with alchemy in medieval times, through the efforts in the last century to develop a "culinary science." The book also describes the way innovation takes place in the kitchen and explains the impact of nouvelle cuisine and current trends. The book by Oxford historian F. Fernandez-Armesto *Food: A History* (Macmillan, 2001), will satisfy those looking for perspective on how technology has changed our diet. There is a recent book by Harvard professor Richard Wrangham, *Catching Fire: How Cooking Made Us Human* (Basic Books, New York, 2009) where he argues that besides making our food safer and creating rich delicious tastes, cooking increased the amount of energy available, enabling our brains to grow larger. Last, if you are into nutrition, an excellent book is *Introduction to Nutrition and Metabolism* by David A. Bender (4th edition, CRC Press, Boca Raton, Florida).

Magazines such as *Scientific American* or the French version *Pour la Science* contain sections in which scientists explain kitchen phenomena in simple but rigorous terms, such as why jelly hardens when it cools, how to make mayonnaise without curdling it, when to add salt to roasted meat, and other similar gastronomic curiosities. There are a number of journals that contain articles about food and science, including the following:

- *Culinology* is the official publication of the *U.S. Research Chefs Association* (RCA). Their publications contain examples of practical applications for culinology (see Section 10.6), recipe development, and food industry issues that may be relevant for readers (www.culinology.com).

- *Journal of Culinary Science & Technology* covers topics such as science and technology behind the meal planning, aspects of basic and applied research in culinary science, healthy eating and lifestyles, and the development of practical cooking skills. (www.haworthpress.com/store/product.asp?sku = J385).
- *Gastronomica* is a magazine focused on the intersection between food, culture, and society. Published quarterly by the University of California Press, it includes articles and essays from columnists and food critics, historians, artists, and so forth (www.gastronomica.org).
- *Gastronomic Sciences* is a journal published by the University of Gastronomic Sciences in Italy (see Section 10.9). The contributors are mainly professors at the university and therefore the articles cover issues related to the Slow Food movement (www.unisg.it).
- *New Food.* Publishes reports on new technology developments and innovation in the food and beverage industry. Four issues per year (www.russellpublishing.com).
- *International Journal of Gastronomy and Food Science* is a peer-reviewed journal that explores the application of a scientific approach to the fields of applied culinary, new culinary concepts, and the sociocultural aspects of gastronomy. The first issue has just come off the press (www.azti.es/ijgfs). The editorial board includes renowned names that should be familiar to you by now: Harold McGee, Peter Barham, Andoni Luis Aduriz, Heston Blumenthal, and René Redzepi (the chef of Noma, the number 1 restaurant in our list in Section 10.3).

In short, there are books and journals that cover the many facets of foods, including cooking, gastronomy, history, culture, and science. No single taste has been left out.

NOTES

1. Hegarty, J.A., and Barry O'Mahony, G. 2001. Gastronomy: A phenomenon of cultural expressionism and an aesthetic for living. *International Journal of Hospitality Management* 20, 3–13.
2. An article on the "futuristic" kitchen can be found in www.marjorieross.com/archives/1085 (accessed April 1, 2010).

3. I tried this dish in 2002 at the Casino de Madrid, where it was called "The twenty-first century Spanish tortilla (omelette)."

4. See www.seas.harvard.edu/cooking/Adria_Talk.pdf (accessed April 16, 2009). Adrià's visit to Harvard was not the first time a famous chef stepped into a classroom of a prestigious university. Heston Blumenthal, owner of the Fat Duck restaurant near London, received an honorary doctorate from the University of Reading in the United Kingdom in 2006.

5. Ferrán Adrià: el cocinero que inventó el aire. (Ferrán Adrià: The cook who invented air). *Revista El Sábado* de El Mercurio, Santiago, October 31, 2003.

6. http://harvardmagazine.com/extras/next-the-harvard-center-gastrophysics (accessed March 16, 2010).

7. Taken from an article by Arthur Lubow for *The New York Times*, August 10, 2003.

8. Santamaría, S. 2008. *La Cocina al Desnudo. Una visión renovadora del mundo de la gastronomía*. Eds. Temas de Hoy, Madrid.

9. For a complete list, go to www.theworlds50best.com/awards/1-50-winners (accessed July 29, 2011).

10. For greater depth on these issues see Gillespie, C. 2001. *European Gastronomy into the 21st Century*. Butterworth/Heinemann, Oxford, pp. 151–155.

11. Data obtained from an article on the best-paid chefs in the world found at www.forbes.com/celebrities/2004/06/16/celebs04land.html (accessed June 18, 2007).

12. Chef commits suicide after a bad critic. *El Mercurio*, Santiago, February 26, 2003.

13. This is the case, for example, at *Eigensinn Farm*, a restaurant located 150 km from Toronto. More than 90% of the restaurant's ingredients come from a neighboring farm. The restaurant and farm are presented as "a self-sustaining ecological system." It has been said that eating at *Eigensinn Farm* "is one of the top 10 culinary experiences in the world," priced at $275 per person. More about this restaurant at www.theglobeandmail.com/report-on-business/article785268.ece (accessed March 20, 2011).

14. It is said that Enrico Fermi (1901–1954), winner of the 1938 Nobel Prize for Physics, while attending a lecture with many complex equations, took the floor and told the young and arrogant scientist: "Before I came here I was confused about this subject. Having listened to your lecture I am still confused...but on a higher level." Great scientists are able to explain complicated issues in simple terms. Note that it is possible that this quote, though attributed to Fermi, was actually spoken by someone else.

15. Laudan, R. 2000. Birth of the modern diet. *Scientific American* 283(2), 76–81.
16. This, H. 2005. Molecular gastronomy. *Nature Materials* 4, 5–7.
17. In 2004 I attended the last molecular gastronomy conference convened by Hervé This in Erice, a village in Sicily. About 30 people were invited, including the second and third best chefs in the world at the time (H. Blumenthal and P. Gagnaire), as well as H. McGee and P. Barham, authors of books on science and gastronomy (see Section 10.10).
18. The Web site http://blog.khymos.org/links/people/(accessed December 14, 2010), lists a number of restaurants and chefs (whose names are in parentheses) that have been influenced by molecular cuisine, including El Bulli (Ferrán Adrià), The Fat Duck (Heston Blumenthal), Pierre Gagnaire (Pierre Gagnaire), Grand Hotel Villa Serbellione (Ettore Bocchia), Saint Pierre (Emmanuel Stroobant) in Singapore, French Laundry (Thomas Keller), Alinea (Grant Achatz), Restaurant L (Pino Maffeo), Moto (Homaro Cantu), Tapas Molecular Bar (Jeff Ramsey) in Japan, Mandarin Oriental Boston (Damian Zedower), Oud Sluis (Sergio Herman), Room 4 dessert (Will Goldfarb), and DOM (Alex Atala) in São Paulo.
19. An interesting report on the modern French macaroon can be found in this article by Meyers, C. 2009. The macaron and Madame Blanchez. *Gastronomica* 9(2), 14–18.
20. An article entitled, Deconstructing molecular gastronomy, in the journal *Food Technology* (June 2008) has been replicated by Hervé This in the same journal.
21. Banay, S. 2005. World's most expensive restaurants 2005, at www.forbes.com/2005/10/12/restaurants-mostexpensive-world-cx_sb_1013feat_ls.html (accessed January 1, 2009).
22. Cassi, D., and Bocchia, E. 2005. *La Ciencia en los Fogones: historia, técnicas y recetas de la cocina molecular italiana.* (Science in the stoves). Ediciones Trea, Gijón.
23. According to *The Concise Larousse Gastronomique*, the title was conferred by Emperor William II saying, "I am the Emperor of Germany, but you're the Emperor of Chefs." Escoffier was awarded France's Legion of Honor in recognition of his contribution to the enhancement of the prestige of French cuisine around the world. Throughout culinary history, there has not been another chef with such an extensive career (64 years).
24. Escoffier, A. 1968. *Mi Cocina*, 3rd edition. Ediciones Garriga S. A., Barcelona, pp. 271–272.
25. With the advent of the Internet, access to scientific information has become globalized and democratized, in the form of complete abstracts from scientific articles as well as partial access to full texts. The Web

sites of major publishers, such as ScienceDirect (www.sciencedirect.com) from Elsevier, provide convenient summaries of publications (and in some cases complete text in pdf format). Another important source of scientific information for nutrition data is PubMed (www.pubmed.com).

26. The case of "polywater" is an example. In the early 1960s, an unknown chemist working in a small institute in a Russian province reported having discovered a special type of water called "anomalous water" or "polywater," which did not freeze or boil like ordinary water. After 5 years and more than 500 publications, it was demonstrated that contamination of laboratory equipment caused all of the unusual results. More details can be found in the book by Franks, F. 1981. *Polywater.* MIT Press, Cambridge, MA.

27. There is limited information about Hamburger University at McDonald's Web sites www.mcdonalds.com/es/usa/work/burgeru.html and www.aboutmcdonalds.com/mcd/corporate_careers/training_and_development/hamburger_university.html.

28. A revised edition is the *Concise Larousse Gastronomique*, Hamlyn, London, published in 2003.

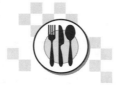

CHAPTER 11

The Science That Fascinates Chefs

Many chefs have been fascinated with science and technology as ways to expand the scope of their creativity. New ingredients, equipment, processes, and even the scientific method have entered the kitchen. The combination of science and imagination boldly gives rise to new and remodeled structures for diners to enjoy. Here are some of the novel ingredients and ideas with which chefs are experimenting

11.1 CHEFS AND INNOVATION

High-level chefs must continually generate new ideas for their menus. The motivation behind all of that innovation is in the words of a respected modern chef: "the excitement and delight in discovering new ways to cook and bringing satisfaction and emotion to the table." Another reason for innovation is protection against plagiarism, which is inevitable in this business and requires constant vigilance. When the ideas of the most talented and successful chefs are copied by lesser chefs, one benefit (though not for the gifted ones) is that their innovations spread. Using an analogy from economics, this phenomenon produces a "trickle-down effect" in which ideas and concepts flow to cooks who may have fewer resources and capacities but reach a broader clientele.

The top chefs usually follow a formal and structured innovation process, with stages that are similar to the development of commercial products.[1] To generate new ideas, they look to other restaurants, traditional recipes, new raw materials and ingredients, patents, and concepts like deconstruction, minimalism, "decontextualization." They make use of the "technical-conceptual search" to develop new products and processing methods. They perform an informal analysis of the ideas, and based largely on intuition, they select those that merit investigation. The phase of developing a culinary concept is essentially to define the concrete message that will be communicated, and this depends on the experience and cooking style of the individual chef. Some chefs have found that science gives them knowledge, methodologies, and a new way of looking at the design of dishes and meals during this stage. One way in which this process differs from industrial product development is that chefs do not typically concern themselves with cost analysis, because they compete in a highly segmented market and are able to pass on higher costs to the menu prices. Finally, using quality ingredients is an important part of the development and marketing process, as "excellent food is made from excellent ingredients." This requires training for the kitchen staff in order that they understand the standards and expectations, so that the dishes served are consistent in quality, taste, and appearance.

Another difference between restaurant food and industrially produced products is that intellectual property protection does not exist in the world of restaurants. But the restaurant business has some important advantages over industry. The use of authorized nontraditional ingredients is left to the discretion of the chef, whose reputation is at stake. With regard to technology, chefs work with small volumes, almost at the laboratory level, which allows them to avoid problems of scale, such as the environmental impact inherent in industrial production. Vacuum impregnation and osmotic dehydration (see Section 11.13), for example, are both beneficial and proven technologies in the lab, but they are difficult to implement on an industrial scale because they generate high volumes of dilute solutions that must be recycled or disposed of, with the associated energy costs or damage to the environment.

Innovative chefs always arouse the suspicions of those who prefer traditional and "natural" raw materials. Many new ingredients, however, are just as natural as traditional ones, such as the cornstarch that has been used for centuries, which is extracted with a "chemical" process (sulfur dioxide is added to the steeping water to suppress detrimental microbes from growing) and then dried, in the same manner that alginates and carrageenan are derived from seaweed. Soybean oil, used for decades, is removed from the grain with an organic solvent similar to aircraft fuel.[2] As mentioned previously, there are natural products that can become toxic and other natural foods from which our bodies cannot efficiently extract nutrients during digestion. If desired, the use of refined ingredients on a menu does not preclude the use of premium natural products as well, such as organically grown fruits and vegetables from small orchards that use good agricultural practices. Many chefs are well aware of the importance of using indigenous foods and local products and developing links with small farmers and artisanal fishermen, as well as the baggage that comes along with combining regional cooking techniques with cutting-edge culinary techniques.

Discussed below are two of the areas that have recently seduced chefs in their quest to develop flavorful new structures that are surprising and even playful: the almost limitless possibilities of the new ingredients and some innovative ways to transform traditional food structures or to create new formats for them.[3]

11.2 THE NEW INGREDIENTS

The massive growing market for restaurant and take-out food, as well as the demand for convenient and low-cost, high-quality food options has led to remarkable growth in the variety of available food ingredients. Signs of this abundance can be seen at food expos, like the one conducted annually by the U.S. Institute of Food Technologists (IFT), where hundreds of companies exhibit products in almost 100 ingredient categories. Some of the categories and the number of companies offering items (in parentheses) who attended the 2009 IFT exhibition included colorants (51), emulsifiers (64), thickeners (57), antioxidants (78), dough conditioners (41), egg substitutes (20), non-nutritive sweeteners (57), taste maskers (40), and preservatives (45). A sampling of some of the favorite ingredients used by the processed foods and restaurant industries, as well as in a number of modern cuisines, is described in Box 11.1.

Gone are the days when the only available thickener was starch (or flour) and when all gels were made with gelatin. Today there are hydrocolloids such as xanthan gum, which give dishes a high viscosity but also exhibit great fluency under agitation (so the product can be mixed). Modified starches (Section 1.13) have an unequaled resistance to freeze-thaw cycles, and therefore can be used in sauces for frozen prepared meals, avoiding any exudation of fluid. Some of the gelling agents in use today, such as agar-agar, have a long history of use in the East but have only recently been introduced into Western cuisine. The majority of the ingredients listed in Box 11.1 come from natural ingredients (fruits, plant exudates, seaweed, legumes, etc.). Most are extracted with methods that have been used in the food industry for a long time and are subjected to stringent food safety regulations regarding purity and dosage. Most of the criticism about the use of these ingredients arises from situations in which diners are not properly informed of their use in restaurant dishes.

A good reference for verifying ingredients and the allowed conditions for their use is the *European Directive on Food Additives* (see also Section 1.4), which covers the entire food industry in the region. There is always a temptation to exceed these limits in some professional kitchens that are not required to publish ingredient lists. The consequences can sometimes be painful—a high dose of carboxymethylcellulose, for example, has quite a strong laxative effect.

11.3 THREE-D SAUCES

There are more than 200 known sauces that are fundamental accompaniments to many dishes. They have been generously spread over

**BOX 11.1   SOME OF THE INGREDIENTS
THAT ARE INCREASINGLY USED
IN COMMERCIAL PRODUCTS AND
GASTRONOMY (WITH THEIR E-CODE)**

Agar-agar (E-406). A polysaccharide extracted from algae such
as *Gelidium* and *Gracilaria* used for centuries in Japan (where
it's known as kanten) to make molded jellies. Heated solutions at very low concentrations (e.g., 1%) form strong gels
when they cool.

Sodium alginate (E-401). Corresponds to the sodium salt of
polysaccharides derived from *Macrocystis pyrifera*, a species
of kelp (large brown algae). It is a cold gelling agent that
requires the presence of calcium ions and is used among
other things to make artificial caviar ("spherification").

Carboxymethylcellulose (CMC) (E-466). A derivative of cellulose
that is soluble in water. It is used to adjust the texture of many
products as a binder, emulsifier, thickener, and so on.

Carrageenans (kappa, iota, and lambda) (E-407). A family of
sulfated polysaccharides extracted from red algae (e.g.,
Chondrus and *Furcellaria*), which have been used as food
additives for hundreds of years. They are utilized as thickeners, gelling agents, or emulsifiers in dairy products, meats,
desserts, salad dressings, and so forth.

Microcrystalline cellulose (E-460). This is composed of small
crystals produced by hydrolysis of pure cellulose. Used in
low-calorie versions of products like desserts and ice cream,
and as a carrier for aromas.

Gelatin. A water-soluble protein obtained from bone or skin
collagen (mainly from pigs). It is used to prepare hot and
cold gelatin and as an emulsifier in foams.

Gellan gum (E-418). A polysaccharide produced by bacteria. It
can form hard and brittle gels, and gives a melting sensation
in the mouth.

Guar gum (E-412). This is obtained from the endosperm of
crushed seeds of the legume *Cyamopsis tetragonolobus* and

consists mainly of high molecular weight polysaccharides. It is used as a thickener and stabilizer in emulsions, and is soluble in cold water.

Xanthan gum (E-415). An extracellular polysaccharide (i.e., secreted into the medium) that is obtained by fermentation mediated by *Xanthomonas campestris.* It is widely used as a natural thickener and emulsifier, and for its thermal stability.

Egg white powder. The powder is spray-dried egg whites that can be used as a substitute for fresh egg whites.

Isomalt (E-953). An alcohol derived from a disaccharide. Used in a wide variety of foods and drugs, it has the same taste, texture, and appearance as sugar, but with half the calories. It's nonsticky because it is not hygroscopic, and it has applications in candy and baked goods.

Soya lecithin (E-322). A mixture of phospholipids that is used as an emulsifier and to make foams. The molecule's characteristic of partly dissolving in water and partly in fat part gives lecithin a versatility that is attractive to chefs, as evidenced by Ettore Bocchia "lecithin gnocchi" that are smooth yet resistant.[4]

Gold (23 carat or 96% pure) and edible silver. They are sold in sheet form, as well as flakes and dust.[5] They are supposed to be inert and excreted from the body without transformation. The Italians (and the Japanese) have a long tradition of using edible gold in their cuisine. In the sixteenth century there was already a dish called *Risotto d'oro con basilico e parmigiano* (gold risotto with basil and Parmesan cheese).

Soy proteins. They are powders with various concentrations of protein: defatted flours (50%), concentrates (70%), and isolates (90%). They are used to make textured meat substitutes, gels, and to stabilize emulsions; also utilized as fortifying proteins and ingredients in baked goods.

Whey proteins. A spray-dried powder made from sweet whey. They are used as a protein source to form gels with heat, among other things.

> *Transglutaminase.* An enzyme that can attach peptides and proteins together. It is used for restructuring tough meat, gel production, texture control in yogurt, and so forth.
>
> *Trehalose.* A disaccharide consisting of two glucose molecules. It is used as a cryoprotectant in surimi.

foods since the fourteenth century, some say in order to hide or divert attention from what is underneath. Nowadays sauces can have a third dimension, surpassing the two-dimensional restriction to merely cover a surface, by converting them into foams (Section 2.7). In addition to their aesthetic benefit, foam bubbles give lightness to otherwise viscous and dominating liquids. Foams are prepared by whisking or siphoning a sauce, puree, or liquid that contains a foaming agent. For example, a juice or a drink can be transformed into a foam by adding *quillaja* (soapbark) extract plus a gum to increase viscosity, then agitating the mixture or dispersing a pressurized gas into it. We have done this to foam a whisky sour.

The technology behind food foams is a hot topic, as there is an ongoing search for products that combine low caloric density with the sensory properties from gas bubbles. There are innovations in the use of foaming agents and gases that can produce different foam structures, as well as new techniques for dispersing gas, such as ultrasound and porous membranes, and in the future, microfluidics.[6]

11.4 EDIBLE FILMS

Several natural polymers can form edible films, including many proteins and lipids, polysaccharides (like cellulose, starch and its components, amylose, and amylopectin), and chitosan, a polymer derived from chitin that gives shrimp and crab shells their rigidity. Some of them are translucent and even transparent, like their cellophane and polyethylene films counterparts. In many cases, the property of water vapor barrier of a film is deficient, so the polymer must be combined with hydrophobic substances. In other cases the films are rigid and brittle so a plasticizer such as glycerol is needed. In the future edible films may cover fresh commercial products like fruits and vegetables, slowing water loss and protecting them from microorganisms. It will also be possible to "waterproof" food structures that should remain dry, like pizza crusts and sandwich bread slices, to protect them from the juices of the fresh ingredients with which they come in contact (lettuce, tomatoes, etc.).

The technology needed to manufacture these films is simple. Some only require the air drying of a thin layer of a properly formulated polymer solution, so chefs have not lagged far behind industry in using them. Chefs have designed an "artificial skin" to cover pieces of a large fish, made from collagen extracted during cooking the same fish and some commercial gelatin. The film is transparent, becomes flexible with moisture so that it conforms to the shape of the pieces, and can be decorated on the outside.[7] In his Chicago restaurant *Moto*, chef Homaru Cantu presents the menu in one of these films that is printed with edible inks. After reviewing the menu and taking notes, the waiter invites diners to eat it. Edible film strips can serve as vehicles for freshening the mouth between courses or to release aromas and special flavors.[8]

11.5 SPHERIFICATION

Much has been written about sturgeon egg caviar, but the truest thing that has been said about this *non plus ultra* of food is that it's "a dream." In Spanish, the expression "it's a caviar" describes something that is exquisite to the palate.[9] Several decades ago, scientists from the former Soviet Union set out to develop synthetic caviar, and there are now several patents for gelled alginate beads. Chefs rediscovered this process of making small gel spheres, which they call *spherification*. Juices, purees, and extracts of various kinds can be dissolved into a solution of 1% to 3% sodium alginate. The mixture is placed in a syringe, from which droplets drip into a calcium solution (usually calcium chloride) where they transform almost instantly into semisolid beads (Figure 11.1). A spoonful of the extract and sodium alginate solution can also be added directly to the calcium solution, thus forming a "skin" around the liquid, which is how "egg yolk"-like culinary creations are made.

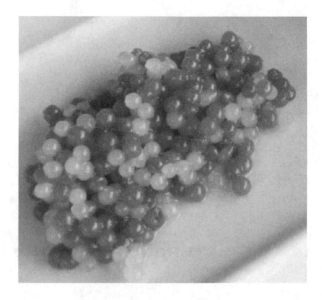

FIGURE 11.1   "CAVIAR" WITH THREE TYPES OF SPHERES CONTAINING TOMATO, ONION, AND PARSLEY EXTRACTS THAT HAVE BEEN GELLED WITH CALCIUM ALGINATE. (PHOTO COURTESY OF IGNACIO GUNDELMAN.)

11.6 SMOKE AND AROMA

Smoke is a mixture of tiny particles and aromas that are generated by the combustion of different woods. Smoke is used more for its effect on a food's taste and appearance than for its limited preservation effect as in the past. Smoke (generated *in situ* or added in liquid form) gives certain dishes unique flavors and aromas associated with native woods and forests. The PolyScience company offers a smoking cannon that chefs can use to infuse smoke flavors into the food at room temperature.[10] A New York chef uses it to smoke lettuce leaves, which he then wraps around raw oysters. Some of the components of smoke, such as benzopyrene, have exhibited under certain experimental conditions mutagenic and carcinogenic effects.

Aromas come from volatile molecules that provoke agreeable olfactory sensations (Section 7.3). For cooking purposes, the goal is to be able to recover an aroma from an ingredient or dish and then concentrate it, in order to add it later as desired. In laboratories, the rotavapor (spinning evaporator submerged in a hot water bath) is used to distill liquid mixtures. Some chefs have used the rotavapor to generate their unique aromas, and even to "distill" clay in order to capture its "earthy essence," which is then converted into foam. Extracts that are temperature sensitive and water immiscible can be distilled with a simple steam distillation apparatus. In this process the sample (leaves, flowers, etc.) is exposed to steam, and those compounds that boil at a lower temperature escape with the water vapor.[11] The mixture is then cooled and condensed into a two-phase liquid, and the oils are isolated from the liquid water (coming from the steam) by phase separation (decanting).

11.7 STRUCTURES THAT SOUND

Some foods generate noise as they break when you bite into them and chew them. Food texture specialists talk about the "acoustic signature" of a food, which is the group of characteristic sound signals that can be picked up by a microphone when a food breaks (Section 2.14). Panels of sensory experts tend to use words like *crumbliness, crispness, crunchiness,* and *crackliness* to describe the textures of food by the sounds that are emitted when they break, although there are no exact definitions for these terms. Crumbly foods tend to break easily into aggregates or granules (e.g., a granola bar). In general, crunchy foods are fragile and fracture easily (with minimal deformation beforehand) and with little effort, while it requires more force to break crispy foods. The category of crispy products includes moist foods like apples and celery, as well as dry foods like potato chips and soda crackers. The crunchiness of a moist food derives from the cell turgor and the breakdown of the cell walls during chewing (Section 2.1), while with dry crunchy foods the sound originates from the vibration of the thin walls of the air cells as they break during mastication. One possible difference between crisp and crunchy foods may be the manner in which the sound sensation reaches the cochlea of the inner ear: through air and the outer ear in the case of crisp foods, or through direct bone conduction from the teeth with crunchy foods. But it's not yet completely clear. My friend Zata Vickers of the University of

Minnesota has spent over 30 years trying to understand the noises produced by food. In any event, chefs are keen to develop structures that will fracture with lots of sound. For this reason chefs tend to overuse frying, which produces a tasty product that also makes satisfying noises.

Perhaps it is the simultaneous occurrence of the tactile sensations in the mouth with the sounds in the ear that makes crisp and crunchy foods so pleasant to eat. In a controversial culinary experiment performed by chef Heston Blumenthal at The Fat Duck, each guest could hear the sounds they produced by chewing amplified through headphones. Very few customers found this experience enjoyable, probably because the excessive role of sound disturbed the balance of sensations.

11.8 EXPLOSIVE AND BUBBLY MATRICES

Unusual or bizarre experiences and playfulness may be an important part of certain tasting menus. The "explosive" and noisy sensations that Pop Rocks® candy produces in the mouth have appeared in restaurant dishes. The effect comes from CO_2 that is trapped under pressure inside small bubbles within a solid matrix of sugar (Figure 11.2). The matrix begins to dissolve upon contact with saliva, and eventually the thin and fragile walls surrounding the bubbles fracture from the pressure, abruptly releasing the gas and causing the characteristic sizzle. General Foods patented this product idea in 1956.[12] The explosive candies are made from a mixture of the matrix ingredients (e.g., sucrose, lactose, and starch) which is heated until the components melt. Carbon dioxide is then injected under pressure (about 40 atm or 4 MPa), the resulting foam is cooled, and the solid is ground into small pieces. One challenge is to find other types of matrices that trap gases (and why not aromas?) to produce the same effect. The violent release of gas that occurs as the matrix dissolves in a liquid has also been exploited to produce foams, as in the case of instant cappuccino powder.

Carbonated fruits ("fizzy fruits") are created by placing pieces of fruit and dry ice (solid carbon dioxide at –78.5°C, also called "carbon dioxide snow") together into a covered jar. After several hours in the

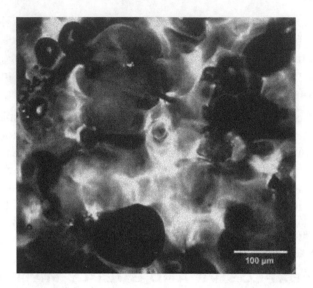

FIGURE 11.2   INTERIOR OF A POP ROCKS PARTICLE SHOWING THE ROUND BUBBLES CONTAIN-
ING PRESSURIZED GAS AND SURROUNDED BY THE SOLID SUGAR MATRIX.

refrigerator the gas sublimates (goes directly to vapor) and pressurizes the container, introducing gas into the fruits. The fruits retain their same taste, but they produce a tingling effect on the tongue with chewing. The effect lasts about 15 minutes, so the fruits must be served quickly. Several chefs use these carbonated fruits, and they have also been used in some school lunches as a novel and entertaining way to encourage consumption of fresh fruits.

11.9 KITCHEN CRYOGENICS

Liquid nitrogen (LN) boils at −196°C under atmospheric pressure. Freezing with LN is based on the principle that the heat needed for evaporating the LN is supplied by the products that are being frozen, so that they cool rapidly to very low temperatures. LN is used in chemistry and physics laboratories, by dermatologists, and to freeze sperm and embryos of livestock. It's very pure and it can be used in direct contact with food. LN should be stored in Dewar flasks, handled only while using insulated gloves and protective eyewear, and applied with care. When freezing with LN, abundant nitrogen gas escapes into the surrounding air, which may affect some people.

When LN is poured onto a food product or the piece is immersed in LN, the food quickly freezes to a very low final temperature, a process unmatched by any other method for freezing foods. Chefs use LN to transform creams into ice creams with velvety smooth textures, or to create frozen "crusts" over warm cream fillings. In the words of chef Joel Robuchon, often a critic of molecular cuisine, "the use of LN allows for the creation of sublime sorbets and sumptuous textures thanks to the high speed of the cooling process which prevents the formation of (large) ice crystals." In our laboratory we developed a "coulant" by dipping a sphere of hot chocolate into LN for a few seconds, until a thin icy crust formed on the outside (Figure 11.3). When the icy crust was broken at the table, the hot chocolate oozed out, with its consistency and aroma intact. This special effect works only if the concoction is served immediately, as eventually the heat of the hot chocolate in the center will melt the outer frozen crust. Some chefs use LN in small tidbits of food for an even more playful trick—the "dragon" effect. The diner is told to place the morsel into his or her mouth, wait a bit while the gas evaporates, and then expel the gas

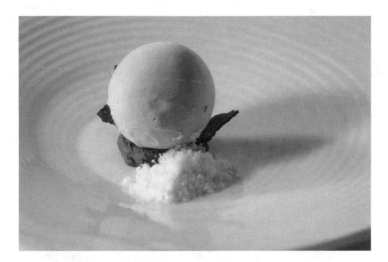

FIGURE 11.3   CHOCOLATE "COULANT" MADE WITH LIQUID NITROGEN. THE COLD OUTER CRUST HIDES THE WARM CHOCOLATE CENTER THAT WILL FLOW OUT AS SOON AS THE SPHERE IS BROKEN.

out through the nose. It's the perfect moment for a photograph—the diner looks like an angry dragon. Another interesting application for LN has to do with the fact that materials frozen with it become very brittle. If citrus slices (cuticles removed), are frozen at less than –130°C and then struck with a hammer, individual juice sacs are created. These little sacs have been used in ice cream and to decorate desserts. Any other ideas?

11.10 COLD REDUCTIONS

Chefs frequently use the term *reduction*. This term comes from recipes that instruct cooks to "reduce" the volume of stocks and juices to a fraction of their original amount, thus thickening and intensifying their flavors. In the classical reduction process a liquid mixture such as a soup, wine, or juice is heated to boiling so that water evaporates, producing desirable aromas but also the loss of volatile substances that escape from the natural product with the water vapor. Heating fruit juices in this way can create strange flavors and damage some vitamins and bioactive compounds, however. Evaporation under vacuum is one alternative used in industry and in laboratories. Water boils at lower temperatures in a vacuum (water's boiling point is 80.6°C at 0.5 atm, for example), and the volatile aromas that escape with the steam can be condensed and reintroduced to the concentrate. Some chefs already have rotary evaporators in their kitchen laboratories that can operate under vacuum, which they can use to prepare nice reductions and concentrates.

Water can also be removed by separating it as ice at temperatures below 0°C (see Section 8.1). When a solution is cooled, the water freezes at temperatures a few degrees below 0°C. For example, in a solution of 12% sucrose (w/w) equivalent to 12°Bx (12 g sucrose/100 g solution), such as that in apple or orange juice, the first ice forms at about –0.8°C (Figure 11.4). If the temperature is lowered to –4.8°C, almost half of the water will be ice and the solution will now have a concentration of approximately 45% sucrose. This is what happens when you remove a bottle of soda that has been left inadvertently in the freezer: you find a core of ice surrounded by syrup. This process is another way to concentrate broths and juices at low temperatures, and it is known as freeze concentration.[13]

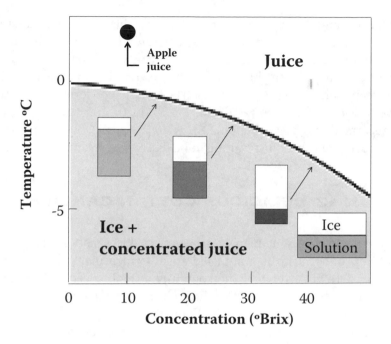

FIGURE 11.4   SEPARATION OF A CONCENTRATED JUICE SOLUTION AND ICE AS THE
TEMPERATURE OF A JUICE DESCENDS BELOW THE FREEZING POINT. AS MORE ICE FORMS THE
REMAINING SOLUTION BECOMES INCREASINGLY CONCENTRATED (REDUCTION), WITHOUT
THE USE OF HEAT.

This concentration method will not produce a 100% concentrated solution, as some of the syrup remains occluded in the ice, but the concentrate retains good color and contains most of the original flavors
and aromas. The best results are obtained if a vacuum is applied to the
frozen mixture in order to recover more syrup, just like when children
suck the sweet liquid and colorant from frozen ice pops, leaving the ice
attached to the popsicle stick.

11.11 STRUCTURING BY FREEZING

Freezing a product that contains some liquid water has also been used
to "texturize" gels. In the production of *kori-tofu*, pieces of gel are frozen
at –10°C, then allowed to rest at –2°C for several weeks. The mixture

is thawed, and the exuded water is removed. The result is a tofu with a more cohesive texture and a porous structure (the pores are the spaces previously occupied by the ice crystals). Chewy, fibrous textures can also be obtained with this method of texturization by freezing. First a protein solution is frozen in such a way that it forms alternating layers of ice and concentrated solution, and then the protein phase is transformed into a gel (Section 2.8). There are some patents on freeze-structuring out there just waiting to be discovered by innovative chefs.

11.12 DELICIOUS COTTON CANDIES

If you look closely at a machine that produces cotton candy, you will notice that it heats granulated sugar (which melts above 150°C, Section 2.4) while rotating the container at high speed. Fine strands are expelled by centrifugal force through various holes, and the strands are then rolled onto a stick. The filaments cool rapidly as they come in contact with the ambient temperature, so that sugar solidifies into the glassy state. The patent for these machines dates from circa 1900, when a candy manufacturer joined forces with a dentist in Nashville, Tennessee—another example of food and science collaboration. Cotton candy has a short life span because it becomes very sticky when exposed to humid air, which causes it to pass from the glassy into the rubbery state (Section 2.3).

Some restaurants serve cotton candy to satisfy the sweet tooth and to recall childhood experiences. Others use it as a base for combining sweetness with contrasting flavors, creating things like cotton candy coated with *foie gras*. They are so much fun to eat. It's amazing that such a simple device for melting solids and forming solid-state glass strands can awaken the imagination in such a way. To experimentation!

11.13 IMPREGNATION UNDER VACUUM

Many fruits and vegetables have large pores in their microstructure that penetrate into the tissues and are normally filled with air. The apple is the most notable. Interconnected pores account for about 20% of an apple's volume. The properties of fruits and vegetables that have been preserved in vinegar come from the ability of their structures to absorb the acetic acid solution. Vacuum impregnation involves immersing pieces of fruits and vegetables in a solution, then using a vacuum to remove some of the gases from the pores. When the fruit returns to atmospheric pressure, the solution fills the pores in place of the air.[14] The solution may contain flavors, vitamins, or bioactive compounds, so it's possible to obtain innovative and nutritious products in this way.[15] You could use this method to impregnate strawberries or watermelon pieces with liquor or extracts of exotic foods.

Will it be possible to use any solution? Gastrovac® is a "vacuum pot" with its own heating source that is used by chefs to perform vacuum impregnation. It also allows for cooking and frying under vacuum, which reduces the temperature and attenuates the undesirable reactions that can occur with heating.

11.14 *SOUS-VIDE* COOKING

Cooking under pressure (like with a pressure cooker) keeps water liquid at temperatures above 100°C and speeds up the cooking process, but what happens when air is removed and the pressure is below atmospheric pressure? Products packaged in impermeable flexible films and sealed under vacuum have been around for over 50 years, and abound in the supermarket, especially sliced meats in the deli section. Others, such as sausages, are heat treated (pasteurized) under vacuum in heat-resistant packaging. The novelty is to use vacuum when cooking fruits, vegetables, meats, and fish. Chef Thomas Keller of The French Laundry in California and Per Se in New York City is at the forefront of this culinary innovation. He reveals his secrets for *sous-vide* (French for "under vacuum") cooking in a book.[16]

The vacuum cooking process begins by putting the food in a plastic bag, creating a vacuum so that it fits snugly over the food, and then sealing it tightly. The second step is to place the bag of food into a hot water bath whose temperature is precisely controlled to an accuracy of 1°C.[17] For this, the chefs utilize the same thermostated circulating water baths used in laboratories, but they call it a Roner.

The star application of this method is for cooking tough meats, where the goal is to soften the tissues without losing the juices (Section 6.8). The myth of "sealing" the meat prior to placing it in the water does not actually help to retain more juices.[18] The proteins that make up the structure of the muscle fibers begin to shorten and release juices at around 54°C and reach maximum shrinkage at temperatures above 75 to 80°C. Moreover, the collagen in connective tissue that toughens the red meats have a denaturation point (solubilization) that depends on the age of the animal and type of meat, but that fluctuates around 70°C. The collagen in fish is softer and dissolves at 50 to 55°C. Many meats soften and remain juicy if they are cooked *sous-vide* for long periods at a temperature between 60 and 85°C (the exact conditions for the various cuts and portions must be determined). Here are some examples: steak, 59.5°C and 45 min; tongue, 70°C and 24 hr; pork leg and shoulder: 82.2°C and 8 hr. In summary, vacuum cooking offers the advantages of delicate textures and decreased loss of the juices and flavors characteristic of the raw materials, along with the possibility of reheating the food before serving in the same closed bag.

11.15 COOKING WITH GLUCONO-δ-LACTONE (GDL)

Glucono-delta-lactone (GDL) is an ester derivative of glucose that hydrolyzes when heated, forming gluconic acid. The use of GDL is permitted in foods, and it's used when a slow release of acid that can be controlled by temperature is required, like when curing raw meats or in the production of some dairy products. The *modus operandi* is similar to the way in which baking powder generates CO_2. GDL is used for gelling casein or soy proteins, with the added benefit that the pH of the gel depends only on the amount of GDL used and the heating temperature.[19] GDL can be used to make yogurt substitutes, avoiding the need to manipulate microorganisms in order to decrease the milk's pH and form gels. GDL is also used to make *tofu*, by gelification of soy protein in combination with calcium.[20]

NOTES

1. A study of the process of culinary innovation, which involved following 12 German chefs with Michelin stars, can be found in Ottenbacher, M., and Harrington, R.J. 2007. The culinary innovation process: A study of Michelin-starred chefs. *Journal of Culinary Science & Technology* 5, 9–35.
2. In fact, the ancient practice of soaking the corn for tortillas in a solution of a chemical called calcium hydroxide (known as *nixtamalization*) produces better bioavailability of the essential amino acids lysine and tryptophan and provides the calcium necessary for absorption of vitamin B3 or niacin.
3. There are a number of Web sites dedicated to unusual modern dishes created by chefs, including POPSCI. See Kamozawa, A., and Talbot, A. 2009. Blowing up cheese with nitrous oxide. www.popsci.com/category/category-badges/kitchen-alchemy.
4. Taken from the article Cassi, D. 2004. Science and cooking combine at gastronomic physics lab in Italy. *Physics Education* 38, 108. Cassi is a physics professor at the University of Parma.
5. You can purchase any of these ingredients at amazon.com. For example, take a look at www.amazon.com/Edible-Gold-Leaf-Chocolates-Leaves/dp/B0006GSQYK (accessed February 4, 2011).
6. Microfluidics is one of the microtechnologies most likely to be applicable for food. Microfluidics involves manipulating fluids (gas or liquid) in small tubes less than 100 microns in diameter, which can produce tiny bubbles or droplets that are very small and homogeneous. For further detail, consult Skurtys, O., and Aguilera, J.M. 2008. Application of microfluidic devices in food engineering. *Food Biophysics* 3, 1–15.
7. The procedure is described in detail in this article by Arboleya, J.C., Olabarrieta, I., Aduriz, A.L., Lasa, D., Vergara, J., Sanmartin, E., Iturriaga, L., Duch, A., and Martínez de Marañón, I. 2008. From the chef's mind to the dish: How scientific approaches facilitate the creative process. *Food Biophysics* 3, 261–268.
8. When you order steak, always ask for the sauce on the side, so that you can easily see the quality of the meat.
9. Take care when using the word exquisite (exquisito) to refer to a delicious meal in Brazil or Portugal, let alone as a compliment to a hostess after a dinner, as it means "odd" or "strange" in Portuguese.

10. The company PolyScience (www.polyscience.com) sold nearly a million dollars worth of equipment to chefs in 2007, including thermostated baths, rotary evaporators, freezers for sauces and purees, and other equipment.
11. In fact, the steam does not physically "drag" aromas but removes them at a temperature below their boiling point, preventing these delicate molecules from breaking down.
12. The history of the development of Pop Rocks (Peta Zetas) and the story of the candy's inventor is told in the book by Rudolph, M. 2006. *Pop Rocks: The Inside Story of America's Revolutionary Candy*. Specialty, Sharon, MA.
13. An updated review of the freeze concentration process can be found in Sanchez, J., Ruiz, Y., Auleda, J.M., Hernandez, E., and Raventos, M. 2009. Review. Freeze concentration in the fruit juices industry. *Food Science and Technology International* 15, 303–315.
14. When using vacuum the maximum attainable pressure difference (which is what matters most because it is the driving force for the process) is almost 1 atmosphere and you need a good vacuum pump in order to achieve this. When applying pressure the maximum attainable pressure differential depends on the strength of the equipment (as there are very powerful pumps available). The process of using high pressure to pasteurize food (Section 8.4) involves pressure differences that may reach several thousand atmospheres.
15. An excellent review of these technologies and their applications for fruits and vegetables is presented in Zhao, Y., and Xieb, J. 2004. Practical applications of vacuum impregnation in fruit and vegetable processing. *Trends in Food Science & Technology* 15, 434–451.
16. Keller, T. 2008. *Under Pressure: Cooking sous vide*. Artisan, New York. In the foreword, Harold McGee celebrates the fact that the most important variable in cooking, heat, can finally be controlled precisely through the temperature of the heating medium (hot water bath).
17. A thorough overview of cooking under vacuum is presented in the article Baldwin, D.E. 2012. Sous vide cooking: A review. *International Journal of Gastronomy and Food Science* 1, 15–30.
18. This has been demonstrated experimentally many times, even by chefs on television shows. For a more complete explanation see This, H. 2006. *Molecular Gastronomy: Exploring the Science of Flavor*. Columbia University Press, New York, pp. 23–25.
19. An extensive background study of the use of GDL in food can be found at www.omri.org/GDL.pdf (accessed December 12, 2009).

20. The preparation of a tofu-like substance made with GDL is presented in Campbell, L.J., Gu, X., Dewar, S.J., and Euston, S.R. 2009. Effects of heat treatment and glucono-δ-lactone-induced acidification on characteristics of soy protein isolate. *Food Hydrocolloids* 23, 344–351.

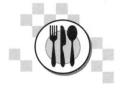

CHAPTER 12

Healthy Habits

We cannot forget that we are products of evolution. A dangerous imbalance can occur when ancient genes must operate with overly powerful fuel and reduced physical activity to burn it. It's best to develop healthy eating habits early on, but it's still possible to acquire them later in life, although through significant effort. Unfortunately, these days time is not on our side and eating quickly is here to stay, unless ... Science and technology have much to contribute to creating healthier food, but individuals have a great responsibility for how it is consumed.

12.1 THE MARK OF THE PAST

It is convenient to analyze aspects of biology from the perspective of evolution.[1] Humans and their ancestors were able to emerge and develop in nearly every ecosystem on earth and in very different climatic conditions consuming various types of food. Even today, there are Arctic populations who still consume diets based on animal foods and others in the highlands of the Andes that primarily subsist on root crops and cereals.[2] It therefore seems unlikely that there is one perfect human diet, but some are probably better than others.

We don't need to go back to the ultimate origin of our species some 6 million years ago in order to review the major changes in human diet. We can begin when humans became hunter-gatherers, approximately 2 million years ago. Their diet was based on the collection of fruits and vegetables, which provided more than half their calories (Figure 12.1). They also hunted wild animals for meat, which required great physical effort. With the domestication of plants and animals that occurred about 10,000 to 12,000 years ago, many groups of hunter-gatherers adopted a more sedentary lifestyle and became members of a primitive agriculturalist society. The presence of valleys irrigated by rivers or the construction of irrigation systems allowed these groups to develop a complex social and cultural activity called *civilization* and the first cities appeared some 5,000 years ago. The big change in the diet of these agricultural societies was the introduction of cereals, which people ate without removing the bran. The industrial revolution introduced

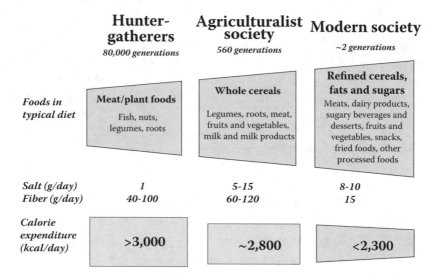

FIGURE 12.1   PREDOMINANT DIETARY FOOD GROUPS (AS WELL AS SALT AND FIBER) DURING THE DIFFERENT STAGES OF HUMAN EVOLUTION UP TO MODERN SOCIETY. THE GROWING AREAS OF THE RHOMBUSES AT THE TOP REPRESENT THE INCREASE IN THE AMOUNT OF FOOD CONSUMED. THE BOTTOM SHOWS THE CALORIC EXPENDITURE DEMANDED BY PHYSICAL ACTIVITY (AND THE AREAS OF THE RHOMBUSES DECREASE). THE FIGURES ARE APPROXIMATE AVERAGES COMPILED FROM VARIOUS SOURCES, BUT THE RELEVANT FEATURES ARE THE TRENDS.

major social and economic changes 260 years ago, and food began to be produced on a large scale. After World War II, and coinciding with a greater abundance of food, a modern society emerged in which the predominant human settlement is within large cities. Alongside, supermarket chains proliferated simultaneously and people increasingly ate outside of the home.[3]

Eighty thousand human generations were hunter-gatherers, followed by approximately 560 generations that depended on agriculture. Ten generations have lived since the beginning of the industrial age, and only two generations have experienced modern society. A generation is about 25 years, which means that human beings have had to fight for their food 99.9% of the time that has elapsed since the appearance of hunter-gatherers. During the last 100 years humans have enjoyed a relatively stable supply of nutrients, and only during the past 50 years some of us have had the benefit of an abundance of food. If the top of this page represented the 12,000 years since the dawn of agriculture, the last century would be the size of one letter. The major differences between the diets of people living in modern urban societies and their ancestors include the types of food consumed and the degree of processing, the amount ingested including that of some specific nutrients, and the difficulty of balancing calories consumed with caloric expenditure due to decreased physical activity. It is not easy to compare the diets of hunter-gatherers, agriculturalists, and individuals in a modern society (e.g., Western diet) given the multiple feeding patterns existing within each group and the conflicting data available. Results of this exercise are presented in Figure 12.1. Surprisingly, the diet of hunter-gatherers appears to be based on meat (and some fish) rather than on collected plant foods, at an approximate ratio of 60/40, which is even higher than the present ratio between both food groups in the dietary energy supply of European countries.[4]

Other things jump out when we analyze the way we live today from the perspective of evolution. Hominids had to develop an ability to withstand famine and food shortages, forcing them to subsist on small sporadic intakes of food.[5] One questions the reasoning behind current dietary recommendations for eating four times a day (including two large meals), when from the viewpoint of calorie reduction it would be desirable to eat less or to just skip a meal. For example, the Incas ate one meal early in the morning and another in the afternoon just before dusk, and did not eat anything in between. Yet they still managed to build a great civilization in only a couple of centuries.[6] Perhaps the true "paleontological diet" should be eating a varied diet in small amounts only when hungry, which in the present situation of abundance and diversity of foods translates into eating what we like (assuming that our preferences include all groups of foods). Another evolutionary aspect to consider is that the purpose of natural selection was to survive only long enough to transfer genes to the next generation. Today's postreproductive period, which seems to make no sense from an evolutionary standpoint, has been extended considerably. This new situation requires an understanding of the nutritional requirements for aging, something mankind has not experienced previously.

Anthropologists have proposed many different hypotheses about why members of the genus *Homo* evolved differently from other primates. Many suggest that it was largely due to the nutritional quality of their diet and how efficiently they were able to find nutrient sources. In an evolutionary context, we are what we have eaten.[7] Evolutionary nutrition is a little known but quite widespread field developed by anthropologists, biologists, geneticists, and physicians. The two basic premises of this group are that the human genome was slowly selected in the past under conditions very different from today, and that changes in lifestyle and diet are occurring these days in an accelerated manner that does not allow for genetic accommodation. The theory is that this mismatch causes some of the degenerative diseases that are currently prevalent.[8] For example, several studies indicate that human beings evolved on a diet with a ratio of omega-6 to omega-3 essential fatty acids of approximately 1, whereas in modern diets the ratio is around 15/1, a ratio that is believed to promote the pathogenesis of many diseases, including cardiovascular disease (CVD), cancer, and inflammatory diseases (see Section 1.2 for fatty acid nomenclature).

A final aspect related to the nutrition of the past has to do with the fact that we require amino acids in the correct proportions in order to make the proteins in our body. These proteins are synthesized from a set of 20 amino acids, and 10 of them must be supplied by the diet (Section 1.2). Many plant foods are deficient in certain essential amino acids. Most cereals are poor in the amino acid lysine, and legumes are short of the sulfur amino acids like methionine and cysteine. Since the beginning of agriculture, all civilizations have managed to develop staple diets that contained a combination of cereals and legumes, providing the complementary essential amino acids necessary to make human proteins. This could have been accidental, but it occurred in the diet of rice and lentils in India, rice and soybeans in China and Southeast Asia, wheat and chickpeas in the Middle East, and corn and beans in Latin America.[9]

12.2 WHAT OUR GENES SAY

What do our genes say about all of this? A *gene* is a segment of DNA (deoxyribonucleic acid) located in some part of a chromosome, whose nucleotide sequence specifies the order of amino acids in a protein. The collection of genes that make up our genetic heritage is called the *human genome*. The interaction of our genome with the environment determines the physical and behavioral traits of living things, and the resulting gene expression is called the *phenotype*. As the enzymes that catalyze most of the reactions in a cell are proteins and they derive from the expression of the genes, cell metabolism is affected by the enzymes present.

The study of the relationship between nutrition and the human genome is called *nutrigenomics*. The most familiar example of how diet can affect the expression of genes comes from honeybees, where the differentiation between the queens and worker bees depends on nutrition. The larvae of worker bees and queens are genetically identical, but when larvae receive a special diet of royal jelly, it becomes a queen bee that is larger, fertile, and can live longer than the worker bees.[10] Similar phenomena have been documented in humans. One study conducted over a 50-year span in California showed that the second and third generations of Japanese residents were significantly taller than their predecessors, which was attributed to nutritional changes that influenced the expression of genes related to height.

Our genes have not changed significantly for at least the last 40,000 years.[11] Less than 1% of the nearly 20,000 protein-coding genes that make up the human genome have changed since the lineage of apes and humans diverged about 6 million years ago. Our bodies have nearly the same genetic hardware as before, but the fuel provided by the foods we eat as well as our levels of physical activity have recently "mutated."

The relationship between genes and certain diseases is being established quickly and often conclusively. There is also evidence that the expression of some genes depends on certain molecules related directly or indirectly with food. One might infer that nutrition affects our bodies not only in the short term (for example, nutritional deficiencies), but also in the long term. Some scientists propose that the recent increase in breast cancer is largely the result of environmental and lifestyle changes, and only occasionally due to genetic abnormalities. The fact that the rate of occurrence of this type of cancer in Third-World societies is only a small fraction, the high incidence in the United States may support that proposition.[12]

In the coming decade it may become possible to cheaply obtain the genetic profile of any individual, identify any genes related to high-risk diseases, and make personalized recommendations about potentially beneficial or harmful foods and nutrients. This concept of food "therapy" is based on the idea that certain foods may promote the action of protective genes while others tend to cancel those effects. However, using nutrition as a means to prevent or cure disease will be much more complicated than drug therapy, because we eat throughout our lifetime (and may not even know what we are eating), we eat numerous different nutrients (which may also interact with one another), and there are many genes involved in metabolism. This concept of *personalized nutrition* has already been applied with delactosed foods (such as lactose-free milk), which are produced for people who have a genetic variation that prevents them from being able to metabolize lactose. Lactose is a disaccharide formed by the union of glucose and galactose (Section 1.2), and in lactose-free milk the lactose has been hydrolyzed with the enzyme lactase, converting it to its two sugars, which can be easily metabolized.

Genetic polymorphism occurs when two or more variants of a gene exist within the same population. Some polymorphisms have been linked to chronic diseases. It is estimated that at least 150 variants of genes are involved in type 2 diabetes and that more than 300 are associated with obesity.[13] Another type of variability in the genetic material comes from epigenetic modifications, which do not involve changes in the DNA sequence but instead occur when alterations of the DNA molecule (e.g., methylations) affect the expression of a gene. Considerable evidence is accumulating that suggests that nutritional imbalance during pregnancy can induce epigenetic mechanisms, causing babies to be more prone to obesity, type 2 diabetes, and metabolic syndrome. It is expected that in the coming years scientists will discover new relationships between the operation of genes and the effect of nutrition.

12.3 THE WEIGHT OF HEALTH

We all want to live longer and achieve a healthy old age, enjoying a high quality of life well into our late years. Psychology research correlates longer life with experiencing a sense of well-being and feeling "happy" by being healthy, well-fed, comfortable, safe, knowledgeable, respected, non-celibate, and loved.[14,15] But how do we achieve this when certain factors involved are beyond our control, like genetics and the environment?

Biologists claim that, at least in animals, a balanced low calorie diet is the surest way to prolong life and to live healthier. One explanation behind this theory is that certain protective genes that were critical when humans had to survive periods of famine are triggered by a low caloric intake. In practical terms, caloric restriction means eating about 30% less than what is considered normal.[16] But it is quite likely that this kind of low food intake would make those who enjoy eating quite unhappy, therefore negating the psychological effect of happiness that also correlated with longevity.

According to the World Health Organization (WHO), there is a growing global epidemic of obese and overweight people (see definitions below) called *globesity*, which could cause serious disruption to the health of about 1,500 million people by 2015. More worrying is that obesity rates are highest among the poor, reaching the same levels as in the affluent classes. U.S. statistics show that overweight and obese adults make up 66% of that population group. At the time, the costs of treating of obesity are higher than for the war in Afghanistan (about $90 billion annually).[17] In Mexico, where even as recently as 1990 it was relatively uncommon to see obese adults, an overweight/obesity rate of almost 70% exists, and diseases related to this excess weight are requiring public health spending of about $15 billion annually. One concern in the developing world is nutrition transition, in which the problems of obesity have become more important than the problems traditionally associated with poverty, like undernutrition and famine.

The sustained prevalence of obesity affects public health. It appears that obesity is associated with an inflammatory condition that links excess body fat and diseases such as type 2 diabetes, hypertension, dyslipidemia (high fat and cholesterol in the blood), cardiovascular disease, gallbladder disease, gout, osteoarthritis, and certain cancers. Some experts think that obesity is only one of the relevant factors responsible for the escalating epidemic of these diseases worldwide. They prefer to hold the metabolic syndrome responsible for these ailments, a condition where excess body fat around the waist is present in conjunction with increased blood pressure, high blood sugar levels, and abnormally high cholesterol levels. The public measures proposed to curve this trend might become extreme. In order to reduce a public health system deficit that amounted to 41 billion euros in 2004, the German Finance Minister suggested that obese people pay more taxes as well as higher insurance rates. Some doctors approved the proposal.[18]

The other side of obesity is related to physical inactivity. As incomes rise and the population becomes more urban, physical activity, defined as any bodily movement produced by skeletal muscles that require energy expenditure, diminishes. Therefore, physical inactivity is now identified as the fourth leading risk factor for global mortality. More time spent traveling by motorized transport, better technologies, less housework, and more passive leisure activities make modern life more sedentary. Some researchers estimate that the daily energy expenditure (adjusted for weight) of modern man is only 65% of that of a Paleolithic human (Figure 12.1). According to international standards, almost 60% of the population is sedentary, or spending less than 30 minutes three times a week on physical activity. WHO has stated:

Conclusive scientific evidence, based on a wide range of well-conducted studies, shows that physically active people have higher levels of health-related fitness, a lower risk profile for developing a number of disabling medical conditions, and lower rates of various chronic noncommunicable diseases than do people who are inactive.[19]

The problem is that when it comes to physical activity, governments and pressure groups have no one to blame except the individuals themselves, which is not the most politically correct approach these days. In summary, healthy adults should undertake at least 150 minutes of moderate-intensity aerobic physical activity per week. Governments are urged to inform their population about the frequency, duration, intensity, types, and total amount of physical activity necessary for good health, and provide multiple strategies aimed at creating supportive environments for physical activity to take place.

"Staying within a healthy weight range is more important for long-term health than all of the concerns about what you eat," says Walter C. Willett of Harvard University. He goes on to say that three aspects related to weight significantly influence the likelihood of experiencing or dying from a heart attack, developing diabetes, or being diagnosed with some form of cancer (breast, colon, or kidney): the height-weight ratio, waist circumference, and weight gain over 20 years.[20] The *body mass index* (BMI) is a parameter widely used to assess the relationship between weight and height, and it is calculated according to the following formula:

$$\text{BMI} = \frac{(\text{weight in kilograms})}{(\text{height in meters})^2}$$

Table 12.1 shows the relationship between BMI and healthy weight, overweight, and obesity. The recommended BMI that is associated with a longer life expectancy is between 20 and 25, while a BMI under 18.5 is a sign of malnutrition. But like many things related to nutrition and health, there is no unanimous agreement on the negative consequences

TABLE 12.1
Relationship between Body Mass Index (BMI) and Healthy Weight,
Overweight, and Obesity

Below 18.5	18.5–24.9	25–29.9	30–34.9	35–39.9	Over 40
Under normal weight	Healthy weight	Overweight	Slight obesity (Class I)	Moderate obesity (Class II)	Morbid obesity (Class III)

of fat accumulation and its direct relationship with various diseases and life expectancy. Critics of strict weight control come mostly from outside the medical profession and argue that mistakes in the statistical processing of obesity data result in an exaggeration in the definition of what it means to be overweight, and finally, an underestimation of the beneficial effect of fat accumulation in cases of diseases that require long-term treatment.[21]

There are easy ways to reduce calorie intake, especially for those with some "give" in their caloric balance. Sugary soft drinks are an invention of the modern food industry that exploit the need to drink fluids, the desire for sweet taste, and the tingly feeling that popping CO_2 bubbles make in your mouth. Coca-Cola was "invented" in 1886 using the cheapest and most common sweetener that existed at the time, refined sugar. But if Coke was developed today, there would probably only be a diet version. Sugary soft drinks are often responsible for up to 8% to 10% of daily energy intake, and each 350 cc can of soda has about 240 kcal, equivalent to 10 cubes of sugar.[22] Someone who consumes one of these sugary drinks every day could lose more than 2 kilos in a year just by replacing it with a drink containing a noncaloric sweetener such as stevia, which is also a natural product (or by drinking water). Weight control in this case only requires a small sacrifice in taste, as well as a certain confidence in the scientists and regulators who studied and approved the artificial sweetener. It seems that the battle is being won: sales of low-calorie carbonated beverages in U.S. supermarkets rose at rates of 10% in 2003 to 2004, while those containing sugar declined by 4.2%.[23] However, statistics also show that three out of four cans of soda that were consumed in the United States during that same period contained sugar (or corn syrup), and that Americans still consume about 560 cans of soda a year per capita. If we examine the diets of some of our ancestral populations who subsisted on very basic diets, such as the Turkana of Kenya and the Incas of the Peruvian highlands, we learn that both the Turkana, who are primarily carnivores, and the Incas, who derive a large proportion of food energy from plants, had a low caloric intake (1500 to 2000 kilocalories per day), which is sufficient for performing most physical tasks.[24] The human species has an impressive resistance to starvation, particularly in adulthood, which should not be surprising given the long periods of hunger that our ancestors had to endure. Healthy individuals of normal weight can lose up to 25% of their original weight without risking their lives. In 1952 the French physician and biologist Alain Bombard crossed the Atlantic in an inflatable raft to prove that castaways could survive an ocean crossing without supplies. Over the course of 65 days he ate only raw fish and occasionally drank seawater, losing 25 kilos in the process. He died in 2005 at the age of 80 years. Several years ago a group of inmates between 30 and 38 years of age went on a hunger strike for 64 days and lost about 20 kilos each. According to medical reports the prolonged fast did not cause any irreversible consequences for them. Adults who have been lost for several days in the wilderness recover quickly without any permanent sequelae, if they survive hypothermia and have water to drink.

12.4 HABITS AND DIETS

A habit is a behavior that is regularly repeated. Your dietary habits consist of the types of foods you eat most often and how you eat them, which in turn are influenced by lifestyle as well as beliefs and traditions. The word *diet* is used to describe the range of food consumed by a population, culture, or individual. Both terms (habits and diets) are at the center of the healthy lifestyle concept, which encompasses eating a nutritionally balanced diet, maintaining proper weight, exercising regularly, not smoking, drinking alcohol in moderation, managing stress, having stable and satisfying work, avoiding drug use, and having good family and social relationships.

The traditional food habits of various countries and cultures are threatened by new forms of nutrition that have found a niche in the fast pace of modern life, especially in urban centers. Even the French, who epitomize people adhering to food traditions and passion for good eating, are "alarmed" by the progressive disintegration of their food habits prompted by the "ever-growing population of working women, uninterrupted days at office, increased urbanization and the important amount of the household budget spent on leisure activities."[25]

Take-away food (a form of fast food) is not just an invention of modern times. The tour guides in Pompeii always stop to show the places where people bought their meals before retiring to their homes, where they did not have cooking facilities. For many centuries in large European cities there were public kitchens where you could buy prepared foods, and food vendors have long existed in most urban environments. In Bangkok, street vendors have been feeding millions of workers for the past 200 years, especially couples with children who have neither the space nor the time to prepare their own meals. Nowadays in Thailand this is a lucrative business with yearly sales of $1,600 million. Some 24,000 registered vendors offer local specialties with varied flavors and textures five times per day.[26]

It seems, then, that the problems with modern fast food include the loss of culinary traditions, the extinction of the relaxing social meal, and above all, the adoption into the diet and exaggerated consumption of foreign food products that are high in saturated fat, sugar, and salt. But the burgers, fries, hot dogs, pizza, ice cream, and sugar-sweetened beverages are considered appetizing by millions of consumers around the world, who, in this era of globalization, consume them freely because of their convenience and low cost. In order to buy a Big Mac, which is identical everywhere on the planet, one must work 185 minutes in Nairobi, 79 minutes in Lima, 52 minutes in Santiago de Chile, and only 12 minutes in New York, and it frees a lot of scarce time (to earn the money to buy it, for example). Ferrán Adrià, the great Spanish chef, recognizes that there are many people in the world who cannot spend more than $3 per day on food, and he is therefore not opposed to fast food: "I go to McDonald's four times a year and have never heard anyone who eats at these places speak badly of fast food. Only those who do not eat fast food speak ill of it."[27] What is at stake, however, is an entire culture of dishes, flavors, and traditional tastes.

Many people prefer to regularly eat traditional meals and fresh "natural" foods without additives, which are produced with agriculture methods that are more environmentally friendly. This concept of "slow food" has emerged in response to fast food. In the words of its founder and president, Italian Carlo Petrini, the Slow Food movement has two key strategies for stopping the "degeneration of taste": education on food and taste, and the protection of food biodiversity through a sustainable agriculture. One big criticism is that Slow Food is more expensive and elitist. In a world where 7 billion individuals need to eat daily, and where a significant percentage of the population lives in large urban centers, all this talk about "eat local," organic food, and artisan products seems a bit unrealistic as a global solution. Moreover, young people are no longer interested in agriculture and migrate to the cities, even as urban living conditions deteriorate, thus the idea of promoting school gardens to bring children closer to food is great. Nevertheless, the philosophy behind Slow Food is very worthy and shared to a different extent by everyone who cares about foods and eating well. In Petrini's words: "the gastronome who is not aware of the environmental implications of his food is stupid. An environmentalist who is naïve of gastronomy is sad."[28] Like what happened with ecology, every future alternative to the food problem will have a place for "slow food."

It is said there are no good foods or bad foods, only good and bad eating habits. Of course there are some foods that are healthier than others, which generally include those with less salt, sugar, and fat. "Junk food," however, contains a high proportion of these components that we associate with food that tastes good, but which are not adequate for good nutrition and health if frequently consumed. Some contend that tasty, convenient, and inexpensive junk food is "not so bad" if consumed in moderate amounts and sporadically.[29] At least this was the conclusion reached by British researchers who questioned the myths surrounding junk food and even dared to claim that junk food products contain some key nutrients.[30] It's important to keep in mind that a burger and fries typically has about 1300 kcal, or 70% of the daily caloric requirement of a child, and is equivalent to the main meal of the day. Experts agree that consumption of hamburgers, hot dogs, and pizza every 15 days is not intrinsically bad, but that getting into a habit of eating these foods more frequently is the problem. Could anyone call "junk food" to traditional products like fried chicken or Chilean "sopaipillas" if they are only consumed occasionally?[31] At the other extreme, foods that appear to be healthier, like bottled fruit juices, may contain as many calories as soda and very little nutrients. Two hundred cc's of clarified apple juice have 165 kcal, and contain fewer vitamins and none of the beneficial fiber found in the whole fruit (see also Section 12.6).

The other meaning of the word *diet* denotes a restriction in dietary intake of calories or of a certain food group, either voluntarily or by prescription. There are thousands of weight-loss diets, as well as the belief that they are a definitive solution. The apple diet, the carrot diet, the shock diet, the moon diet, the cabbage diet, and even the high calorie diet or anti-diet are some of the most renowned (see Box 12.1). The least appealing ones are those based on recipes and menus elaborated by nutritionists and proposed in their books, because they are just playing at being chefs. At the end all weight-loss diets come down to consuming fewer calories, so the only effective diet is the thermodynamic diet, which translates into eating less.

There are diets that propose drinking lots of water, which is great for the bottled water business, which exceeds $15 billion per year worldwide. A liter of bottled water can cost more than 100 times the value of a liter of regular drinking water, but this does not make it more pure. Even in developed countries the standards for bottled water are no more stringent than those governing potable water. A U.S. study revealed that of 108 brands of bottled water, 15% contained more bacteria than allowed by the standards of microbiological purity, and a fifth of the samples contained industrial chemicals like toluene, styrene, and so forth, though at fairly low levels.[32]

Weight-loss diets are usually boring and only have a short-term effect. They do not create good eating habits and do not allow for the enjoyment of the full range of culinary variety. To paraphrase the Jews returning from Egypt, restricted diets "dry our souls" (Section 9.1). Diets can become somewhat impractical when dieters must separate themselves from those who are not dieting at meals, put more effort

---

**BOX 12.1   THE "PRINCIPLES" BEHIND
CERTAIN WEIGHT-LOSS DIETS**

Low-fat diets. The rationale is that fat provides more than double the calories of protein and carbohydrates. These diets
drastically restrict excess fat intake but do not distinguish
between "good" and "bad" fats (Section 1.2). One downside
is that fat consumption may provide a satiety effect that
helps to moderate caloric intake.

Low-carbohydrate diets. The premise is that by reducing the
amount and type of carbohydrate consumed the insulin
level is kept steady and less sugars enter your cells. Thus,
energy comes from stored fat.

Low-calorie diets. The idea is that a calorie is a calorie regardless
of its source (see Section 6.4). Therefore if you reduce the
total caloric intake and increase caloric expenditure (exercise) you will gradually lose weight. It requires counting
calories and taking control over portion sizes.

High-protein diets. These are based on the satiating effect of
proteins and a higher energy expenditure in their digestion.
They also require a low carbohydrate intake.

---

into shopping and cooking, and sometimes spend more money. There
are also possible health consequences due to too much (e.g., protein) or
too low (e.g., essential fatty acids) intake of specific nutrients. Finally, it
has been shown that 95% of dieters regain the weight they lost within
6 months of ending the diet, as these kinds of diets do not create permanent eating habits.

Many healthy eating habits are formed during childhood, so education
about foods and nutrition at home and in schools is very important.[33]
But eating habits change over time due to work and social environments, trends, and mainly because of the rapid pace of modern life. So
far there is no evidence that there is a better diet for mind and body
than one that is varied, tasty but frugal, and shared in a social environment. Those who are waiting for a miracle pill to help them lose weight
without any sacrifice or side effects were born a bit too early.

12.5 TIME IS NOT ON OUR SIDE

In 1964 the Rolling Stones recorded the song "Time Is on My Side" which included the lyrics: "you're searching for good times, but just wait and see." In reference to food consumption, for some people the good times mean not having to worry about what and how much they eat. After a little while they will see their bellies bulging and later on the consequences of obesity. The problem with "good times" nowadays is that the day still has 24 hours and we have to pack an ever-increasing amount of activities into this period. As we are often reminded, time is our scarcest resource.

According to the Bureau of Labor Statistics (www.bls.gov) in 2010 the American population on average spent 8.7 hr sleeping, 5.2 hr on leisure and sports (including 2.7 hr watching TV and only 0.35 hr in exercise), 3.5 hr dedicated to working, 1.25 hr on eating and drinking, and 0.56 hr on food preparation (for a total of 1.81 hours on food-related activities). Figures had not changed much from 2003. Of course these values are only referential and depend on definitions (e.g., like what is considered "work") and how the surveys were conducted (see original reference for details).

For a better appreciation of how time is used by a greater proportion of the population—those who live in large urban centers in developing and emerging countries—let's revise the statistics for the 6 million population who live in a megacity like Santiago de Chile.[34] To start, people spend more time sleeping and in personal care activities (11.8 hr versus 9.5 hr in the United States). Working or studying takes 7 hr. Moving around the city requires a daily average of 1.5 hr, which increases to 2.2 hr if only transportation to work is considered. Sitting in front of the TV and using the Internet take an amazing 2.6 hr. Adding all this up, we already have 22.9 hr, and these "average" individuals haven't eaten yet. Statistics show that a total of 1.3 hr is spent on food preparation, which probably also includes eating and drinking. And here is the problem: the data tell us the day has 24.2 hours.

Slower mobility through longer distances and smaller places to live (city densification) is the trend. The cornucopia of modern "leisure activities" and other technological distractions grow every day and take lots of our time: video games, the social networks, affordable cable TV, and so forth. Would the hundreds of millions of people in these huge cities exchange some of their scarce free time to cook their food, not to mention to grow it, given the present eating alternatives? Could they? Should they? I leave the answers to sociologists and other experts on human behavior. But one thing is for sure: When it comes to buying, preparing, and eating food, time is not on the side of the "stressed" residents of the urban metropolis. The hope is that *the times they are a-changin'* for better.[35]

12.6 "HEALTHY DIETS"

It's not easy to define what constitutes a healthy diet, probably because there is no "one" healthy diet that works for everyone. Most nutritionists agree that a balanced and healthy diet consists of a wide variety of foods, predominantly fruits and vegetables, whole grains, and protein sources like poultry, fish, eggs, legumes, and dairy products. It should be low in fat (especially saturated fat), salt, and sugar. The Harvard School of Public Health prefers to refer to *healthy eating habits*, which include physical exercise, caloric equilibrium, and attention to weight changes. These same good habits include the consumption of plenty of fruits and vegetables, whole grains, fish, milk (for calcium), and healthy fats (like olive oil and canola oil), with a reduced amount of red meat, refined grains, sugary drinks, and fries. Finally, a daily multivitamin pill and moderate consumption of alcohol are recommended as well. Physical exercise is a very important component of healthy living.[36]

In 2004 the WHO approved its *Global Strategy on Diet, Physical Activity and Health*, which resulted in a series of recommendations directed toward the food industry. Some of these recommendations included promoting healthy diets and physical activity; limiting levels of saturated fats, trans fat, sugar, and salt in food products; expanding the pool of healthy and nutritious products available; providing appropriate and understandable information to consumers; practicing responsible advertising (especially with ads directed at children); providing packaging information enabling consumers to make informed choices; and supplying government agencies with information on the composition of products.[37] Ten multinational food companies with annual sales totaling more than $350 billion and accounting for almost 80% of food advertising have committed to these objectives, forming the International Food and Beverage Alliance (IFBA).[38]

Much of the interest in nutrition and healthy diets derives from studies that positively correlate "better" diets with a lower incidence of chronic noncommunicable diseases such as cancer, cardiovascular disease, diabetes, and so forth. It has been postulated that an ideal diet may prevent up to 30% of cancers. The *Mediterranean diet* (MD) is a varied and tasty option that is based on the traditional diet of the European countries of the Mediterranean Sea basin. There are four other areas in the world with similar climatic conditions, conducive to the production of many of the foods that make up a large part of the Mediterranean diet: California, central Chile, southwest Australia, and the coastal areas of South Africa. The benefits of the Mediterranean diet were noted some 40 years ago, after an epidemiological research project called the Seven Countries Study demonstrated that there was a much lower incidence of acute myocardial infarction in the rural areas of the Mediterranean. The MD is low in saturated fat and high in polyunsaturated fats, with a good balance between omega-3 and omega-6 fatty acids, low in animal protein, and rich in antioxidants (vitamins and polyphenols), complex carbohydrates, and fiber. The main components of the diet include a relatively high intake of fish and white meats, whole grains and legumes, fruits and vegetables, virgin olive oil (high in monounsaturated fatty acids), and moderate consumption of dairy products and wine.[39]

The fact that the United States and France share similar per capita consumption of fats and cholesterol, but that the incidence of CVD is significantly lower in France is known as the *French Paradox*. One likely explanation, based on the analysis of the typical diets, is that the French consume a moderate amount of wine. This drink has two positive effects on the risk of cardiovascular disease: the effect of the alcohol itself (shared by all alcoholic drinks) and those of the antioxidant polyphenolic compounds derived from grapes. Multiple studies have shown that moderate consumption of wine (especially red) reduces the risks associated with CVD. The benefit is not just associated with the MD; the consumption of red wine is still beneficial as a complement to a Western-style diet (Section 12.7).

As pointed out, current scientific evidence suggests that most of the benefits of the MD derive from the antioxidant compounds found in wine, fruits and vegetables, and virgin olive oil (Section 1.8). *Oxidative stress* leads to reactions of free radicals (highly reactive atoms or molecules with unpaired electrons) with lipids, proteins, carbohydrates, and DNA, which triggers irreversible physiological damage (Section 7.9). Oxidative damage in biological molecules is associated with pathologies such as cancer, atherosclerosis, as well as aging. By elevating the antioxidant capacity of blood plasma, the MD may protect against oxidative damage. Many fruits, vegetables, and wine contain high amounts of polyphenols, a group of compounds with very active antioxidant properties. Polyphenols are also present in tea, coffee, and chocolate. Berries have the highest total content of polyphenols, and apples are close behind.[40]

Industrial processing, particularly heating, greatly reduces the concentration of polyphenols in fruit juices and decreases the antioxidant capacity.[41] When the cell structures are broken to release the juice, the polyphenols are liberated from the fruit matrix and become free to participate in oxidation reactions and be transformed into polymerized brown pigments before they enter your mouth. Freshly squeezed juice is therefore more beneficial than juice that has been reconstituted from a processed concentrate. In a recent study (surprisingly there aren't many on this important topic), heating during blanching of fruits and hot filling of a bottled blackberry juice reduced the values of anthocyanins by 52%, and the total antioxidant capacity dropped by 47%.[42] This undesirable process may occur also when making jams or fruit compotes for desserts. This is another example of getting less nutrition than we should (and pay for), as discussed in Section 7.8.

What about vegetarian diets? Vegetarians eat plant products with or without the addition of eggs and dairy products. They are likely to have a low BMI (Section 12.3) and tend to consume plenty of fruit and vegetables. The current position of the American Dietetic Association is that "appropriately planned vegetarian diets" are healthful and nutritionally adequate, and could even contribute to the prevention of certain diseases. It's important for vegetarians to understand what "appropriately planned" means. Some potential shortcomings of vegetarian diets include: (a) marginal amounts of omega-3 fatty acids (EPA and DHA), that's why a microalgae supplement is recommended; (b) inorganic iron in fruits and vegetables is much less absorbed than the heme iron found in meat and fish (i.e., as part of hemoglobin or myoglobin), and its absorption may be inhibited by phytates and polyphenols present in vegetables, tea, coffee, and cocoa derivatives; and (c) insufficient calcium, which can lead to osteoporosis. Vegetarians must obtain calcium from milk, green vegetables, or foods fortified with this mineral.[43]

In conclusion, everything seems to indicate that what we eat has both immediate and prolonged repercussions for our health. Importantly, the modern concept of "diet" emphasizes regularly eating a large variety of foods, with no predominance of certain foods or specific nutrients over others.

12.7 NUTRITIONAL ENGINEERING

The pyramid collapsed. It's not an archeological disaster though—it's just the food pyramid that the U.S. Department of Agriculture (USDA) proposed in 1992 as a guide for people to choose a healthy diet. The pyramid had different levels (from the base to the apex) representing the proportion of each food group that should make up total daily consumption. The base, the largest section of the pyramid, included complex carbohydrates, whole-grain bread, rice, breakfast cereals, and pasta. The top of the pyramid contained foods that should be consumed in smaller amounts or occasionally, such as fats and oils. In between there were (in descending order of importance) fruits and vegetables; meat, poultry, and eggs; and milk and dairy products.[44]

Why did the original food pyramid fall in 2005? It was partly out of a desire to simplify the recommendations, but mainly because new epidemiological evidence (and practical experience) showed that a varied diet is not only more appealing but also healthier. It recognized also that certain types of fats are essential to good health and they come in foods mixed with "not so good" fats. Also, a high carbohydrate intake may not always be beneficial, both in terms of calories and sugar load. In the new food pyramid, called *MyPyramid*, all food groups extended from the base to the apex in order to show that eating a variety of foods was best (Figure 12.2).

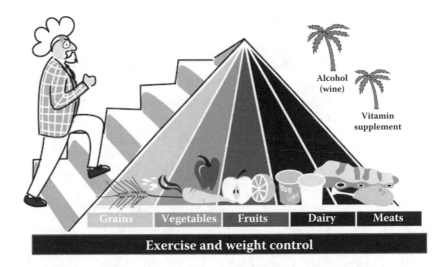

FIGURE 12.2   MYPYRAMID, THE 2005 FOOD PYRAMID OF THE U.S. DEPARTMENT OF
AGRICULTURE (USDA). ONE DIET DOES NOT FIT EVERYBODY, SO FOOD CHOICES AND PORTIONS
DEPEND ON EACH INDIVIDUAL. MYPYRAMID HAS RECENTLY BEEN REPLACED BY MYPLATE.
(FROM USDA.)

MyPyramid was built on a foundation of daily exercise and weight control. It promoted the use of vegetable oils (mono- and polyunsaturated), whose positive effect on cholesterol control had been proven in epidemiological studies, as well as the consumption of products made with whole grains (like whole-wheat bread and high-fiber cereals). It recommended that the diet should include plenty of fruits and vegetables, as well as nuts and legumes. Certain foods should be consumed in limited amounts: red meat, butter, white rice, white bread, potatoes, pasta, and sweets. The new pyramid did not stand alone but was surrounded by palm trees, representing recommendations for the use of vitamin supplements and moderate consumption of alcohol when not contraindicated.

These pyramids were an exercise of "nutritional engineering," usually put into practice by governments, aiming to induce a collective action on attitudes and social behaviors related to food consumption. For instance, if everyone followed the recommendations, it is argued, obesity rates would slowly decrease. Substituting half of your daily intake of refined grains (like bread and polished rice) with whole grains, eating plenty of fruit and vegetables, and exercising 30 to 60 minutes a day would be enough to improve your energy balance and help you to lose weight if necessary.

How long did MyPyramid last? Not very long. In June 2011 the USDA replaced MyPyramid with MyPlate. When it comes to food, a plate is a more positive and understandable image than a pyramid. What about the new recommendations? The *MyPlate* guidelines are simpler and more direct: enjoy your food while eating less, avoid oversized portions, eat more fruits and vegetables, choose foods with less salt, and opt for water instead of sugary drinks[45]—not unlike what has been presented in this book so far.

Nutritionists may have oversimplified the recommendations once again. There is growing evidence that not all starches are nutritionally equal. Starches that are more resistant to digestive enzymes generate less sugar, decreasing their association with type 2 diabetes (Section 7.7). It's also very likely that the health benefits associated with drinking alcohol are not from the alcohol per se, but derive from other components of alcoholic beverages such as polyphenols, which are abundant in wine and act as antioxidants. There are other nutritional recommendations being implemented in parallel, such as the "Five a Day" plans that exist in over 40 countries, which promote the consumption of five servings of fruits and vegetables per day for their supply of vitamins, minerals, fiber, and phytochemicals. But all this is just one side of the equation; we are born to run after our food and no concrete actions emerge for an increase on physical activity.

12.8 INFORMATION OVERLOAD

If you only listened to the news media it would be difficult to know what to eat and what to avoid, because there is too much information and the information is very often contradictory. One day margarine is good and butter should be avoided. A few years later, these recommendations were reversed and butter was declared healthier because margarine contained unhealthy trans fatty acids (see Section 1.3). Similar situations have arisen with eggs, certain sweeteners, and many additives, among other things. People become confused, incredulous, and sometimes deceived. The problem is partly because the original information is written by scientists and intended for other scientists, rather than for the media and the general public (Section 10.8). The media extracts information from scientific papers that might be of interest to the public, interprets and translates it into simple language, then distributes the information in the form of straightforward messages, with attention-grabbing headlines and omitting any scientific details that might "confuse" the public. In this process the media almost always loses track of assumptions, methodological subtleties, and special circumstances that may have been a vital part of the paper. In the end, people have difficulty understanding the real issue and making decisions.

To appreciate why these problems occur we must understand the methods used by medical doctors and nutritionists to test hypotheses about whether certain dietary factors are beneficial or harmful. It is not easy to perform experiments with humans, and controlled experiments (with "volunteers") must comply with strict ethical protocols, making them more complex and costly. In addition, there is great variability in individual response (that is, people differ in their reactions to similar foods, see Section 5.3) and so it is difficult to assemble groups of homogeneous individuals from which extrapolations can be made in order to draw conclusions that are valid for an entire population. Finally, it takes time to determine whether results are clearly beneficial or harmful. The types of studies that examine the impact of nutrients on health are briefly described in Box 12.2.

The claim that diets rich in antioxidants reduce the risk of some degenerative diseases comes from data acquired from various studies similar to those outlined above. Epidemiological studies were used to describe the French Paradox (Section 12.5), which linked the lower incidence of cardiovascular mortality in France with the regular, moderate consumption of wine (known to contain powerful antioxidants). Many longitudinal studies have corroborated a study that found that daily consumption of fruits, vegetables, and tea was positively associated with the cardiovascular health and longevity of over 800 seniors. There is also evidence from several clinical intervention trials, such as one that involved thousands of elderly people who were given vitamin E over 6 years, which demonstrated a reduction in the incidence of Alzheimer's disease compared to the control and placebo groups.

BOX 12.2   SOME SOURCES OF INFORMATION AND TYPES OF STUDIES THAT ARE USED TO EVALUATE THE IMPACT OF DIFFERENT FOODS ON NUTRITION AND HEALTH

Epidemiological studies analyze a large amount of existing medical information to find possible factors that affect a health condition. Obviously, the interpretation and conclusions depend on the quality of the information.

Longitudinal studies follow during a period of time and observe a large and homogeneous group of people. Participants may have to record what they eat, which is not easy. Also, people usually eat a wide variety of things, making it very difficult to single out the effect of a specific nutrient.

Clinical intervention trials are studies in which a controlled intervention is performed in the diets of a group of people. One subgroup receives a specific diet, another receives a placebo, and a third control group continues with their usual diet. Effects of the target group after the intervention is over are rarely observed, as habits are not created.

Animal experiments were very common in the past but today they are universally challenged on ethical grounds, especially when they involve species close to humans. Animal experimentation produces results that are not always transferable to other species (from rats to humans, for example).[46,47] The confinement and isolation of caged animals increases stress, influencing their response to treatment.

Finally, several animal studies gave encouraging results for a variety of food antioxidants, as one study in rats that showed that phenolic extracts from apples protect the gastric mucosa.

These types of studies abound in the scientific literature, but the results are not always as apparent and consistent as with the above example of antioxidants. In many cases the items that appeal to the press come from prospective investigations that are not yet conclusive and only serve to generate new working hypotheses. The press adds enticing headlines (such as "a new food that cures cancer!"). Studies that monitor a group of people who are showing a positive response during the intervention are particularly vulnerable to this problem. Most of the positive outcomes of these studies are only sustained as long as the individuals are still research "subjects." Thereafter control of the information is lost and interpretations of the data give rise to varied recommendations by food professionals and dieticians, or even self-prescription and self-treatment.[48] A recent newspaper article titled "Junk food can be as addictive as tobacco and drugs," was based on a scientific publication in which rats were fed cafeteria food such as sausages, cheesecake, and coffeecake. Not once did the authors of the paper refer to diet administered to the rats as "junk food."[49]

Consumers obtain abundant nutritional information directly from the packaging on processed foods. Nutrition labeling provides the total amount and energy contributed by the basic components, lists the main ingredients (in descending order contained by the product), and provides nutrition messages such as "sugar free," "light in sodium," or "reduced cholesterol."[50] These messages are not easy to understand, unless we happen to have previous information with which to compare. For example, "low calories" means the food must have "less than 40 kcal per reference amount customarily consumed," a phrase that is not very helpful. Nutritional information is often based on 100 grams of dry product, as in the case of spaghetti. To calculate the calories and nutrients in what you are eating, you would have to weigh a portion of cooked noodles and then estimate how much water they absorbed.

Although people read the nutrition information labels on packaged foods more often than ever before, the vast majority of shoppers report that they do not understand at least one of the ingredients listed. This is not very surprising as some lists are long and many of the ingredients are complex substances with very specific functions (see Section 1.4). Some of this information can only be understood by people who have studied nutrition in school or have researched it on their own. Marketing is not specifically intended to clarify things. Nectar was the drink of the gods in Greek mythology, but according to a food manufacturer, "nectar" is a product made of fruit pulp, water, sugar, citric acid, chemical preservative, and a stabilizer. Very few consumers are aware that a bottle with the word "NECTAR" written on it in large letters next to a picture of a provocative fruit contains citric acid, sodium benzoate, potassium sorbate, xanthan gum, natural-identical flavoring (*sic*), and colorant, as stated in a small box somewhere on the label. All of this is clearly misleading to the consumer.

In summary, it's necessary to have a good understanding of the assumptions, methods, and designs of the clinical and laboratory trials, as well as the statistical concepts behind the conclusions (Section 5.6) in order to correctly interpret nutritional studies. Much of the information we receive is based on poorly documented inferences from extrapolations made onto other populations (from small animals to humans, for example), or is simply the product of sensationalist pseudo-science.

12.9 EDUCATING CONSUMERS

If you were to test a group of students on their knowledge of food and nutrition, the results would be disastrous. Clearly this subject is neglected in the elementary and high school curriculum, and the little information that is covered is often incorrect. It's hard to guess how many students will need to solve quadratic equations in their lives, but it is certain that they will all need to eat. In chemistry class, high school programs prefer to cover the experimental classification of soils based on their properties and the steps in the production of sulfuric acid, rather than matters that are directly related to personal well-being and quality of life.[51] Meanwhile, one-third of school-age children in the United States are overweight or obese.[52]

Although ideally kids would receive good nutrition at home, schools provide much of what children eat between ages 4 and 18, a critical period for forming good eating habits. What needs to be done? First, units on nutrition and food chemistry, even on cooking and gastronomy, should be incorporated into the curriculum materials.[53] Next, the quality of school lunches should be improved to include more fruits, vegetables, legumes, and fish, and fewer high-fat products. This may be more costly but should be considered an investment against likely future spending on public health for problems associated with poor nutrition. The food industry should be challenged to develop foods that are cheap and healthy, and especially convenient and attractive to school-age children. School lunchtime should be an opportunity to encourage good nutritional habits and basic food appreciation, highlighting the benefits of traditional diets and emphasizing tastes and textures. Local foods should have a "story" that makes them more attractive and provides a place for them in modern life, which is where creative chefs have an important role to play. The *collation* (a term from the eighteenth century for the sweet dishes that were served at the end of the evening) that children bring to school is often unnecessary from a nutritional standpoint and creates bad habits like snacking.[54] Finally, the snacks (candy, cookies, etc.) that are sold from school snack bars should be mostly "healthy," with less salt, sugar, or fat, or simply banned. The traditional school stores in the United Kingdom are unfortunately still called "candy shops."

Physical education in schools is inadequate and falls short of 3 hours per week, which is not enough to meet the physiological adaptations required by the increased food consumption. Almost half of the children fall into the category of sedentary, especially girls. Students should be encouraged to walk or bicycle to school, and better safety measures should be enacted to support this practice.

The food industry should also contribute to the education of consumers by providing information about their research, issuing truthful advertising, and promoting healthier products. A multinational food company brings hundreds of millions of products to the world market daily, and the packaging for these products represents thousands of square meters of space that could convey health messages to consumers. Some companies have formed consortiums with universities to study how consumer behavior, especially that of children, responds to healthier products.[55]

12.10 MBA: MASTER'S DEGREE IN BETTER *ALIMENTATION*

All of the scientific and empirical evidence that has been presented in the preceding pages can be distilled into three fundamental rules for establishing a relationship with food that provides a high degree of personal well-being and a healthy, vital life: first, eat a nourishing and varied diet; second, maintain a healthy weight and refrain from eating in excess; and third, exercise. These tasks are listed in order of increasing difficulty. Eating a varied diet (something grandmothers have always told their grandchildren) is not very complicated these days with the superabundance of food that's available. In order to eat a nourishing diet you must learn to distinguish good foods from less nutritious foods, know how to taste, and try new things. Maintaining weight within certain limits requires dedication, perseverance, and one more factor that is rare these days: "will power." As far as physical activity is concerned, the most important thing is to simply make time for exercise, by establishing routines that are flexible and enjoyable. In adults, the most appropriate way to meet daily physical activity requirements is to walk at least 20 to 30 minutes per day, instead of always traveling by car.

People already have the tools for better nutrition right in their hands (or in their mouths and pockets), yet incomprehensively the problem keeps moving away from individual responsibility toward government intervention and regulation. If people read and understood the information about food and nutrition, would it really be necessary to add warnings to the packaging of high-fat foods like cheese (what would the French say?) or ban all advertising of "junk food"? Do we also need to be protected from overdrawing our checkbooks and from ads and e-mails inviting easy credit? The vast majority of people know the personal consequences of mishandling money and irresponsible borrowing.

Speaking of money and finances, many people aspire to earn a Master's in Business Administration (MBA). But there is another MBA degree, a *Master's in Better Alimentation*. Although the word *alimentation* exists in English and refers to the act of giving or receiving nourishment, its use is not as extended as in French or Spanish. This MBA is an invitation to improve your eating habits and increase your physical activity over the course of 1 year. It is clear that there are shorter "courses" out there called diets, but they are boring, only provide short-term effects, and do not create good habits. This MBA degree is based on the empirical fact that in order to radically change eating habits in today's world, the transformation must be gradual and the individual must internalize the new habits, to minimize the dropout rate. This MBA is a self-taught course and there are no prerequisites or tuition costs (in fact you may actually save money), and if completed, the course will change your quality of life. Like other master's programs, it requires daily dedication and a minimum of two semesters to complete. Admission to the MBA program does require consultation and approval from your physician. As there are neither professors nor course evaluations for this MBA, it is performed by self-assessment and the exams are self-graded. To pass Physical Activity I, you must double your current exercise amount or reach the equivalent to 2 1/2 hours of moderately intense walking per week. In the second semester, you must add some light jogging. The Food Accounting course involves learning the approximate caloric content of every food that you eat and how to interpret nutritional labeling, in order to develop the habit of carrying a daily mental tally of calories ingested. Any excess calories must be detracted from the following day's allotment; no late assignments will be accepted. The Food Habits course covers the basics of learning to eat better by reducing portions, cutting back on high-fat foods, replacing sugary drinks with sugar-free options, and eating more fruits and vegetables. One strategy for eating less is to apply a 10% tax on your food portions, either by leaving food uneaten, or serving less. Those who are accustomed to eating more calories (hence overeating) can self-impose a higher tax rate. You must gradually cut back on trips to "junk food" outlets and fast food restaurants and replace them with home-cooked meals. The Food and Nutrition course involves learning the basics of these subjects, which are available in many books and online. The monthly exams are weight checks and waist measurements.

The course lasts 1 year and by the end of the year you will see results. Not only will you have reduced your weight and waist circumference, but you will have also developed better, healthier habits. You might even consider a PhD, which involves more profound and interesting courses such as processing of foods, kitchen laboratories, advanced nutrition and health, history of cuisine and gastronomy, introduction to marathons, and prolonged field trips to the gym or hiking in the mountains.

12.11 DESIGNING FOODS

Our intuition tells us that eating as our grandparents did may be the most desirable and healthiest way. But there are several things that were different in those times. Grandmothers did not work outside their home, so they had time to shop in fresh markets and cook at least twice a day. As few of them had access to refrigerators and freezers, food was prepared with fresh ingredients. Housework, walking to do daily shopping, and taking care of children demanded more physical activity than it does today. Their children (our parents) played in the street and walked to school, while children of this generation are entertained with video games and are picked up by a bus. Scientific knowledge about food and nutrition was quite limited, and many of the old beliefs, like the idea that fat children were healthier, have since fallen by the wayside. So, a simplistic plan for returning to the home-cooked diet of the past is quite an attractive proposal. It's probable that this could be a plausible option for the most privileged populations in developed countries, but it's unlikely that it would be feasible for the hundreds of millions of people around the world living in urban areas where time is the scarcest commodity (Section 12.5). Moreover, though there have been astounding scientific and technological advances in the last two decades which have revolutionized several different spheres of our daily life, few of them have had an impact on food and nutrition.

Having reached this point in the journey from prehistory to the present day, and having jumped from genes to cells and the molecules in food structures, a very pertinent question emerges: Could it be that some of today's most popular processed foods (i.e., those that most people enjoy eating) simply don't meet the requirements imposed by modern life? Many were never actually designed but were probably first prepared by an illiterate cook. These convenience foods whose textures and flavors we now like too much are quick to prepare and consume and are affordable, but they are too high in calories. They can become harmful if we do not have the desire to limit their consumption or to burn off the excess calories we consume. Now that we have reached the twenty-first century, with more innovation and changes occurring in the area of food and nutrition than we've ever experienced in the past, this could be the time to mobilize science and technology to design or redesign some key processed foods.

Design means to create with an ultimate goal. For example, the houses, cars, electronics, and clothes we use are designed to meet current requirements. This design is constantly revised and improved as needs change, and technology provides more convenient alternatives. But our food has never been designed in this way. There are no blueprints for french fries, schematics of ice cream, or prototypes of hamburgers. Chefs and nutritionists talk about "menu design" or the selection of dishes to satisfy the sensory demands of diners or specific nutritional needs, respectively.

One might argue that over millions of years of trial and error, it's unlikely that nature made a mistake in the solutions that have evolved, and that it is advantageous to use them. But this assumption is not always correct when it is necessary to address problems that appear suddenly. When people first dreamed of air travel, Leonardo da Vinci was stumped by the problem of copying bird flight. The propulsion of aircraft is based on very different physics than that used by birds. Nature will continue to be an endless source of inspiration for cooks and scientists, but you can't always look to nature to find solutions to problems it has never faced.

We put artificial parts and tissues into our bodies to replace or repair the natural function of certain organs that modern life has exhausted or destroyed.[56] If the dysfunction in our bodies comes from an uncontrollable urge to eat certain foods, and we have the capability for making better, healthier foods, why not give consumers the choice? If people are eagerly and often irresponsibly searching out pseudo-drugs or surgery to resolve the consequences of obesity, why not apply twenty-first century scientific knowledge toward providing more low-risk food alternatives instead? These healthier food choices would definitely be less risky for the consumer than buying miracle supplements or other false panaceas that are offered openly on the Internet and do not meet government safety standards.

What detractors of the food industry call "reengineered" or "designed" products are largely reformulations of traditional foods containing smaller or greater amounts of a target component. In fact, industry should be blamed for not using all the available scientific knowledge to provide innovative healthy alternatives for some foods, beyond just *low-fat, reduced-sugar, no-trans oils*, and *hi-fiber* versions. The current goals for designing processed food products include reducing the content of sugar, salt, and unhealthy fats, as well as reducing total calories and inducing a more prolonged feeling of fullness. We have already discussed the technique of replacing some of the natural molecules with designed molecules (Section 1.13) and "boosting" portion size with structures that trap water or air (Sections 2.7 and 2.8). Sensory aspects are fundamental in developing any designed product, because above all people must want to eat the food.

The processed food industry has always been regarded as traditional and slow to innovate, but today it should stand ready to provide products that result in better health and well-being. It is likely that the twenty-first century will bring some important new designed foods to the market, which will have as large an impact as mayonnaise, chocolates, french fries, and others did when they "appeared" a couple of centuries back. These older processed foods still satisfy the palate and the brain today, but have a negative effect on health when consumed in excess. Along the way there will be hurdles to overcome, concerning both how ingredients and products depart from "natural" ones, and over what is considered safe and healthy. The task is not easy and the challenges are enormous.

NOTES

1. Dobzhansky, T. 1973. Nothing in biology makes sense except in the light of evolution. *The American Biology Teacher* 35, 125–129.
2. Alaskan Eskimos have a daily energy intake of 3000 kcal, of which nearly 50% comes from fat, 30% to 35% from protein, and less than 20% from carbohydrates (mostly in the form of glycogen).
3. Abundant information on urbanization in countries with low and middle income levels can be found in Cohen, B. 2004. Urban growth in developing countries: A review of current trends and a caution regarding existing forecasts. *World Development* 32, 23–51.
4. Cordain, L., Eaton, S.B., Brand Miller, J., Mann, N., and Hill, K. 2002. The paradoxical nature of hunter-gatherer diets: Meat-based, yet non-atherogenic. *European Journal of Clinical Nutrition* 56, S42–S52.

5. Cordón, F. 1980. *Cocinar hizo al Hombre*. (Cooking Made Mankind). Tusquets Eds., Barcelona, p. 109. Apparently there is an English version: Cordon, F. 1980. *Introduction to the Biological Basis for Feeding*, Elsevier, London.

6. Bollinger, A. 1993. *Así se alimentaban los Inkas*. (So the Inkas Were Fed). Los Amigos del Libro, Cochabamba. There is only a German version of the book under the title of *So Nährten sich die Inka*.

7. Leonard, W.R. 2002. Food for thought: Dietary change was a driving force for evolution. *Scientific American* 287(6),106–115.

8. Eaton, S.B., and Cordain, L. 1997. Evolutionary aspects of diet: Old genes, new fuels. In *Nutrition and Fitness: Evolutionary Aspects, Children's Health, Programs and Policies* (A.P. Simopoulos, ed.), Karger, Basel, pp. 26–37.

9. A simple article that explains complementary amino acids and the quality of dietary protein: Vitz, E. 2005. Amino acid complementarity: A biochemical exemplar of stoichiometry for general and health sciences chemistry. *Journal of Chemical Education* 82, 1013–1016.

10. Kucharski, R., Maleszka, J., Foret, S., and Maleszka, R. 2008. Nutritional control of reproductive status in honey bees via DNA methylation. *Science* 319, 1827–1830.

11. Cordain, L., Gotshall, L.W., Boyd Eaton, S., and Boyd Eaton III, S. 1998. Physical activity, energy expenditure and fitness: An evolutionary perspective. *International Journal of Sports Medicine* 19, 328–335.

12. Nesse, R.M., and Williams, J.C. 1998. Evolution and the origins of disease. *Scientific American* 279(5), 86–89.

13. Underwood, A., and Adler, J. 2005. Diet and genes. *Newsweek*, January 17, pp. 40–48.

14. Frederickson, B.L. 2003. The value of positive emotions. *American Scientist* 91, 330–335.

15. About being happier, the quote is from S. Pinker and cited in Bloom, P. 2010. *How Pleasure Works: The New Science of Why We Like What We Like*. W.W. Norton, New York, p. 8.

16. Sinclair, D.A., and Guarente, L. 2006. Unlocking the secrets of longevity genes. *Scientific American* 294(3), 48–51, 54–57.

17. More on the consequences of obesity can be found at Centers for Disease Control and Prevention. Overweight and obesity: Causes and consequences. www.cdc.gov/obesity/causes/health.html (accessed February 8, 2012).

18. Taxes not paid. *Irish Examiner*, September 11, 2004.

19. The contents of the book *Global Recommendations on Physical Activity for Health* can be downloaded at www.who.int/dietphysicalactivity/publications/9789241599979/en/index.html.

20. Willett, W.C. 2003. *Eat, Drink and Be Healthy*. Free Press, New York.
21. Wayt Gibbs, W. 2005. Obesity: An overblown epidemic? *Scientific American* 292(6), 48–55.
22. Malik, V.S., Schulze, M.B., and Hu, F.B. 2006. Intake of sugar-sweetened beverages and weight gain: A systematic review. *American Journal of Clinical Nutrition* 84, 274–288.
23. Anonymous. 2005. Cruising the center-store aisle. *Food Technology* 59(10), 28–39.
24. Leonard, W.R. 2002. Food for thought: Dietary change was a driving force for evolution. *Scientific American* 287(6), 106–115. In addition, both the Turkana and the Incas have low levels of total cholesterol (between 140 and 150 mg/dL).
25. See Poulain, J.P. 2002. The contemporary diet in France: "De-structuration" or from commensalism to "vagabond feeding." *Appetite* 39, 43–55.
26. A report on street food vendors in Thailand appeared in *The New York Times* on May 27, 2009.
27. "Ferrán Adrià: el cocinero que inventó el aire." Interview in *Revista El Sábado* de El Mercurio, Santiago, October 31, 2003. Adrià and his associates (NH Hotels) opened in 2004 a restaurant chain under the name of Fast Good that offered "healthy and high quality fast food." The restaurants were closed in June 2011.
28. Quote adapted from Halwell, B. 2004. *Eat Here: Reclaiming Homegrown Pleasures in a Global Supermarket,* W.W. Norton, London, p. 148.
29. For those seriously interested in "junk food," see Smith, A.F. 2006. *Encyclopedia of Junk Food and Fast Food*. Greenwood, Connecticut.
30. Feldman, S., and Marks, V. 2005. *Panic Nation: Exposing the Myths We're Told about Food and Health*. John Blake, London.
31. A *sopaipilla* is a round piece of deep-fried dough served with hot molasses.
32. See article by Shermer, M. 2003. Bottle twaddle. *Scientific American* 289(1), 33.
33. Currently many children worry about ecology and the environment because they have been taught about these issues both at home and in schools, a fundamental combination.
34. Data obtained from Sistema Integrado de Encuestas de Hogares. 2008. Encuesta Experimental sobre uso del tiempo en el Gran Santiago. www.ine.cl/canales/sala_prensa/noticias/2008/mayo/pdf/presentacion300508.pdf (accessed February 12, 2012).
35. Part of Bob Dylan's song "The Times They Are A-Changin'" that goes: "for the loser now/will be later to win/for the times they are a-changin'."

36. More information about healthy diets can be found at Harvard School of Public Health. The Nutrition Source: Knowledge for Healthy Eating. www.hsph.harvard.edu/nutritionsource/ (accessed February 12, 2012).

37. For more information see the original WHO document, which can be found at www.who.int/dietphysicalactivity/strategy/eb11344/strategy_ english_web.pdf (accessed April 14, 2010).

38. The Web site of the International Food and Beverage Alliance is www.ifballiance.org.

39. There are many publications, scientific and popular, on the Mediterranean diet. Maybe one can start with the book by Cloutier, M., and Adamson, E. 2004. *The Mediterranean Diet*. Avon, New York. There is also the Web page www.mediterraneandiet.com/.

40. The average values of total polyphenols are between 300 and 600 mg/100 g in blueberry varieties, and 100 mg/100 g in apples.

41. Mattivi, F. 2004. Antioxidantes polifenólicos naturales en la dieta. In *Dietas Mediterráneas: la evidencia científica* (F. Leighton and I. Urquiaga, eds.), Universidad Católica de Chile, Santiago, pp. 100–111. Available only in Spanish.

42. Gancel, A.-L., Feneuil, A., Acosta, O., Pérez, A.M., and Vaillant, F. 2011. Impact of industrial processing and storage on major polyphenols and the antioxidant capacity of tropical highland blackberry (*Rubus adenotrichus*). *Food Research International* 44, 2243–2251.

43. For more information on vegetarian diets, see Anonymous. 2009. Position of the American Dietetic Association: Vegetarian diets. *Journal of the American Dietetic Association* 109, 1266–1282.

44. Information about the USDA food pyramid is available at www.mypyramid.gov/ (accessed April 28, 2011).

45. See the Web site at www.choosemyplate.gov/.

46. As an example, in a 1988 study, the effect of carcinogens on animals as genetically close as rats and mice matched in only 70% of cases. See Barnard, N.D., and Kaufman, S.R. 1997. Animal research is wasteful and misleading. *Scientific American* 276(2), 80–82.

47. Animal studies are controversial even within the scientific community, and animal rights groups, as expected, are opposed to them. Safety trials for a new pesticide may require 10,000 animals of different species, if it has been shown to reach the bloodstream.

48. An interesting case was Linus Pauling (1901–1994), winner of two Nobel Prizes (Chemistry and Peace), who recommended taking high doses of vitamin C (about 10 grams per day) to counteract the oxidation caused by aging, and in particular the common cold. In his words "if I don't live

to be one hundred years old, it's because I didn't begin to take megadoses of vitamin C until I was sixty-five, when my body was already old" (but he meant, "already oxidized"). Pauling lived 93 years.

49. Johnson, P.M., and Kenny, P.J. 2010. Dopamine D2 receptors in addiction-like reward dysfunction and compulsive eating in obese rats. *Nature Neuroscience* 13, 635–641.

50. Definitions of the U.S. Food and Drug Administration (FDA) for nutrient content claims as of October 2009 can be found at www.fda.gov/Food/GuidanceComplianceRegulatoryInformation/GuidanceDocuments/FoodLabelingNutrition/FoodLabelingGuide/ucm064911.htm (accessed January 24, 2012).

51. The Chilean Ministry of Education Web site http://aep.mineduc.cl/images/pdf/2005/Em_quimica.pdf (accessed March 1, 2010), details seven key themes with various subjects, all of which fall within the remit of a teacher in Chile who must teach chemistry at the middle-school level. The word "food" appears once in the 11 pages of the text, and in relation to food additives.

52. Michelle Obama recently announced that one of her principal legacies will be to end childhood obesity. See www.letsmove.gov/ (accessed February 28, 2012).

53. Hervé This wrote a book for children which is available in French (*La Casserole des Enfants*, Belin, Paris, 1998) in which he refers to molecules, starches, and emulsions. Celebrity chef Heston Blumenthal has developed a series of experiments and demonstration videos of the chemistry involved in food and cooking. See Lister, T., and Blumenthal, H. 2005. *Kitchen Chemistry*. Royal Society of Chemistry, London, pp. 101–102.

54. A survey of Chilean schoolchildren between the ages of 8 and 15 years old from 10 public and private schools gives an idea of the impact of snacks and food purchases from school kiosks. Half of the students bring food to school, the average purchase was $1, and 61% of the purchases corresponded to chips and other snacks, candy, and cookies. *El Mercurio*, Santiago, Thursday, August 2, 2007, p. A11.

55. During a state visit to the Netherlands, the national delegation headed by President Bachelet took the opportunity to visit the *Restaurant of the Future* at the University of Wageningen, one of the most important universities in Europe for food research. The day of the visit, researchers were studying children's reactions to vegetables prepared in different ways. See www.restaurantvandetoekomst.wur.nl/UK/ (accessed April 18, 2011).

56. A recent article by Khademhosseini, A., Vacanti, J.P., and Langer, R. 2009. Progress in tissue engineering. *Scientific American* 300(5), 64–71, reported that some 50 million Americans, most older than 65 years, are currently alive thanks to artificial organs. Engineered biological tissues are created to fit and produce a noticeable change in the quality of life for patients with dysfunctional organs.

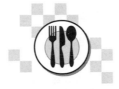

CHAPTER 13

Final Comments

After this long journey, everything seems to be fitting into place. Never before have we been so easily able to follow our ancestral instincts for eating a healthy varied diet and taking pleasure from food, as nutritious food has become much more accessible to most people. But our planet, its population, and people's lifestyles have changed, which will necessarily have an impact on how we produce and eat our food. In order to evolve into *Homo gastronomicus* we must know what we eat, enjoy it, avoid excess, choose foods from a variety of sources, and exercise. Otherwise we risk becoming *gastronators*—mindless consumers of empty structures.

13.1 LESSONS FROM A FAILED EXPERIMENT

The last two generations of human beings have unknowingly served as guinea pigs in the largest nutrition experiment ever known. The hypothesis for this experiment: if people are given an ample variety of affordable foods, they will choose well, eat healthily, and enjoy their meals. The subjects of this research, people living in urban centers around the world, were provided with well-stocked refrigerators at home and a varied, quite affordable supply of readily available foods. But the results of this experiment differed from what was expected and have proven the hypothesis false. The projection for 2015 is that 1.5 billion people in the world will be overweight or obese, and as a consequence many of them will suffer a variety of chronic diseases that severely affect the quality of their lives.

What went wrong and why? One simplistic explanation is that humans do not know how to deal with abundance, and the present pace of technology is too fast for our biological adaptations: we are products of evolution not revolution. And what a revolution it has been—to have such an abundance of tasty food. Our bodies and brains are wired for scarcity and survival, not for superabundance. A similar global experiment is being carried out now, this time focused more on the quality of interpersonal relationships. With ample access to communication and information the results should be available shortly.

But, let's get back to food and another global experiment. The theory was that this abundance of food would trickle down from the rich to the poor, and that hunger and malnutrition would disappear in a globalized world. The painful reality is that there are still 850 million people who are malnourished and 250 million suffering from hunger. These people are still poor, and resources have not "trickled down" from the wealthy to help them—another failed experiment.

The results of these failed science experiments were not reported and have been relegated to the bottom desk drawer. But in the case of the nutrition experiment, the evidence is too hard and glaring to hide. A lesson can be learned from every mistake, however, and in this case it has to do with the millions of people on this planet who do benefit from the modern food supply, and consequently enjoy longer and better lives. They have found ways to make healthy satisfying choices from the abundance and variety of food available, and have managed to overcome the limitations imposed by their human hardware. I have denominated this group of individuals *Homo gastronomicus*. Here are their secrets:

1. They are aware that food is a very important part of their lives. They have made the effort to learn the basics of food science and nutrition, which allows them to access the information available in the twenty-first century and make informed decisions. They can distinguish the "wheat from the chaff," and they do not fall for "bait and switch" tricks relating to food. They don't follow gurus, worship particular nutrients, or demonize certain foods outright. They eat sparingly from a variety of foods, enjoying every bite.

2. They believe in the laws of thermodynamics. They know that maintaining a proper weight is the basis for good health, and that it involves a delicate balance between calories consumed and calories expended. They follow a proper fitness routine to help burn off extra calories and stay vigorous. They have found their own balance, without resorting to crash diets or absurd deprivations, limiting their consumption of foods that are high in sugar, some fats, and salt, adjusting portion size, and almost unconsciously keeping mental account of the calories they eat and burn off.

3. They are realistic and confident but cautious. Human life on this planet has changed, including how and what we eat, and where our food comes from. They are aware that regulatory agencies do their job of protecting public health better than they could do it themselves, and demand accurate and timely information on any risks involved. They believe there is some truth in the assertion that "there are no bad foods," but know that some foods are better than others when consumed routinely. They rely on science's efforts to understand food production and preservation processes, and their complex impact on nutrition and health.

4. Their nutrition choices are evidence-based, or as they say today, based on "intuitive intelligence." A varied diet similar to what humans have eaten since ancient times is a good starting point—it's advantageous to our genes and "familiar" to our bodies. They understand that we are made to eat a small amount of food and that our "software" (our will and judgment) should prevail over our "hardware" (biological wiring). But each person is different and what may be optimal for one person may not be appropriate for another.

5. They value the pleasure of eating well, which does not mean eating too much or only eating sophisticated or expensive foods. They are curious about gastronomic advances and trends, experiment with new ideas, and often cook at home. They have learned to taste food using all five senses, to drink slowly and with moderation, and they take time to enjoy their meals. They avoid eating alone, because they believe that eating is part of what it means to be human and should be a social activity, not merely an activity for survival.

6. These individuals are aware that they live on a planet with limited resources and that in the future we will become more particular and demanding about the way food is produced, especially animal products and those harvested from the sea. They understand the impact of waste on the environment and the use of scarce resources like energy and water.

13.2 *HOMO GASTRONOMICUS* AND GASTRONATORS

Let's recapitulate. This apparent polarization of consumption patterns among those who have access to abundant food sources is surprising. On one side are those who eat to satisfy a basic need, and on the other there are a few who are concerned with obtaining the best of everything that they eat. Most people simply swallow their food greedily, but a few taste it thoughtfully in search of delight, delicacy, and remembrance. There are those who know little or nothing about how food and physical activity contribute to their health and well-being, and those who want to know more about it and put their knowledge into practice. In summary, people in the first group are the *gastronators*, those who devour food almost unconsciously, in excess, and without really tasting it. They suffer the consequences of their voracity in the form of the many problems that come with obesity.

The new *virtual branch* on Homo gastronomicus, or those who have "evolved" into a higher state of well-being through eating habits that

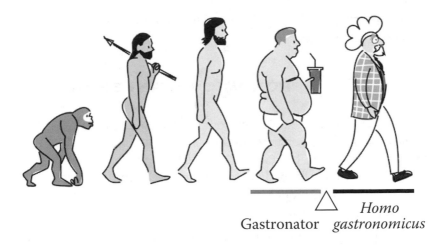

Homo
Gastronator   *gastronomicus*

FIGURE 13.1   HUMAN EVOLUTION AND THE HYPOTHETICAL EMERGENCE OF THE *GASTRONATOR*
AND *HOMO GASTRONOMICUS* IN THE TWENTY-FIRST CENTURY.

are compatible with most of the six items described above. Whether
an individual becomes a gastronator or joins the ranks of the *Homo
gastronomicus* is, for the most part, a personal decision. (Figure 13.1).

The *Homo gastronomicus* is not necessarily a gourmet. He or she is just
a lucky inhabitant of the twenty-first century who values the fruits
of agriculture and the modern food industry and, above all, well-
prepared food that is eaten socially. I run into Homo gastronomicus
everywhere, as they come from all walks of life: in a university cafeteria in Italy, in a small *cevichería* in Lima, and in the streets of Paris
carrying a baguette and a bottle of wine. But I am sure most of the time
they prefer preparing food and eating at their homes. I have also met
them hiking in the Andes and jogging in the park, as they all tend to
have routines that liberate time for exercising. Some of them don't eat
meat, others distrust synthetic colors, and several are concerned with
"food miles"—all of which is perfectly fine. Most of them like buying
at the fresh food market on weekends, trying new foods and ingredients, cooking at home, and eating socially. The tastes and attitudes of
Homo gastronomicus about food are like "votes," and the food industry,

the restaurant business, and the government are listening and slowly responding to suit their preferences.

13.3 GASTRONOMIC ENGINEERING

Over the last several years I have come to the conclusion that *gastronomic engineering* is a separate discipline much in the same way that molecular gastronomy (science and molecules in the kitchen), neurogastronomy (study of food sensations in the brain), and gastroeconomics and gastroanthropology are separate disciplines in the study of foods and their relation with humans.[1]

Gastronomic engineering is the application of the science of food materials and principles of engineering to: (a) understand the mechanisms by which molecules are organized at different scales into recognizable elements that give foods and dishes their desirable properties; (b) visualize and characterize food structures so they can be related to sensorial and physiological responses; (c) be able to control the physical and chemical transformations during processing and cooking, in order to design structures that are appealing, tasty, safe, and more nutritious; (d) understand the role that food structure plays in the release and absorption of nutrients (bioavailability) inside our bodies; and (e) utilize the fascinating examples of the engineering taking place inside foods during processing and cooking to teach students and chefs, and bring people closer to the engineering in foods.

The role of food structure is becoming more relevant as focus moves from single foods to complete diets and from specific nutrients to the aggregated effects of all components of a meal. Food structure can play an important role in redesigning traditional foods to have fewer calories, making foods (e.g., certain vegetables) more acceptable to children, and developing textures in special diets for the growing population of elderly people, to name a few examples. As mentioned earlier, emphasis has shifted away from the issue of nutrient deficiency in favor of the bioavailability and interactions of nutrients inside our bodies within the presence of a food matrix. Gastronomic engineering will provide a substantial foundation in this area, helping scientists, food producers, and chefs to develop new innovations in the early twenty-first century.[2]

13.4 A TIME FOR FOOD (STRUCTURE)

The previous chapters have proposed a scientific perspective that focuses on food structures rather than molecules. Although the nutrients our bodies need are molecules, we ingest them in the form of appetizing food structures, not as chemical powders or nutrition pills. Molecules behave differently when confined within structures, and because food is made up of many types of molecules, the situation is even more complex. Moreover, although the way food molecules react once they are released from their matrices is quite well understood (food chemistry), the interactions that occur when they are inside our bodies are still mostly unknown.

Viewing and characterizing food structures has become fairly routine in most research labs over the last 30 years, and it's increasingly possible to study them at the nano and micron levels using physical and chemical techniques, even in real time. Thus, most of the natural food structures as well as those acquired during processing are quite well established. The link between the structural architecture and the properties of foods is still missing, however, partly because it is often difficult to define desirable or undesirable attributes. This important issue must be resolved if we are to further understand the food we are eating.

But this is not enough. This "micro" approach to understanding foods also has to meet the macro needs of people and be inserted in a larger perspective. We all enjoy eating, and we develop both good and bad habits relative to our food. Currently our big problem is that there is too much energy in what we eat compared to the physical activity we spend to burn it. Thermodynamics tells us that these extra calories will be stored as fat while evolutionary traits (defined by our genes) mandate our bodies to respond (e.g., by gaining weight) in ways that make us unhealthy and depressed. We also must rely on processed foods to feed the 7 billion inhabitants of this planet, but the messages about what is healthy or unhealthy (for our bodies and minds) in these foods are still quite confusing.

Nutritionists, medical doctors, food technologists, social scientists, psychologists, and neurobiologists are increasingly interested in the axis that connects our brain and our cells and passes through our digestive tract. The focus of this research has shifted away from individual nutrients and moved toward the whole structure of food and meals as the unit of analysis for our eating patterns. We are just starting to understand how the same material may take different forms when it becomes structured, and can therefore elicit different sensorial and nutritional responses and interactions once it is broken down in our mouths and digestive tracts.

If the technological advances introduced by cooking food helped to develop our brains several thousands of years ago, it may well be that present technologies have some answers for our bulging bodies. Most of the processed foods that we like (and which are here to stay) were developed without any scientific support or knowledge about their health effects. Despite significant advances in science, the technological alternatives that have been proposed to improve these foods (except in the case of noncaloric sweeteners) have been disappointingly simple: increase fiber, lower fat, add more water, and so forth. These alterations generally come at the expense of taste. And even though technology has invaded our lives in many ways, taking up our limited time and even entering our bodies, we are still quite skeptical about technological solutions when it comes to food.

There is another twist in the tail. The structures of processed foods do not spontaneously and capriciously come to be in the kitchen; they respond to the same well-known basic phenomena as any other material in human creation. The good news is that once we understand what is happening with food structures, we will have the ability to modify and even design them, wisely, for the first time.

There is a potential gourmet inside each one of us, and the ample variety of foods available today has brought new opportunities for everyone. Collaboration between chefs and scientists is resulting in many new culinary advances, which will enrich our meals and our daily lives. Chefs know how to make meals attractive and people tend to follow their lead, as demonstrated by numerous newspaper columns and TV shows. Scientists, on the other hand, will take their research knowledge and mobilize it to turn these gastronomic creations into products. The time has come to serve our plates with novel food structures (in the correct amounts), alongside the best of our traditional foods, to create diets that are nutritionally adequate and also enjoyable. So, let's start walking ... literally.

NOTES

1. See also a chapter called Aguilera, J.M. 2009. In *An Integrated Approach to Food Product Development* (H.R. Moskowitz, I.S. Saguy, and T. Straus, eds.), CRC Press/Taylor & Francis, Boca Raton, FL, pp. 317–328.
2. In fact, the Spanish version of this book is entitled *Ingeniería Gastronómica* (Gastronomic Engineering). It was published by Ediciones Universidad Católica in 2011 (more information at http://ediciones.uc.cl/).

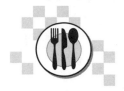

APPENDIX

ABBREVIATIONS

ADI: acceptable daily intake
BHA: butyl hydroxyanisol
BHT: butyl hydroxytoluene
BSE: bovine spongiform encephalopathy
CFU: colony forming units
CVD: cardiovascular diseases
D: diffusion coefficient, diffusivity
DHA: docosahexanoic acid
DNA: deoxyribonucleic acid
DSC: differential scanning calorimetry
EFSA: European Food Safety Authority
EPA: eicosapentanoic acid
FA: fatty acid
FAO: Food and Agriculture Organization of the United Nations
FDA: U.S. Food and Drug Administration
GDL: glucono-delta-lactone
GI: glycemic index
GM Food: genetically modified food
GMO: genetically modified organism
GR: glycemic response
GRAS: generally recognized as safe
HDL: high density lipoproteins
HFCS: high-fructose corn syrup
HLB: hydrophile-lipophile balance
HPP: high pressure processing
IQ: intelligence quotient
LD_{50}: median lethal dose

LDL: low density lipoproteins
LN: liquid nitrogen
MD: Mediterranean diet
MRI: magnetic resonance imaging
MW: molecular weight
NASA: National Aeronautics and Space Agency (U.S.)
NGO: non-governmental organization
NMR: nuclear magnetic resonance
PCB: polychlorinated biphenyl
PCR: polymerase chain reaction
PUFA: polyunsaturated fatty acid
PVC: polyvinyl chloride
RDS: rapidly digestible starch
RFID: radiofrequency identification
RH: relative humidity in the air (%)
RMR: resting metabolic rate
RNA: ribonucleic acid
ROS: reactive oxygen species
RS: resistant starch
SCFE: supercritical fluid extraction
SDS: slowly digestible starch
TBHQ: terbutyl hydroquinone
Tg: glass transition temperature
TTI: time-temperature indicators
UHT: ultra-high temperature
USDA: United States Department of Agriculture
WHO: World Health Organization

UNITS

cc: cubic centimeter (or mL)

dL: deciliter (or 0.1 liter)

g: gram

kcal: kilocalorie

kg: kilogram

L: liter

mg: milligram

mL: milliliter

mm: millimeter

mmol: millimol

μm: micrometer or micron

nm: nanometer

ppb: parts per billion

UNDERSTANDING THE FORMULAE OF LIPIDS

Triglyceride (fat) = Glycerol + 3 fatty acids

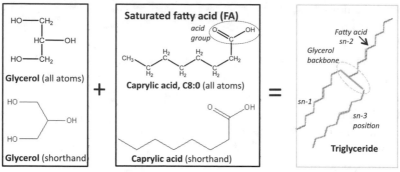

Glycerol (all atoms)

Glycerol (shorthand)

+

Saturated fatty acid (FA)

acid group

Caprylic acid, C8:0 (all atoms)

Caprylic acid (shorthand)

=

Fatty acid sn-2

Glycerol backbone

sn-1

sn-3 position

Triglyceride

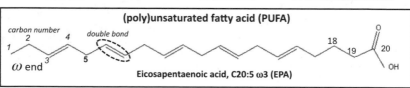

(poly)unsaturated fatty acid (PUFA)

carbon number 2 4 *double bond*

1 3 5

ω end

18 19 20

Eicosapentaenoic acid, C20:5 ω3 (EPA)

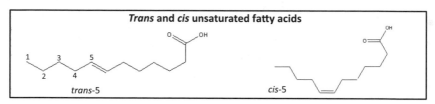

***Trans* and *cis* unsaturated fatty acids**

1 3 5
2 4

trans-5

cis-5

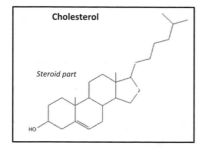

Cholesterol

Steroid part

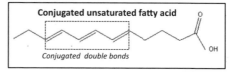

Conjugated unsaturated fatty acid

Conjugated double bonds

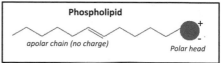

Phospholipid

apolar chain (no charge)

Polar head

INDEX

fried, 273
poached, 208
white, 20, 128, 190
yolk, 71, 79, 131, 190, 332
Eicosapentaenoic acid (EPA), 5
Elastin, 70
Electron cryomicroscopy, 113
Electron microscopy, 112
Emulsifier, 12, 76, 306
Emulsions
    butter, 76, 159
    cream, 76
    mayonnaise, 76, 94, 247
    oil/water, 210
    W/O/W, 77
Energy
    adhesion, 63
    entropy, 205
    free, 205
    homeostasis, 215
    infrared, 223
    input into intenive agriculture, 143
    nuclear, 33
    solar, 2–3
Enzymatic browning, 10, 18
Enzymes, 4
    amylases, 11
    digestion, 117
    hydrolytic, 60
    inhibitors, 33
    lingual, 247
    lipases, 11
    pancreatic, 248
    pepsin, 247
    polyphenol oxidase, 18
    proteases, 11
    rennin, 91
    transglutaminase, 333
EPA, *see* Eicosapentaenoic acid
Equilibrium, 208–210
    barriers, 210
    characteristics making food unique, 208
    degrees of doneness, 208, 209

egg white, 209
frying, 284
metastable, 65–66
oil/water emulsion, 210
transient period before equilibrium, 209
variables affecting equilibrium, 308
Essential amino acids, 4
Experience economy, 163
Experimental design, 194

F

FA, *see* Fatty acids
Failed experiment, lessons from, 387–390
    biological wiring, 389
    caution, 389
    importance of food, 389
    intuitive intelligence, 389
    largest nutrition experiment, 387
    laws of thermodynamics, 389
    limited resources, 390
    pleasure of eating well, 390
    results of failed science experiments, 388
    revolution, 388
    subjects of research, 388
Fats
    digestion, 247
    globules, 79, 80, 88, 134, 159
    saturated, 5, 152, 251, 280, 366
    substitutes, 43
    triglycerides, 5, 11, 42, 73, 254, 397
    unsaturated, 5
Fatty acids (FA), 4–5
    saturated, 5
    trans, 1, 307
    unsaturated, 5, 6, 7, 73, 366
FDA, *see* U.S. Food and Drug Administration
Fermentation
    cheese, 32–33
    gases produced during, 84